New Aspects in Diabetes

New Aspects in Diabetes

Treatment Strategies with Alpha-Glucosidase Inhibitors

Third International Symposium on Acarbose

Editors: Pierre J. Lefèbvre and Eberhard Standl

Walter de Gruyter
Berlin · New York 1992

Editors

Prof. Dr. P. J. Lefèbvre
Centre Hospitalier Universitaire
Département de Médecine
4000 Liège 1
Belgium

Prof. Dr. E. Standl
Städtisches Krankenhaus Schwabing
III. Medizinische Abteilung
Kölner Platz 1
8000 München 40
Germany

Die Deutsche Bibliothek – CIP-Einheitsaufnahme

New aspects in diabetes : treatment strategies with alphaglucosidase inhibitors / Third International Symposium on Acarbose. Ed. P. J. Lefèbvre and E. Standl. – Berlin ; New York : de Gruyter, 1992
ISBN 3-11-013469-1
NE: Lefèbvre, Pierre J. [Hrsg.]; International Symposium on Acarbose < 03, 1991, München >

Typesetting: Arthur Collignon GmbH, Berlin. – Printing: Gerike GmbH, Berlin. – Binding: Mikolai, Berlin. – Printed in Germany.

List of first-mentioned contributors

Dr. H. de la Calle
Hosp. Ramón y Cajal
Ctra. Colmenar Km 9,1
28034 Madrid
Spain

Dr. R. F. Coniff
Miles Pharmaceutical Division
Medical Department
400 Morgan Lane
West Haven, Ct. 06516
USA

Prof. Dr. S. H. Croog
University of Connecticut Health Center
Framlington, Ct. 06032
USA

Prof. Dr. Yoshio Goto
Tohoku Kosei-nenkin Hospital
Aza Fukumoru Takasago
Sendai 983
Japan

Prof. Dr. Yuichiro Goto
Tokai University
Int. Med. I
Bosei-dai, Isehara
Kanagawa 259-11
Japan

Prof. Dr. M. Hanefeld
Klinik für Innere Medizin
Medizinische Akademie
„Carl Gustav Carus"
8019 Dresden
Germany

Dr. H. Hobler
Bayer AG
Pharma Forschungszentrum
Aprather Weg
5600 Wuppertal
Germany

Dr. P. Hollander
International Diabetes Center
5000 West 39th Street
Minneapolis, M. N. 55416
USA

Prof. Dr. Y. Ikeda
The Jikei University School of Medicine
Internal Medicine II
3-25-8, Nishi-Shinbachi
Minato-Ku
Tokyo
Japan

Dr. R. Josse
St. Michael's Hospital
38 Shuter Street, Suite 213
Toronto M5B 1A6
Canada

Prof. Dr. H. E. Lebovitz
State University of New York
Health Science Center at Brooklyn
450 Clarkson Avenue
Brooklyn, N. Y. 11203-2098

Prof. Dr. P. J. Lefèbvre
Centre Hospitalier Universitaire
Départment de Médecine
4000 Liège 1
Belgium

Prof. Dr. H. Lithell
Uppsala University
Department of Geriatrics
Box 12042
75012 Uppsala
Sweden

Prof. Dr. H. Meyer
Bayer AG
5090 Leverkusen
Germany

Prof. Dr. J. L. Pinquier
Eclimed, IRT
Hospital Universitaire Cochin
27, Rue du Faubourg
St. Jacques
75679 Paris
France

Dr. F. X. Pi-Sunyer
Obesity Research Center
St. Luke's/Roosevelt Hospital Center
Amsterdam Ave. at 114th Street
New York, N. Y. 10025
USA

Prof. Dr. S. A. Raptis
II. Med. Universitätsklinik
Propädeutik „Evangelismos"
P. O. Box 14127
11510 Athen
Greece

PD Dr. G. Rohr
Universität Heidelberg
Klinikum Mannheim
6800 Mannheim
Germany

Prof. Dr. C. Rosak
J. W. Goethe Universität
Zentrum für Innere Medizin
6000 Frankfurt a. M.
Germany

Prof. Dr. N. Sakamoto
Third Department of Int. Med.
Nagoya University School of Medicine
Nagoya
Japan

Dr. D. S. Schade
The University of New Mexiko
School of Medicine
Div. of Endocrinology & Metabolism
2211 Lomas N. E.
Floor 7 South
Albuquerque, N. M. 87131
USA

Dr. M. Spengler
Bayer AG
Pharma Forschungszentrum
Aprather Weg
5600 Wuppertal
Germany

Prof. Dr. E. Standl
Städtisches Krankenhaus Schwabing
III. Medizinische Abteilung
Kölner Platz 1
8000 München 40
Germany

Dr. K. Tawara
Medicine & Development Division
Bayer Yakuhin, Ltd.
5-18, Doshomachi, 1-chome
Chuo-ku, Osaka 541
Japan

Dr. M. Toeller
Diabetes-Forschungsinstitut
an der Universität Düsseldorf
Auf'm Hennekamp 65
4000 Düsseldorf 1
Germany

Prof. Dr. G. L. Vega
University of Texas
Southwestern Medical Center
5323 Harry Hanes Boul
Dallas, Texas 75235/9052
USA

Dr. S. Waadt
Max-Planck-Institut für Psychiatrie
Klinische Abteilung
Kraepelinstraße
8000 München
Germany

Dr. J. Wernecke
Universitätskrankenhaus Eppendorf
I. Med. Klinik
Martinistr. 52
2000 Hamburg 20
Germany

Prof. Dr. Willms
Fachklinik für Diabetes und Stoffwechsel
Kirchberg 21
3422 Bad Lauterberg
Germany

Prof. Dr. P. Zimmet
International Diabetes Institute
260 Kooyong Road
Caulfield South, 3162
Australia

Contents

H. Meyer
Introduction 1

I New aspects in diabetes mellitus

P. Zimmet, S. Serjeantson
The epidemiology of diabetes mellitus and its relationship with cardiovascular disease 5

H. E. Lebovitz
Syndrome X: fact or fiction? 23

R. G. Josse
Strategies for the treatment of hyperglycemia in Syndrome X 35

H. Lithell
Treatment strategies of Syndrome X – hypertension and vascular complications 51

G. L. Vega
Lipid metabolism: metabolic consequences of moderate hypertriglyceridemia 59

P. J. Lefèbvre, A. J. Scheen
Update on the treatment of NIDDM 71

E. Standl, H. U. Janka, H. Stiegler, H. Mehnert
Hyperinsulinemia and macrovascular complications in NIDDM 87

II Quality of life in diabetes mellitus

S. H. Croog
Diabetes and quality of life: some current issues in definition and research 99

S. Waadt, G. Duran, M. Waadt, P. Herschbach, F. Strian
Quality of life in patients with type II diabetes mellitus 111

M. Toeller
Well-being in non-insulin-dependent diabetic patients (NIDDM) – a long-term follow-up 127

III Studies with acarbose

M. Hanefeld
Acarbose monotherapy in non-insulin-dependent diabetes mellitus – the German experience 147

B. Willms
Acarbose in non-insulin-dependent diabetes mellitus: combination with sulfonylureas and interaction with diet 163

Yuichiro Goto, Yoshio Goto, S. Nakagawa, H. Orimo, Y. Ikeda, N. Sakamoto, I. Fukui, S. Tarui, S. Baba, T. Kaneko, G. Mimura
Clinical efficacy of BAY 5421 (acarbose) in non-insulin-dependent diabetes mellitus (NIDDM) – a placebo-controlled double-blind comparative study 177

N. Sakamoto, N. Hotta, N. Koh, F. Sakakibara, T. Haga, M. Kobayashi, H. Kakuta, T. Sano, H. Yamada, H. Matsumae, S. Kitazawa
Effects of long-term administration of acarbose in patients with NIDDM – a double-blind study with placebo 191

Y. Ikeda, A. Tsuruoka, K. Izumi, M. Yoshida, Y. Nakata, Y. Omori, M. Sanaka, T. Kitagawa, Y. Miyamoto, H. Fujita, M. Kondo, T. Sato, A. Takeda, A. Tanae, K. Matsuoka, K. Murakami, S. Yamamoto
Effects of acarbose on blood glucose control in insulin-dependent diabetes mellitus 201

S. A. Raptis
European experience in the treatment of IDDM with acarbose in combination with insulin 213

Round table discussion on open questions and future aspects 227

IV Abstracts

R. F. Coniff
A multi-center, double-blind, placebo-controlled study of the long-term efficacy and safety of acarbose (BAY g 5421) in the treatment of obese patients with NIDDM treated by diet alone 233

R. F. Coniff, R. J. Innerfield
A multi-center, double-blind, placebo-controlled study of long-term efficacy and safety of acarbose (BAY g 5421) and sulfonylureas in the treatment of NIDDM inadequately controlled by maximal doses of sulfonylureas 234

F. X. Pi-Sunyer
A multi-center, double-blind, comparative study of the long-term efficacy and safety of acarbose (BAY g 5421) vs. placebo in the treatment of patients with insulin requiring type II diabetes mellitus 235

D. S. Schade
Prospective, multi-center studies of the efficacy and safety of acarbose (BAY g 5421) in the treatment of type I diabetes mellitus 237

P. Holander, R. F. Coniff
Two multi-center, double-blind, placebo-controlled studies of efficacy and safety of acarbose treatment of type I diabetes 238

J. Wernecke, M. Dreyer, R. Fisch, G. Michels, M. Lührs, H. G. Dammann
Clinical study of reduced postprandial hyperglycemia by acarbose and glycemic impact of fructose and sucrose in insulin therapy 239

M. Spengler, G. Hänsel, K. Boehme
6 months monotherapy of NIDDM with acarbose or glibenclamide 243

H. Hobler, M. Spengler
Decreased insulin requirement and postprandial insulin plasma concentrations under treatment with the α-glucosidase inhibitor acarbose 247

Yoshio Goto, T. Toyota, S. Oikawa, Y. Maruhama, M. Tamura, K. Komatsu, H. Fujiya, R. Abe, H. Kikuchi
Long-term treatment of BAY g 5421 (acarbose) in non-insulin-dependent diabetes mellitus 251

H. de la Calle, F. Escobar, D. Figuerola, E. Gíl, J. L. Herrera-Pombo, A. Jiménez, A. de Leiva, L. F. Pallardo, F. Piñón, J. Soler, J. Tebar, V. A. Vásquez
Clinical efficacy and tolerability of acarbose in IDDM treatment 258

A. Calle, C. Rodríguez, E. Gíl
Effects of acarbose on the glycemic index of different foods 262

G. Rohr, I. Schmidt, U. Schwedes, K. H. Usadel, Chr. Norenberg, M. Spengler
Effects of acarbose on the release of gastrointestinal, pancreatic and hypophysial hormones including somatostatin in type II diabetics 266

C. Rosak, B. O. Boehm, P. H. Althoff, H. Hobler, K. Boehme
Influence of acarbose on the release of gastrointestinal, pancreatic and hypophyseal hormones including somtostatin in healthy volunteers 274

K. Tawara, N. Mochizuki, A. Donkai, Y. Hikima
Acarbose: an intestinal tract α-glucosidase inhibitor – pharmacological effects on insulin and glycemia in response to a sucrose load 277

M. Spengler, M. Cagatay
Assessment of efficacy and tolerability of acarbose (Glucobay®) by clinical data pool 280

M. Spengler, H. Hobler, M. Cagatay
Long-term tolerability of acarbose 285

M. Spengler, M. Cagatay
Assessment of efficacy and tolerability of acarbose in diabetic patients 5 – 16 years of age 289

J. L. Pinquier, J. Y. Pello, E. Rey, D. De Lauture, P. D'Athis, G. Strauch, G. Olive, I. Morer, F. Prunièras
Effect of acarbose repeated dosing on antipyrine test in healthy volunteers 292

Introduction

H. Meyer

Every compound in pharmaceutical research and development has its ups and downs, but acarbose certainly has more than average. The explanation is very simple – the innovator takes the higher risk. As with many other innovations, acarbose does not emerge from one of the established companies in these respective disease areas, but from a company with limited experience in diabetes. Starting out with the highly innovative concept of selective inhibition of intestinal glucosidases, new models in biochemical, animal and clinical pharmacology had to be developed. Standard toxicology models had to be refined, resulting in a considerable increase of development time. Regulatory authorities have changed the guidelines for the assessment of clinical efficacy in the meantime and the clinical development program had to be refocussed. We have to convince the Scientific and Medical Community of the importance of this new therapeutic principle. It took confidence in the value of the product and the tenacity and perseverance of a company like Bayer to give this story a happy end.

Today we are certain that acarbose with its new and independent mechanism will represent an important alternative and addition in the treatment of diabetes. Let me take this opportunity to thank the inventors, the scientists and the clinical investigators for their efforts and wish the symposium every success in defining new targets for the further development of acarbose.

I New aspects in diabetes mellitus

The epidemiology of diabetes mellitus and its relationship with cardiovascular disease

P. Zimmet, S. Serjeantson

Introduction

The literature on the epidemiology of diabetes continues to expand rapidly, reflecting the appreciation that many aspects of the aetiology and natural history of both insulin-dependent diabetes mellitus (IDDM) and non-insulin-dependent diabetes mellitus (NIDDM) may be elucidated through well planned epidemiological studies. In addition, such studies are now providing a more detailed perspective of the global distribution and social, economic and public health impact of the disease. Apart from this, the putative risk factors for NIDDM are becoming clearer, thus presenting opportunities for the development of primary prevention programmes aimed at reducing the huge morbidity and mortality from diabetes [60].

The emergence of high rates of NIDDM in developing countries has created a major public health problem [10]. Vaughan et al. [49] have recently reviewed this subject and noted that while studies conducted in developed countries confirm the high economic burden of diabetes and its complications, information on the magnitude of this burden in developing countries is almost non-existent. They believe that the prevention of diabetes alone is not a viable policy option but rather that the priority lies with a broad approach to the prevention of a whole range of non-communicable diseases (NCD), including diabetes, and to improved case detection and management. This fits with the current World Health Organization approach to the prevention and control of NCD [42]. Vaughan and his colleagues stress that a major priority should be for further research on the incidence, aetiology and prevention of IDDM and NIDDM in developing countries [49].

Recent epidemiological studies have added to our knoweledge of the aetiology and natural history of glucose intolerance and its inter-relationship with other cardiovascular disease risk factors [59], an area of great interest at the present time. Non-insulin-dependent diabetes tends to cluster with other cardiovascular disease risk factors [59], and this clustering also is seen with impaired glucose tolerance (IGT), raising the issue of a common aetiology for abnormal glucose tolerance and the other components of the cluster, such as dyslipidaemia, hyperinsulinaemia, central obesity and hypertension. These and other aspects of the epidemiology of diabetes will be addressed in this review.

The epidemiology of insulin-dependent diabetes mellitus

Incidence and prevalence

There is now a large body of data on the incidence and prevalence of IDDM in various countries [2, 39, 55]. Whilst this information is of importance in adding to our knowledge of the public health implications of IDDM, these epidemiological studies thus far contributed relatively little to our understanding of the aetiology of this disorder. The interested reader is referred to an extensive review of the major global studies of IDDM prevalence and incidence [39].

The most notable finding from the many recent IDDM studies is the wide variation in the geographic and ethnic distribution of IDDM. There is a greater than 55-fold difference between Finland, with the highest incidence, and Korea with the lowest [55]. A north to south gradient in incidence, with lowest levels found in countries nearest the Equator has also been noted [55]. It has been suggested that this may result from differences in environmental risk factor levels [55], but it could also reflect the fact that populations with lower genetic susceptibility and/or ascertainment of IDDM reside in tropical areas tend to live in these regions since the highest prevalence and incidence patterns are seen in developed countries with Caucasoid populations [39].

The general impression from African studies has been of a low prevalence of IDDM. However, recent study from Sudan showed a prevalence of 0.95/1000 in school children between the ages of 7 and 14 years [12]. Of 41 children with IDDM, 7 (17%) were previously undetected, suggesting not only that IDDM is not as rare as previously thought but also that there may be significant underascertainment of cases. IDDM was also considered to be rare in Malta but a recent study questions this belief [41]. The age adjusted prevalence for 0–19 year old females was 1.1/1000 and that for males was 0.95/1000. The mean annual incidence between 1980–87 in 0–19 year olds was 13.3/1000. These prevalence and incidence rates are similar to those seen in Denmark which has the lowest rate of the Scandinavian countries [39] whose populations are generally considered to have the highest incidence for IDDM in the world.

There is increasing evidence that the environmental contribution to IDDM aetiology has been underestimated in the past [55]. Bingley and Gale have reviewed studies of the incidence of IDDM in Europe [2]. There was a rising incidence in many northern European countries, with a rate equivalent to a doubling time of 20 – 30 years in some. The rapidity of change suggests that environmental factors are responsible, with the implication that if these factors could be identified, primary prevention of IDDM might become possible [55].

However, Dorman et al. [7] have suggested that geographical and racial differences in incidence of IDDM may be almost entirely explained by genetic differences. These workers found that the lack of aspartic acid at position 57 of the HLA-DQ β-chain (non-Asp 57) is highly associated with susceptibility and that there was a strong positive linear correlation found between the incidence of IDDM and non-Asp 57 gene frequency in healthy control subjects from 5 populations. This hypothesis certainly needs to be tested in other populations, given a recent report suggesting that Japanese people do not fit the relationship [1].

The relative importance of environmental factors is suggested by the large difference in incidence of IDDM observed between Finland and Estonia. The highest incidence of IDDM in the world is found in Finland [39] and Estonia is geographically close to Finland. The population is ethnically and linguistically similar but the incidence of IDDM is approximately one-third that of Finland [26]. This contrast in incidence between populations with an apparently similar genetic background provides an opportunity for specific studies of the environmental risk factors for IDDM.

Similarly, the existence of temporal trends in IDDM occurrence provides considerable support for the importance of environmental determinants of the disease [6]. Nonetheless, with the new genetic data on non-Asp 57 as a marker for IDDM, it would appear that future epidemiological studies will need to take a more balanced approach to assessing the role of both genetic and environmental factors. Such studies, together with more information on other putative aetiological environmental factors, will indeed bring primary prevention of IDDM closer.

The epidemiology of non-insulin-dependent diabetes mellitus

There is now considerable evidence that NIDDM is lifestyle related [56]. Given the dramatic change of lifestyle in many developing populations, epidemiologists have been presented with unparalleled opportunities to study the genetic and environmental determinants of NIDDM through both cross-sectional and longitudinal studies.

Prevalence

There is marked variation in the prevalence of NIDDM between populations [56]. Comparison of prevalence studies should be performed with care for a number of reasons, including the use of different oral glucose loads and diagnostic criteria, and method of population selection [10]. However, comparability has become less of a problem in recent times, with many studies following the recommendations of the 1980 and 1985 World Health Organization reports.

The late Kelly West was one of the first to highlight the large differences in prevalence of diabetes (NIDDM) in his classical study of 12 populations from different parts of the globe [51]. Prevalence ranged from lowest in East Pakistan (now Bangladesh) to highest in American Cherokee Indians.

As early as the mid-1960's workers in South Africa had noted marked interethnic differences in diabetes prevalence between South African Blacks, Whites and migrant Asian Indians [28]. Similarly Prior [36] and later our own group [57] demonstrated low prevalence of NIDDM in Pacific island populations living a more traditional lifestyle while their urban counterparts exhibited much higher prevalence. This information, put together, highlighted the role of both genetic and environmental factors in the aetiology of NIDDM.

Prevalence in Caucasoid populations varies between 3% and 6% of adults, but much higher rates (as high as 35%) are seen in certain Micronesian and Polynesian Pacific islanders, American Indians, Mexican Americans, Creoles in Mauritius and Surinam, Australian Aborigines, and migrant Asian Indian communities [10, 56, 57]. Studies of Asian Indian migrants in several countries, including Fiji, South Africa, Singapore, the UK, Mauritius and Tanzania, have demonstrated much higher prevalence than occurs in the other ethnic groups in those countries or on the Indian subcontinent [10, 56].

High NIDDM prevalence has also been reported in Maltese [40], Saudi Arabians [14], Canadian Indians [53] and Chinese in Singapore, Mauritius and Taiwan [8]. It seems that with progressive modernization and industrialization, many more populations will experience rising NIDDM prevalence. Extrapolation from our own findings in Mauritius gives some indication of the coming pandemic, and will be discussed later.

Certainly, there is mounting evidence that NIDDM is on the increase in Canadian Indians [53]. Young et al. have recently reported on the prevalence of diagnosed diabetes for 74% of the registered Indian and Inuit (Eskimo) population of Canada from case registers maintained by the federal agency responsible for Indian Health Services. The highest prevalence, 8.7% occurred amongst Indians in the Atlantic region, followed by Ontario (7.6%). Manitoba, Quebec, Saskatchewan and Alberta fell into an intermediate range of 3.9 to 5.7%. As these were diagnosed cases, it is likely that the true prevalence is at least double these figures, as in most developing populations, ascertainment is around 50% of total cases [8]. The Indian prevalence was considerably higher than that for all other Canadians (self reported prevalence of 2.4%) [53].

The rising global prevalence of non-insulin-dependent diabetes mellitus

The prevalence of glucose intolerance in Caucasoid populations is the "gold standard" to which studies in other ethnic communities are compared. Thus, the study on prevalence of glucose tolerance in the white population of Wadena, USA is of great interest [17]. Total prevalence of abnormal glucose tolerance (IGT – 15.1% and NIDDM – 8.1%) was 23.2% by WHO criteria. This is consistent with the USA national estimate from the NHANES II study [21]. The prevalence of abnormal glucose tolerance in Wadena and the USA overall is substantially higher than that reported in Australia [18] and estimated in the United Kingdom [33].

While it is unclear whether the difference in the prevalence of glucose intolerance between Caucasian populations of the USA and elsewhere is due to genetic or lifestyle factors (such as nutrition, obesity and patterns of physical activity), evidence exists to suggest that the US population may be more obese than others [19]. It is therefore possible that with increasingly sedentary lifestyle practices, the prevalence of glucose intolerance in other Caucasoid populations and, indeed, many newly-industrialized nations, will eventually reach or exceed that of the USA.

Public health planners in both developed and developing countries must face the prospect of a doubling of rates of abnormal glucose tolerance within 10–20 years. The "double hit" of morbidity and mortality specifically related to diabetes and its microvascular complications, plus the contribution of abnormal glucose tolerance to cardiovascular disease (CVD) must be taken into account.

The prospect of a potential public health disaster in many developing populations is the message from Mauritius, a multi-ethnic island nation in the southwestern Indian Ocean which has one of the world's highest diabetes mortality rates [8]. The prevalence of both IGT and NIDDM was investigated in 5080 Muslim and Hindu Indian, Creole (mixed African, European, and Indian origin), and Chinese Mauritian adults aged 25–74 years. Age- and sex-standardized prevalence of IGT and NIDDM was remarkably across ethnic groups (16.2 and 12.4% in Hindu Indians, 15.3 and 13.3% in Muslim Indians, 17.5 and 10.4% in Creoles, and 16.6 and 11.9% in Chinese, respectively). The high prevalence of abnormal glucose tolerance in Asian Indians in Mauritius has also been reported from other countries to which they have migrated [10, 55, 56], as illustrated in Figure 1. For example, in Asian Indians from Tanzania, the overall age-adjusted prevalence of IGT and NIDDM in subjects aged 15 years and over was recently reported at 21.5% and 7.1%, respectively [30]. NIDDM is already common in some Indian subcontinent communities and the implications for public health in modernizing India from the incipient NIDDM epidemic are enormous [55].

The Mauritius picture also indicates similar possibilities for mainland China and continental Africa. The high prevalence of NIDDM in the Mauritian Creoles

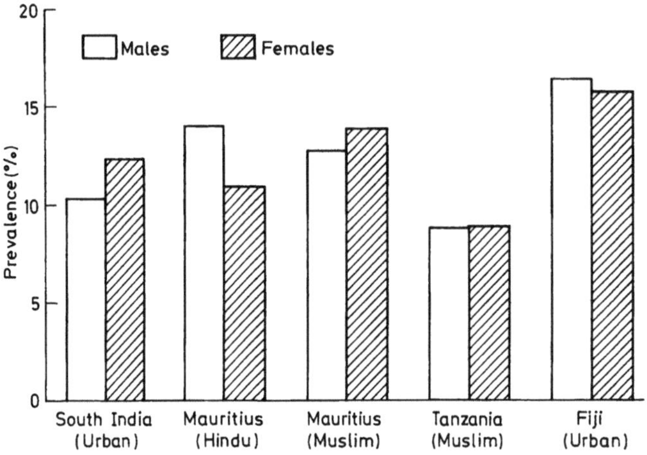

Fig. 1: Comparison of age-standardized prevalence of non-insulin-dependent diabetes mellitus in Asian Indians – aged 25–74 years from the Indian subcontinent and migrant communities overseas.

and Chinese were quite unexpected [8]. The prevalence of NIDDM in mainland China is quite low [56]. The Mauritius study, coupled with evidence that prevalence may be rising in other Chinese populations, indicate the prospect of an epidemic of NIDDM in the People's Republic of China in association with progressive socio-economic development. Similarly, moderate to high NIDDM prevalence is seen in people of African origin in the USA, United Kingdom, Mauritius and in Surinam, suggesting that mainland African populations can also expect to see increasing rates of glucose intolerance in future years [8, 10, 21, 56]. This possibility is supported by the findings of McLarty et al. [31], who assessed the prevalence of diabetes mellitus and IGT in 6299 Africans, aged 15 years and over, in 6 villages in rural Tanzania. The prevalence of diabetes was 0.9% and 7.8% of the subjects had IGT. There were 8 newly diagnosed diabetics for each known case, and the majority of these were symptom free.

Given the high prevalence of diabetes of 8% reported in the US black adult population, the potential exists for these same high rates to be matched in African populations with progressive modernization of life-style [21]. The already relatively high prevalence of IGT in the Tanzanian population points to this eventuality.

Despite overwhelming anecdotal and inferential evidence that NIDDM prevalence is rising in most populations around the world, there is surprisingly little directly comparable data to confirm such increases. There is indirect evidence from the Pima Indian studies that this is happening, but it has been well-documented in the Polynesians of Rarotonga (Cook Islands), where the prevalence of NIDDM in men increased from 5.4% to 10.6% between 1980 and 1987 [56]. In women, the prevalence rate increased from 7.7% to 10.7%. Similarly, there has been an apparent increase in diabetes prevalence in Singapore over the 10-year period since 1979 [47].

In fact, based on data from these and other populations, we have suggested that an "epidemicity index" [10, 11] may be useful as an indicator of the potential for higher future NIDDM prevalence in whole populations.

Epidemicity index – an indicator of future diabetes in a population

The relationship between the prevalence of IGT and NIDDM was studied across populations of the Pacific Ocean region in order to assess whether variability in those two proportions might follow a predictable pattern related to modernization of lifestyle and risk factor levels [10]. The epidemicity index, calculated as the percentage of total glucose intolerance (TGI) made up by IGT (i. e. IGT/TGI), had a strong negative correlation with NIDDM prevalence (Fig. 2). Moreover, when IGT/TGI was plotted against NIDDM prevalence for the genetically homogeneous rural (relatively traditional) and urban (modernized) segments of 5 Pacific island populations there was a clear tendency for IGT/TGI to decline as the prevalence of NIDDM increased [11].

This suggests that the epidemicity index may have some use as an indicator of the potential for higher future NIDDM prevalence in populations, which will

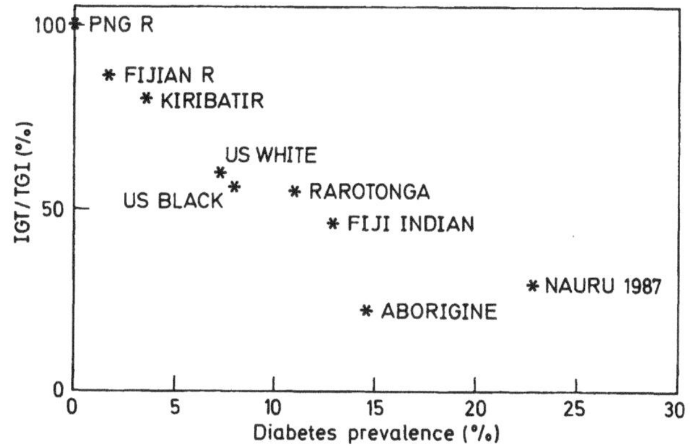

Fig. 2: Epidemicity index (IGT/TGI) versus NIDDM prevalence in rural and urban populations from Kiribati (Micronesian), Western Samoa (Polynesian), Wallis Island (Polynesian) and Fiji (Melanesian and Indian).
Reproduced with permission of Elsevier Science Publishers from G. Dowse and P. Zimmet [10].

probably equilibrate at a certain NIDDM prevalence depending on the strength of their genetic susceptibility to the disease and their degree of exposure to adverse environmental risk factors, including modern diet, physical inactivity and obesity [11].

NIDDM and other cardiovascular disease risk factors

While it is convenient to discuss the epidemiology of diabetes under the headings of the different types (that is, IDDM and NIDDM), it is becoming more difficult to define the limits of NIDDM. NIDDM and, in fact, abnormal glucose tolerance (IGT and diabetes combined) are risk factors for CVD and there is a tendency for cardiovascular disease risk factors to cluster in individuals [59]. By contrast, IDDM is a relatively discrete disorder with respect to clinical and biochemical presentation and its autoimmune aetiology.

Another important question relates to the status of IGT. It has been argued that IGT does not warrant categorization as a separate entity, and that IGT and NIDDM, rather than being considered as discrete and separate states should they be combined and regarded as the spectrum of abnormal glucose intolerance [23, 59].

In addition, given that NIDDM often occurs in association with other risk factors for coronary artery disease (CAD) e. q. dyslipidaemia, hypertension and obesity, the question also arises as to whether NIDDM is a discrete disease or part of a cluster of risk factors for cardiovascular disease such as the recently described "Syndrome X" or similar risk factor linkages [38, 59]. These have been described by a number of workers over the last 40 years including Crepaldi, Vague, Prior, Björntorp, Kissebah, Modan, Hanefeld, Reaven, DeFronzo, Kaplan and others [61]. Kaplan has suggested the rather attractive term "Deadly Quartet" to describe the combination of upper-body obesity, glucose intolerance, hypertriglyceridaemia and hypertension [27]. We do not believe that the components listed for "Syndrome X" [27] reflect the whole spectrum of the risk factor cluster. Table 1 provides a more complete perspective of these components.

How discrete a condition is NIDDM? More epidemiological data are required to allow a firm conclusion and a major issue in respect of this is the relationship between the risk of CVD and glucose intolerance [59, 61]. That is, is there a threshold of hyperglycaemia that is associated with increased risk of cardiovascular disease, either alone or in combination with other risk factors?

Longitudinal epidemiological studies incorporating measures of glucose tolerance and other CVD risk factors provide the opportunity to address this issue. We have studied this in the Mauritian population on a cross-sectional basis. There is a graded increase in levels of several CVD risk factors with increasing glucose intolerance, even at levels below that which defines IGT (Zimmet, P., Dowse, G. – unpublished data). For example, fasting plasma triglyceride and serum insulin concentrations, and also systolic blood pressure rise linearly with increasing glucose intolerance. Thus even the earliest evidence of glucose intolerance is associated with increased CVD risk, as has been demonstrated in the Whitehall (United Kingdom) study [25].

Table 1: Components of Syndrome X and other similar syndromes reflecting increased cardiovascular disease risk

"Syndrome X"	*"Syndrome* X + + +"
Insulin resistance	Insulin resistance
Glucose intolerance	Glucose intolerance
Hyperinsulinaemia	Hyperinsulinaemia
Increased VLDL triglycerides	Increased VLDL triglycerides
Decreased HDL cholesterol	Decreased HDL cholesterol
Hypertension	Hypertension
	Abdominal fat distribution
	Hyperuricaemia
	Physical inactivity
	Ageing

Impaired glucose tolerance and risk of cardiovascular disease

The debate concerning whether IGT is a true entity and its prognostic significance in relation to NIDDM is not purely academic. While it is not possible to answer the question at this point in time, it is clear that persons with IGT have elevated levels of risk factors of CVD and this risk is translated into CVD endpoints in longitudinal studies [25], as has been confirmed yet again in the Paris Prospective Study [16]. Triglyceride, cholesterol and insulin (fasting and 2-hour) concentrations were significantly higher in those who died from coronary heart disease compared to those who did not. Subjects with IGT had mortality rates nearly identical to those of newly-diagnosed diabetics, 2.7/1000 per year and 2.9/1000 per year respectively. In addition, the levels of cardiovascular risk factors in subjects with IGT were more like those in diabetic than in normal subjects.

Perhaps the major justification for the separate category of IGT was the putative risk of CVD [23, 59]. Yet, as Yudkin et al. [54] have recently pointed out, there is still a lack of consensus about the excess risk of CVD in persons with IGT. However, subjects with IGT from a number of populations show hyperinsulinaemia and insulin resistance and increased prevalence of other cardiovascular risk factors [23, 58, 59].

O'Dea et al. studied a small rural Aboriginal community in northern Australia [35] and demonstrated an unexpectedly high prevalence of IGT (7.4%) and NIDDM (11.5%) in adults over 17 years of age, in view of their relative leanness. Insulin response to glucose showed wide variation with the upper tertile mean 2-hour insulin being more than seven times that of the lower tertile mean. Hyperinsulinaemia was associated with IGT, elevated triglycerides and lower HDL cholesterol. This combination has caused great interest and Haffner et al. [20] have asked the key question: "Does the clock for coronary heart disease start ticking before the onset of clinical diabetes?". This has important implications in the study of the genesis of complications of diabetes.

The epidemiology and risk factors for microvascular and macrovascular complications are quite different. Duration of diabetes and degree of hyperglycaemia have been consistently shown to be the major risk factors for microvascular complications [59, 61]. This is not so for the macrovascular complications, and it appears that the explanation lies with the variety of metabolic abnormalities described earlier, plus their interaction with life-style risk factors such as cigarette smoking and physical inactivity [59].

Certainly, the diagnostic criteria for "diabetes" (and hence the definition of the entity itself) have been based on the specificity of the microvascular complications for plasma glucose levels exceeding 11.1 mmol/l following a 75-g oral glucose tolerance test [10].

Data from a number of populations show that hyperinsulinaemia predates NIDDM by many years and that subjects with IGT are also hyperinsulinaemic [58]. Three longitudinal studies have found that hyperinsulinaemia is predictive of subsequent cardiovascular disease [13, 37, 50]. There was a also close correlation between the prevalence of macrovascular disease and daily insulin dose in insulin-treated NIDDM subjects in the Schwabing (Germany) Study [44].

Haffner et al. [20] have assessed the association of hyperinsulinaemia and risk of CVD in the population-based San Antonio Heart Study and documented the CVD risk factor status of 614 initially non-diabetic Mexican Americans. In 43 subjects who subsequently developed NIDDM at 8 year follow-up, there were higher baseline levels of fasting and 2-hour glucose, fasting insulin, total and LDL cholesterol, body mass index and blood pressure, and lower levels of HDL cholesterol than in subjects who remained non-diabetic. The majority of these differences persisted after adjustment for obesity and/or level of glycaemia but were abolished after adjustment for fasting insulin concentration. When subjects with IGT at baseline were eliminated, the more atherogenic pattern of cardiovascular risk factors still persisted. Therefore, it appears that subjects who develop NIDDM are at increased risk of coronary heart disease many years before onset of clinical diabetes [20, 61].

Other epidemiological studies support these data. CVD risk factors and IGT were studied in Hispanic and Anglo subjects participating in the San Luis Valley Diabetes Study in Colorado USA [3]. In both ethnic groups, persons with IGT had cardiovascular risk profiles that were intermediate between subjects with normal glucose tolerance and NIDDM. Similarly, in the study from Rancho Bernardo, California USA, a less favourable CVD risk factor profile preceded the diagnosis of both NIDDM and IGT (49). Adverse CVD risk factor levels among subjects with IGT have also been reported in Australian Aborigines [35], Fijian Melanesians and migrant Asian Indians [5], and in Micronesians from Kiribati [4].

These data are compatible with the findings that subjects with NIDDM have excessive risk of mortality from CVD [15], and raise a number of important issues. Firstly, the concept that macrovascular disease is a chronic complication of NIDDM needs to be reviewed or qualified. The above evidence is consistent with the fact that macrovascular disease is an integral part of the CVD risk factor cluster or syndrome which includes IGT, NIDDM and even lesser degrees of abnormal glucose tolerance [61]. The critical question that arises is to what extent the glucose intolerance contributes independently to risk of CVD, given the presence of the other cardiovascular risk factors. In any case, it can be argued that macrovascular disease is part of the natural history of glucose intolerance (including NIDDM), i. e. part and parcel of the disease itself.

Steiner [45] has recently reminded us [45] of the debt we owe to Joslin who, in 1927, prophetically wrote: "With an excess of fat diabetes begins and from an excess of fat diabetics die, formerly of coma, recently of arteriosclerosis". Moreover, Fontbonne et al. [16] have also provided a timely reminder that while the coronary heart disease/cholesterol debate continues unabated, hypertriglyceridaemia is an important predictor of coronary heart disease mortality in subjects with IGT and NIDDM and that it has a possible role in the excessive occurrence of atherosclerotic vascular disease in persons with abnormal glucose tolerance.

Secondly, given the increased prevalence of cardiovascular risk factors and increased risk of CVD in subjects with IGT, should intervention activities be targeted at this group of "high risk" individuals? There are few studies which satisfactorily address this issue, but to date there is little positive evidence for any benefits of screening for asymptomatic glucose intolerance [9].

Ethnic factors in the relationship between cardiovascular disease and glucose intolerance

Epidemiologists and clinicians have long been puzzled by the variation in patterns of cardiovascular disease in different ethnic populations and it was this phenomenon that led to the WHO Multinational Study of Vascular Disease in Diabetics

[48]. This study, involving 14 national samples, demonstrated marked differences in prevalence of macrovascular disease with much higher rates in Western Europe than in Hong Kong and China. While the prevalence of microvascular disease was similar between countries, the pattern of macrovascular disease in diabetics was similar to those people without diabetes i. e. cultural and ethnic factors appeared more likely to contribute to the variation in macrovascular disease than the diabetic state per se.

The reasons for such differences have been the subject of a number of recent studies. Mitchell et al. investigated why the lower CVD mortality in Mexican Americans compared to non-Hispanic whites was confined to men [29]. Cardiovascular risk factors were compared between the two groups and CVD risk factors scores (including diabetes prevalence) were higher in Mexican-Americans than in non-Hispanic whites of both sexes. Yet while the risk factor scores were higher in Mexican-Americans, these were not translated into higher CVD endpoints. There were lower cardiovascular mortality rates among Hispanic men compared to non-Hispanic white men. They speculated that the less favourable cardiovascular risk profile in Mexican-American men indicates that there might be as yet unidentified (possibly genetic) factors that are protective against heart disease in Mexican-American men despite high CVD risk profiles. However, if genetic factors are involved, they must operate differently in men and women, since relative protection is observed only among men.

American Indians may also be relatively resistant to coronary heart disease. Although the Pima Indians have the world's highest reported prevalence of NIDDM [56], they have a low frequency of CHD. Nelson et al. [34] have recently reported on the incidence of fatal CHD in Pima Indians with NIDDM in comparison to non-diabetics. The Pima Indians, despite their high prevalence of NIDDM had a low incidence of fatal CHD compared with the primarily Caucasian population of Framingham. As no CHD occurred in non-diabetics, diabetes was a major risk factor for fatal CHD in Pimas during the 10 year period of the study.

Risk factors for fatal CHD in diabetic Pima Indians included older age, male gender, duration of diabetes, insulin therapy, proteinuria, renal insufficiency, medial arterial calcification, diabetic retinopathy and ECG abnormalities [34]. The "traditional" risk factors, such as total serum cholesterol, hypertension and smoking did not predict CHD in the diabetic Pimas. Their lesser contribution in this population apparently magnifies the importance of NIDDM as a risk factor for CHD.

However, in this study no data on triglycerides or insulin concentrations were reported so that even this conclusion must be tempered, given the putative impact of these two metabolic factors in the aetiology of CHD [16, 61]. Nevertheless, the lack of fatal CHD among non-diabetic Pima Indians is striking, and this, coupled with the low rates compared with the Framingham populations, raises the possibility of protection by some, as yet unknown factors modulating which, as suggested earlier, may have a genetic basis.

At the opposite end of the spectrum of CVD risk and prevalence are the migrant Asian Indians. McKeigue et al. [30] have recently reviewed reports of CHD in migrant Asian Indians. High CHD prevalence is common in these people from the Indian subcontinent and rates are often higher than those of the indigenous population e.g. Fiji [43], United Kingdom [52] and Singapore [22]. In many of these populations, the high rates of CHD cannot be explained on the basis of conventional risk factors such as cholesterol, cigarette smoking, obesity or hypertension. While it has been suggested that NIDDM may be a major factor [24], it seems feasible and more likely that hyperinsulinaemia/insulin resistance, a well documented feature in Asian Indians [61], may have an important role. This would also explain the low plasma HDL cholesterol, and high triglyceride concentrations and high prevalence of NIDDM in these people.

It has been suggested that this elevated CHD risk has a genetic basis, and the spectre of genetically determined insulin resistance/hyperinsulinaemia as an underlying factor emerges [61]. Should genetic factors be shown to be important in modulating risk of CHD in different ethnic groups, then this will have important implications for primary prevention programs as strategies aimed at lifestyle change will need to be targeted at the "high risk" groups, which may have a major genetic component to their risk.

As was discussed earlier, there are now three longitudinal studies that show high insulin levels constitute a predictor of future cardiovascular disease [13, 37, 50]. It was long considered that increased CHD risk associated with NIDDM was secondary to the diabetes or glucose intolerance. There is now considerable evidence against this and it has been elegantly summarized by Jarrett [24] recently. There is considerable circumstantial evidence to support the fact that CHD and NIDDM are associated disorders.

Evidence summarized earlier suggests that it is hyperinsulinaemia/insulin resistance that may be the common aetiological factor or link. While the art and excitement precedes the available scientific data on this link, this is clearly an area where current prospective studies in a number of unusual populations may shed light in the near future. The results will be very important in relation to future efforts to prevent and control diabetes and its associated macrovascular disorders.

Acknowledgements

Supported by grant DK 25446 from the National Institute of Diabetes and Digestive and Kidney Diseases. We thank Mrs. S. Fournel for the preparation of the manuscript.

References

[1] Awata, T., T. Kuzuya, A. Matsuda et al.: High frequency of aspartic acid at position 57 of HLA-DQ β-chain in Japanese IDDM patients and nondiabetic subjects. Diabetes *39* (1990) 266–269.

[2] Bingley, P. J., E. A. M. Gale: Rising incidence of IDDM in Europe. Diabetes Care *12* (1989) 289–295.

[3] Burchfiel, C. M., R. F. Hamman, J. A. Marshall et al.: Cardiovascular risk factors and impaired glucose tolerance: The San Luis Valley Diabetes Study. Am. J. Epidemiol. *131* (1990) 57–70.

[4] Collins, V., R. Taylor, P. Zimmet et al.: Impaired glucose tolerance in Kiribati. N. Z. Med. J. *97* (1984) 809–812.

[5] Coventry, J., H. King, P. Zimmet et al.: Impaired glucose tolerance in the biethnic (Melanesian and Indian) populations of Fiji. Diabetes Res. *3* (1986) 427–432.

[6] Diabetes Epidemiology Research International Group: Secular trends in incidence of childhood IDDM in 10 countries. Diabetes *39* (1990) 858–864.

[7] Dorman, J. S., R. E. LaPorte, R. A. Stone et al.: Worldwide differences in the incidence of type I diabetes are associated with amino acid variation at position 57 of the HLA-DQ β-chain. Proceedings of National Academy of Science, USA *87* (1990) 7370–7374.

[8] Dowse, G. K., H. Gareeboo, P. Z. Zimmet et al.: The high prevalence of glucose intolerance in Indian, Creole and Chinese Mauritians. Diabetes *39* (1990) 390–396.

[9] Dowse, G., P. Zimmet, K. G. M. M. Alberti: Screening for diabetes and other categories of glucose intolerance. In: K. G. M. M. Alberti, R. De Fronzo, H. Keen et al. (eds.): International Textbook of Diabetes Mellitus, John Wiley, London 1991 (in press).

[10] Dowse, G. K., P. Z. Zimmet: The prevalence and incidence of non-insulin dependent diabetes mellitus. In: K. G. M. M. Alberti, R. Mazze (eds.): Frontiers in diabetes research: current trends in non-insulin-dependent diabetes mellitus, pp. 37–59. Elsevier, Amsterdam 1989.

[11] Dowse, G. K., P. Z. Zimmet, H. King: Relationship between prevalence of IGT and NIDDM in a population – the "epidemicity" index. Diabetes Care *14* (1991) in press.

[12] Elamin, A., M. I. A. Omer, Y. Hofvanger et al.: Prevalence of IDDM in schoolchildren in Khartoum, Sudan. Diabetes Care *12* (1989) 430–432.

[13] Eschwege, E., J. L. Richard, N. Thibult et al.: Coronary heart disease mortality in relation with diabetes, blood glucose and plasma insulin levels. Hormone Metab. Res. *15* (1985) (Suppl) 41–56.

[14] Fatani, H. H., S. A. Mira, A. G. El-Zubier: Prevalence of diabetes in rural Saudi Arabia. Diabetes Care *10* (1978) 180–183.

[15] Finch, C. F., P. Zimmet: Mortality from Diabetes. In: K. G. M. M. Alberti, L. P. Krall (eds): The Diabetes Annual/4, pp. 1–16. Elsevier, Amsterdam 1988.

[16] Fontbonne, A., E. Eschwege, F. Cambien et al.: Hypertriglyceridaemia as a risk factor of coronary heart disease mortality in subjects with impaired glucose tolerance or diabetes: Results from the 11-year follow-up of the Paris Prospective Study. Diabetologia *32* (1989) 300–304.

[17] French, L. R., J. R. Boen, A. M. Martinez et al.: Population-based study of impaired glucose tolerance and type II diabetes in Wadena, Minnesota. Diabetes *39* (1990) 1131–1137.

[18] Glatthaar, C., T. A. Welborn, N. S. Stenhouse et al.: Diabetes and impaired glucose tolerance: a prevalence estimate based on the Busselton 1981 survey. Med. J. Aust. *143* (1985) 436–440.

[19] Gurney, M., J. Gorstein: The global prevalence of obesity – an initial overview of available data. World Health Statistical Quarterly *41* (1988) 251–254.

[20] Hafner, S. M., M. P. Stern, H. P. Hazuda et al.: Cardiovascular risk factors in confirmed prediabetic individuals. Does the clock for coronary heart disease start ticking before the onset of clinical diabetes? JAMA *263* (1990) 2893–2898.

[21] Harris, M. I., W. C. Hadden, W. C. Knowler et al.: Prevalence of diabetes and impaired glucose tolerance and plasma glucose levels in US population aged 20–74 Yr. Diabetes *36* (1987) 523–534.

[22] Hughes, K., P. P. B. Yeo, K. C. Lun et al.: Cardiovascular diseases in Chinese, Malays, and Indians in Singapore. II. Differences in risk factor levels. J. Epidemiol. Comm. Hlth. *44* (1990) 29–35.

[23] Jarrett, R. J.: Do we need IGT? Diabetic Medicine *4* (1987) 544–545.

[24] Jarrett, R. J.: Epidemiology and public health aspects of non-insulin-dependent diabetes mellitus. Epidemiol. Rev. *11* (1989) 151–171.

[25] Jarrett, R. J., P. McCartney, H. Keen: The Bedford Survey: Ten year mortality rates in newly diagnosed diabetics, borderline diabetics and normoglycaemic controls and risk indices for coronary heart disease in borderline diabetics. Diabetologia *22* (1982) 79–84.

[26] Kalits, I., T. Podar: Incidence and prevalence of Type 1 (insulin-dependent) diabetes in Estonia in 1988. Diabetologia *33* (1990) 346–349.

[27] Kaplan, N. M.: The deadly quartet. Upper-body obesity, glucose intolerance, hypertriglyceridaemia and hypertension. Arch. Int. Med. *149* (1989) 1514–1520.

[28] Marine, N., O. Edelstein, W. P. U. Jackson et al.: Diabetes, hyperglycaemia and glycosuria among Indians, Malays and Africans (Bantu) in Cape Town, South Africa. Diabetes *18* (1969) 840–857.

[29] Mitchell, B. D., M. P. Stern, S. M. Haffner et al.: Risk factors for cardiovascular mortality in Mexican Americans and non-Hispanic whites. The San Antonio Heart Study. Am. J. Epidemiol. *131* (1990) 423–433.

[30] McKeigue, P. M., G. J. Miller, M. G. Marmot: Coronary heart disease in South Asians overseas: A review. J. Clin. Epidemiol. *42* (1989) 597–609.

[31] McLarty, D., A. B. M. Swai, H. M. Kitange et al.: Prevalence of diabetes and impaired glucose tolerance in rural Tanzania. Lancet *1* (1989) 871–875.

[32] McPhillips, J. B., E. Barrett-Conner, D. L. Wingard: Cardiovascular disease risk factors prior to the diagnosis of impaired glucose tolerance and non-insulin-dependent diabetes mellitus in a community of older adults. Am. J. Epidemiol. *131* (1990) 443–453.

[33] Nabarro, J.: Diabetes in the United Kingdom: some facts and figures. Diabetic Medicine *5* (1988) 816–817.

[34] Nelson, R. G., M. L. Sievers, W. C. Knowler et al.: Low incidence of fatal coronary heart disease in Pima Indians despite high prevalence of non-insulin-dependent diabetes. Circulation *81* (1990) 987–995.

[35] O'Dea, K., R. J. Lion, A. Lee et al.: Diabetes, hyperinsulinemia and hyperlipidemia in small Aboriginal Community in Northern Australia. Diabetes Care *13* (1990) 830–835.

[36] Prior, I. A. M., F. Davidson: The epidemiology of diabetes in Polynesians and Europeans in New Zealand and the Pacific. N. Z. Med. J. *65* (1966) 375–383.

[37] Pyörälä, K. E., S. Savulainen, J. Kaukola et al.: High plasma insulin as coronary heart disease risk factor. In: E. Eschwege (ed.): Advances in Diabetes Epidemiology. INSERM Symposium No. 22, pp. 143–148. Elsevier, Amsterdam 1982.

[38] Reaven, G. M.: Role of insulin resistance in human disease. Diabetes *37* (1988) 1595–1607.

[39] Rewers, M., R. E. LaPorte, H. King, J. Tuomilehto: Trends in the prevalence and incidence of diabetes: insulin-dependent diabetes mellitus in childhood. World Hlth. Statist Quart. *41* (1988) 179–189.

[40] Schranz, A. G.: Abnormal glucose tolerance in the Maltese. A population-based longitudinal study of the natural history of NIDDM and IGT in Malta. Diabetes Res. Clin. Practice *7* (1989) 7–16.

[41] Schranz, A. G., V. Prikatsky: Type 1 diabetes in the Maltese islands. Diabetic Med. *6* (1989) 228–231.

[42] Shigan, E.: Integrated programme for non-communicable diseases prevention and control (NCD). World Hlth. Statist Quart. *41* (1988) 267–273.

[43] Sicree, R. A., J. Tuomilehto, P. Zimmet et al.: Electrocardiographic abnormalities amongst Melanesian & Indian men of Fiji: prevalence and associated factors. Int. J. Cardiology *19* (1988) 27–38.

[44] Standl, E., H. U. Janka: High serum insulin concentrations in relation to other cardiovascular risk factors in macrovascular disease of type 2 diabetes. Hormone Metab. Res. *17* (1985) 46–51.

[45] Steiner, G.: From an excess of fat, diabetics die. JAMA *262* (1989) 398–399.

[46] Swai, A. B. M., D. G. McLarty, F. Sherrif et al.: Diabetes and impaired glucose tolerance in an Asian community in Tanzania. Diabetes Res. Clin. Practice *8* (1990) 227–234.

[47] Thai, C., P. P. B. Yeo, K. C. Lun et al.: Changing prevalence of diabetes mellitus in Singapore over a ten year period. In: S. Vannasaeng, W. Nitianant, S. Chandraprasert (eds.): Epidemiology of diabetes mellitus: Proceedings of the International Symposium of Epidemiology of Diabetes Mellitus, pp. 63–67. Crystal House Press, Bangkok 1987.

[48] The World Health Organization Multinational Study of Vascular Disease in Diabetics: Prevalence of small vessel and large vessel disease in diabetic patients from 14 centres. Diabetologia *28* (1985) 615 – 640.
[49] Vaughan, P., L. Gilson, A. Mills: Diabetes in developing countries: its importance for public health. Hlth. Policy Planning *4* (1989) 97 – 109.
[50] Welborn, T. A., K. Wearne: Coronary heart disease incidence and cardiovascular mortality in Busselton with reference to glucose and insulin concentrations. Diabetes Care *2* (1979) 154 – 160.
[51] West, K. M.: Epidemiology of diabetes and its vascular complications. Elsevier, New York 1978.
[52] Woods, K. L., A. Samanta, A. C. Burden: Diabetes mellitus as a risk factor for acute myocardial infarction in Asians and Europeans. Br.Hrt. J. *62* (1989) 118 – 122.
[53] Young, T. K., E. J. E. Szathmary, S. Evers et al.: Geographical distribution of diabetes among the native population of Canada: A national survey. Soc. Sci. Med. *31* (1990) 129 – 139.
[54] Yudkin, J. S., K. G. M. M. Alberti, D. McLarty et al.: Impaired glucose tolerance. Is it a risk factor for diabetes or a diagnostic ratbag? Br. Med. J. *301* (1990) 397 – 402.
[55] Zimmet, P., C. Finch, G. Dowse: The epidemiology of diabetes mellitus. In: K. G. M. M. Alberti, L. P. Krall (eds.): The Diabetes Annual/5, pp. 1 – 21. Elsevier, Amsterdam 1990.
[56] Zimmet, P., G. Dowse, A. Kriska et al.: Recent development in the epidemiology of non-insulin dependent diabetes. Diabetes Nutr. Metab. *3* (Suppl. 1) (1990) 3 – 15.
[57] Zimmet, P., G. Dowse, C. Finch et al.: The epidemiology and natural history of NIDDM – Lessons from the South Pacific. Diabetes Metab. Rev. *6* (1990) 91 – 124.
[58] Zimmet, P., G. Dowse, P. Bennett: Hyperinsulinaemia is a predictor of non-insulin-dependent mellitus. Diabete et Metabolisme *17* (1991) 101 – 108.
[59] Zimmet, P.: Non insulin-dependent (type II) diabetes mellitus – does it really exist? Diabetic Med. *6* (1989) 728 – 735.
[60] Zimmet, P.: Primary prevention of diabetes mellitus. Diabetes Care *11* (1988) 258 – 262.
[61] Zimmet, P.: The epidemiology of diabetes mellitus and related conditions. In: K. G. M. M. Alberti, L. P. Krall (eds.): The Diabetes Annual/6. Elsevier, Amsterdam 1991 (in press).

Syndrome X: fact or fiction?

H. E. Lebovitz

Introduction

The concept that non-insulin-dependent diabetes mellitus is one component of a more extensive metabolic syndrome was popularized in 1988 by Reaven [33]. He called this metabolic disorder "Syndrome X" and listed its components as shown in Table 1. He suggested that: (1) this syndrome maybe of great importance in the genesis of coronary artery disease. (2) that the common feature of this syndrome is insulin resistance and that all other abnormalities result from it. Zimmet [43] in a later publication proposed that central obesity be added to the syndrome. Others have proposed broading the link from coronary artery disease to macrovascular disease [38].

Table 1: Syndrome X as described by Reaven [33]

Resistance to insulin-stimulated glucose uptake
Glucose intolerance
Hyperinsulinemia
Increased very-low-density lipoprotein triglyceride
Decreased high-density lipoprotein cholesterol
Hypertension

The fundamental questions underlying Syndrome X are whether it is a unique entity or just an association of several metabolic abnormalities; and, if it is a unique entity, can all of its components be causally related to insulin resistance and/or hyperinsulinemia?

Evidence for the existence of Syndrome X

The evidence for the existence of Syndrome X comes from many excellent clinical studies. Insulin resistance as a basic abnormality in non-insulin-dependent diabetes mellitus has been repeatedly demonstrated by Reaven and his co-workers

Authors studies supported by grants from Roerig Division of Pfister Pharmaceutical Co, Merck Sharp and Dohme and the General Clinical Research Center Branch of the Division of Research Resources of the National Institutes of Health (RR00318).

[31, 32, 33] and confirmed in numerous publications by DeFronzo and his colleagues [6, 7] as well as many other investigators. While considerable controversy continues to exist as to whether insulin resistance is a primary defect or secondary to deficient insulin secretion, several studies which have shown the presence of insulin resistance in non-diabetic relatives of non-insulin-dependent diabetic patients indicate that at least in some individuals insulin resistance must be the primary abnormality [9, 22]. The increased prevalence of hyperinsulinemia in populations which have a high prevalence of non-insulin-dependent diabetes mellitus support the concept that insulin resistance occurs early in the course of NIDDM and is compensated for by hyperinsulinemia [15, 36]. Both the cross-sectional and longitudinal studies in Pima Indians [24] add further support to the concept that insulin resistance is the early abnormality and that decreased insulin secretion occurs late and accounts for the development of frank hyperglycemia.

The evidence to link insulin resistance and/or hyperinsulinemia to increased coronary heart disease is based on data from several large epidemiologic studies. The 11.5 year follow up of the approximately 6900 males in the Paris Prospective study identified fasting and 2 hr post glucose load plasma insulin levels as independent risk factors for death from coronary artery disease [10]. Similar results were reported from the Helsinki Policeman study [29] and Busselton study [41]. Data such as that of Zavaroni et al. [42] who showed that normal weight individuals who have plasma insulin levels higher than 2 standard deviations above the mean of the population have an increased cardiovascular disease risk factor profile (higher fasting plasma triglycerides, lower serum HDL cholesterol, higher systolic and diastolic blood pressures) strengthen the concept that insulin resistance and hyperinsulinemia are associated with a high risk for coronary heart disease. Similar data from the San Antonio Heart Study show that individuals destined to develop NIDDM have marked increases in CV disease risk factors while they still have normal glucose metabolism or impaired glucose tolerance [16].

Data linking hypertension to insulin resistance comes from several sources. Ferrannini et al. [11] studied 13 patients with essential hypertension and found that they exhibited a degree of insulin resistance as measured by the euglycemic insulin clamp that was almost as severe as patients with NIDDM. Additional reports showing that patients with essential hypertension have insulin resistance and hyperinsulinemia have appeared over the last several years [30]. The possible mechanisms for such a relationship have been reviewed by Donahue et al. [8] and include such factors as the role of fat distribution on insulin secretion and blood pressure, insulin's effect on the sympathetic nervous system and insulin's action on sodium transport. Several animal models of hypertension are associated with insulin resistance [30, 33].

The adverse effect of diabetes mellitus in accelerating atherosclerosis and increasing the prevalence of clinical coronary artery, cerebrovascular and peripheral vascular disease have been repeatedly documented in numerous studies [13, 19, 20, 23, 28]. In particular, those studies indicate that NIDDM either directly or through its metabolic changes (hyperglycemia, dyslipidemia, hyperinsulinemia, hypertension, renal disease etc.) causes accelerated macrovascular disease.

Evidence questioning the validity of the concept of Syndrome X

The body of data supporting the existence of Syndrome X as presented above is most impressive and leads to a theory of pathogenesis as noted in Figure 1.

Current concepts of Syndrome X

Insulin resistance
↓
Hyperinsulinemia
↓
Normal glucose metabolism
Hypertension
Elevated VLDL triglycerides
Decreased HDL cholesterol
Macrovascular disease

↙	↘
Loss of beta cell function	Continued exaggerated beta cell function
↓	↓
Diabetes mellitus	Normal glucose metabolism

Fig. 1: The current proposed theory of Syndrome X with insulin resistance as the underlying cause.

Insulin resistance is proposed as the central abnormality. The compensation for insulin resistance would be a secondary hyperinsulinemia. Either the insulin resistance or the hyperinsulinemia would cause hypertension, increased VLDL triglyceride, decreased HDL cholesterol and accelerated atherosclerosis. Hyperglycemia (NIDDM) would only occur in those individuals whose beta cells could not continue to compensate through out life.

If insulin resistance and/or hyperinsulinemia were the underlying abnormality of the components of Syndrome X including central obesity and macrovascular disease, one might expect that populations with an increased prevalence of NIDDM and presumably insulin resistance should show a comparable increase in the prevalence of the components of Syndrome X and those components should be correlated with the insulin resistance.

Relationship of insulin resistance to hypertension

The studies which show a positive relationship between insulin resistance and blood pressure have been performed in white populations or Chinese men in Taiwan [11, 27, 35, 39]. Saad et al. [34] (Tab. 2) studied the relationship between insulin resistance, hyperinsulinemia and blood pressure in 116 Pima Indians, 53 whites and 42 blacks who were normotensive and did not have diabetes [34]. When corrected for age, sex, body weight and percentage of body fat there was no significant relationship between insulin resistance and/or hyperinsulinemia with blood pressure in the blacks or Pima Indians but there was in the whites. Other data showing a weak or no correlation in blacks between plasma insulin levels and blood pressure exist [25, 40]. Plasma insulin levels and blood pressure are weakly related in Mexican American men ($r = 0.3$, $p < 0.001$) but not women ($r = 0.1$) [14]. The relationship between plasma insulin levels and blood pressure is very weak (< 1% of the variance in BP) in the various populations of Mauritius [2] and inconsistent in Pacific Island populations (Micronesians, Polynesians and Melanesians) [5].

Table 2: Correlation of insulin resistance to mean arterial blood pressure in Pima Indians, whites and blacks [34]

Variable	Pima Indians	Whites	Blacks
– Fasting Plasma Insulin			
Mean (pmol/l)	176	138	122
Correlation with BP	−0.06	0.42**	−0.10
– 2 hr Plasma Insulin			
Mean (pmol/l)	850	478	419
Correlation with BP	0.04	0.29	0.18
– Glucose disposal to 40 mU insulin $\cdot m^{-2} \cdot min^{-1}$			
Mean ($mg \cdot kg^{-1} \cdot min^{-1}$)	12.7	17.1	19.5
Correlation with BP	−0.02	−0.41*	−0.04

* $p < 0.001$
** $p < 0.01$

Even among white populations there is considerable variation in the relationship between blood pressure and plasma insulin concentrations. Some authors note a strong correlation and others a weak one. Laakso et al. [21] for example, found that essential hypertension contributes to insulin resistance in the presence of NIDDM only in non-obese white subjects.

A synthesis of the available data suggest that hypertension is associated with insulin resistance and/or hyperinsulinemia primarily in white populations and even there with significant variability. There is little evidence to support a relationship between hypertension and insulin resistance in non-white populations.

Relationship of NIDDM and insulin resistance to macrovascular disease

The relationship between insulin resistance and/or hyperinsulinemia and macrovascular disease varies considerably among different racial and ethnic populations. It was observed as early as 1967 that Pima Indians, who have been found to have the highest prevalence of NIDDM, have a very low frequency of coronary heart disease [37]. Using electrocardiographic evidence of coronary heart disease, Ingelfinger et al. [18] found a prevalence of 1.6/100 in Pima Indians over 40 years of age. This was about ½ the rate of the general population in Tecumseh, Michigan (primarily a white population). These observations are particularly relevant when one considers the fact that Pima Indians are markedly obese, have severe insulin resistance and have plasma insulin levels that are several fold higher than the normal white population. The reasons for the low prevalence of coronary artery disease in Pima Indians are unknown, but it has been observed that their lipid and lipoprotein metabolism differs from that of whites [17] (Tab. 3). It

Table 3: Lipid and lipoprotein metabolism in Pima Indians as compared to a white population

1. In adult non-diabetic Pima Indians, plasma total and LDL cholesterol are lower than in the white population (approximately 0.8 mM for total cholesterol).
2. In adult non-diabetic Pima Indian males, plasma total and LDL cholesterol do not increase with age.
3. In adult non-diabetic Pima Indian men and women, plasma HDL cholesterol is lower than in the white population (approximately 0.1 mM in men and 0.3 mM in women).
4. In non-diabetic Pima Indian men up to age 35 years and Pima Indian women up to age 55 years plasma triglyceride is higher than in the white population (approximately 0.2 to 0.4 mM).
5. The development of hyperglycemia in Pima Indians causes the expected rise in plasma triglycerides and fall in plasma HDL cholesterol.

seems unlikely that these differences can account for the observed differences in prevalence. Insulin sensitivity in non-diabetic Pima Indians is correlated inversely with plasma triglyceride levels and directly with plasma HDL cholesterol levels [1].
A similar dissociation between coronary artery disease and the components of Syndrome X has been observed in Mexican-Americans [26]. Mexican-Americans have a 3 fold greater prevalence of NIDDM than non-hispanic whites. Additionally, they have higher plasma triglycerides, systolic and diastolic blood pressures and body mass index and lower high-density lipoprotein cholesterol than non-hispanic whites. Insulin resistance and hyperinsulinemia are significantly increased in the Mexican-American population. However, coronary artery disease mortality is lower in Mexican-American men than in non-Hispanic white men.

In black Americans with diabetes, the prevalence of coronary artery disease is less than in white Americans with diabetes. This however, may be due to a large percentage of black NIDDM patients having normal insulin sensitivity rather than insulin resistance [4]. Figure 2 depicits data indicating that in black Amer-

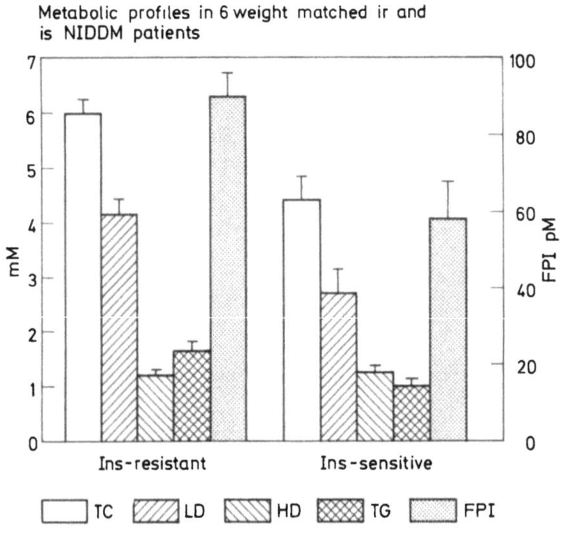

Fig. 2: The relationship of insulin resistance to cardiovascular disease risk factors in black NIDDM patients. The insulin resistant and sensitive groups have a glucose disposals in response to a 1 mU · m^{-2} · min^{-1} insulin infusion of 3.9 ± 0.4 and 6.5 ± 0.1 mg · kg^{-1} · min^{-1} respectively. In these weight matched patients, total plasma cholesterol (TC), low density lipoprotein cholesterol (LD), fasting triglyceride (TG) and fasting insulin (FPI) were significantly greater ($p < 0.05$) in the insulin-resistant group than in the insulin-sensitive group. High density lipoprotein cholesterol (HD) was not significantly different between the two groups.

icans with NIDDM, an increased cardiovascular disease risk factor profile is associated with insulin resistant NIDDM but not with insulin-sensitive NIDDM [3].

Hyperinsulinemia as an independent risk factor for coronary heart disease

A very recent analysis of the 15 year follow up of the 6903 men in the Paris Prospective Study [12] shows that the independent predictors of coronary heart disease death were: systolic blood pressure, number of cigarettes smoked per day, plasma cholesterol level and 2 hour post-glucose load plasma insulin level (above and below 452 pM). Fasting plasma insulin levels were no longer an independent predictor of death by coronary heart disease. The investigators now interpret their data to indicate that insulin resistance but not circulating insulin levels is associated with the increased risk of death.

Conclusions

Figure 3 gives a qualitative assessment of the prevalence of the various components of what is currently thought to be Syndrome X in several well studied racial and ethnic populations. As can be noted, there are numerous dissociations among

	Caucasians	Blacks	Mexican-Americans	Pima Indians
Insulin resistance	+ +	+	+ + +	+ + + +
Hyperinsulinemia	+ +	+	+ + +	+ + + +
Glucose intolerance	+ +	+ + +	+ + + +	+ + + + +
Increased VLDL triglyceride	+ +	+	+ + +	+ + +
Decreased HDL cholesterol	+ +	?	+ + +	+ + +
Hypertension	+ +	+ + +	+ + +	+
Coronary artery disease	+ + +	+ +	+	+
Central obesity	+ +	+ + +	+ + + +	+ + + + +

Fig. 3: Racial variations in the various components of Syndrome X. The prevalence in the populations is semi-quantitative with 1+ being the least and 5+ the most.

the various components in blacks, Mexican-Americans and Pima Indians. Blacks with NIDDM have a lower prevalence of insulin resistance than whites with NIDDM, however the prevalence of hypertension and central obesity are significantly greater. It is unclear whether NIDDM in blacks is associated with a decrease in plasma HDL-cholesterol as it is in whites with NIDDM. Pima Indians have a very high prevalence of insulin resistance, central obesity and NIDDM, but hypertension and coronary artery disease are significantly less than in the white population. Mexican-Americans show a greater prevalence of all of the components of Syndrome X than whites except for coronary heart disease which has a lower prevalence. The prevalence of hypertension is significantly greater in Mexican-Americans than in Pima Indians though insulin resistance occurs more frequently in Pima Indians.

How does one reconcile these observations with the concept that Syndrome X is causally related to insulin resistance and plays a significant role in the genesis of coronary artery disease? One potential explanation as depicted in Figure 4 is that

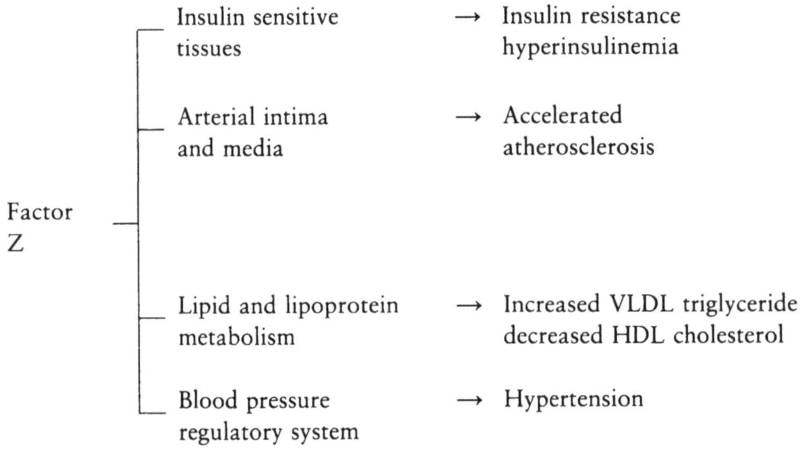

Fig. 4: Hypothesis of the pathogenesis of the chronic metabolic disease syndrome.

Syndrome X is the expression in whites of a much more complex disease process. This complex disease process would be due to a factor which we can call Z. Z can interact with: (1) insulin-sensitive tissues to cause insulin resistance (2) arterial intima and media to accelerate atherosclerosis (3) blood pressure regulatory systems to cause hypertension (4) lipid and lipoprotein metabolism to cause changes in triglyceride and HDL-cholesterol metabolism. The extent to which Z interacts with the various target tissues would depend on the biochemistry and regulatory systems of the particular tissue. These systems would be the result of the specific genetics of the race or ethnic group.

Insulin resistance would be just one component of this syndrome rather than the causative factor. Such a scheme could explain all of the observations noted in Table 3. In whites the expression of all of the components of the chronic metabolic disease syndrome would be very strong, while in other races and ethnic groups their expression could be variable.

If one wanted to hypothesize that insulin resistance is the central defect, then the variable expression of the components of Syndrome X are inexplicable. Furthermore, it would require that all components of the syndrome be highly correlated with the insulin resistance. To date such evidence does not exist.

One can speculate endlessly about the validity and cause of Syndrome X. In the final analysis, proof of its existance and elucidation of its cause and pathogenesis will require intervention studies with specific therapeutic agents.

References

[1] Abbott, W. G. H., S. Lillioja, A. A. Young et al.: Relationship between plasma lipoprotein concentrations and insulin action in an obese hyperinsulinemic population. Diabetes *36* (1987) 897–904.

[2] Alberti, K. G. M. M., G. Dowse, C. Finch et al.: Is blood pressure related to peripheral insulin levels? A community study in Mauritius. Diabetes *38* (1989) Suppl. 92 A (Abstract).

[3] Banerji, M. A., H. E. Lebovitz: Coronary heart disease risk factor profiles in black patients with non-insulin-dependent diabetes mellitus: Paradoxical patterns. Am. J. Med. *91* (1991) 51–58.

[4] Chaiken, R. L., M. A. Banerji, R. M. Pasmantier et al.: Patterns of glucose and lipid abnormalities in black NIDDM subjects. Diabetes Care *14* (1991) 1036–1042.

[5] Collins, V. R., G. K. Dowse, C. F. Finch et al.: An inconsistent relationship between insulin and blood pressure in three Pacific Island populations. J. Clin. Epidemiol. *43* (1990) 1369–1378.

[6] DeFronzo, R. A.: The triumvirate: beta cell, muscle, liver. A collusion responsible for NIDDM. Diabetes *37* (1988) 667–687.

[7] DeFronzo, R. A., D. Simonson, E. Ferrannini: Hepatic and peripheral insulin resistance: A common feature of type II (non-insulin-dependent) and type I (insulin-dependent) diabetes mellitus. Diabetologia *23* (1982) 313–319.

[8] Donahue, R. P., J. S. Skyler, N. Schneiderman et al.: Hyperinsulinemia and elevated blood pressure: cause, confounder or coincidence. Am. J. Epidem. *132* (1990) 827–836.

[9] Eriksson, J., A. Franssila-Kallunki, A. Ekstrand et al.: Early metabolic defects in persons at increased risk for non-insulin dependent diabetes mellitus. N. Engl. J. Med. *321* (1989) 337–343.

[10] Eschwege, E., J. L. Richard, N. Thibult et al.: Coronary heart disease mortality in relation with diabetes, blood glucose and plasma insulin levels. The Paris Prospective Study, ten years later. Horm. Metab. Res. *15* Suppl. (1985) 41–45.

[11] Ferrannini, E., G. Buzzigoli, R. Banadonna et al.: Insulin resistance in essential hypertension. N. Engl. J. Med. *317* (1987) 350–357.
[12] Fontbonne, A., M. A. Charles, N. Thibul et al.: Hyperinsulinaemia as a predictor of coronary heart disease mortality in a healthy population: the Paris Prospective Study, 15-year follow-up. Diabetologia *34* (1991) 356–361.
[13] Fuller, J. H., M. J. Shipley, G. Rose et al.: Mortality from coronary heart disease and stroke in relation to degree of glycaemia: the Whitehall study. Br. Med. J. *287* (1983) 867–870.
[14] Haffner, S. M., D. Fong, H. P. Hazuda et al.: Hyperinsulinemia, upper body adiposity and cardiovascular risk factors in non-diabetics. Metabolism *37* (1988) 338–345.
[15] Haffner, S. M., M. P. Stern, H. P. Hazuda et al.: Hyperinsulinemia in a popoulation at high risk for non-insulin-dependent diabetes mellitus. N. Engl. J. Med. *315* (1986) 220–224.
[16] Haffner, S. M., M. P. Stern, H. P. Hazuda et al.: Cardiovascular risk factors in confirmed prediabetic individuals. Does the clock for coronary heart disease start ticking before the onset of clinical diabetes. J. A. M. A. *263* (1990) 2893–2898.
[17] Howard, B. V., M. P. Davis, D. J. Pettitt et al.: Plasma and lipoprotein cholesterol and triglyceride concentrations in the PIMA Indians: distributions differing from those of Caucasians. Circulation *68* (1983) 714–724.
[18] Ingelfinger, J. A., P. H. Bennett, I. M. Liebow et al.: Coronary heart disease and Pima Indians. Diabetes *25* (1976) 561–565.
[19] Kannel, W. B., D. L. McGee: Diabetes and cardiovascular risk factors: the Framingham Study. Circulation *59* (1979) 8–13.
[20] Krolewski, A. S., J. H. Warram, P. Valsania et al.: Evolving natural history of coronary artery disease in diabetes mellitus. Am. J. Med. *90* Suppl. 2 (1991) 56–61.
[21] Laakso, M., H. Sarlund, L. Mykkanen: Essential hypertension and insulin resistance in non-insulin-dependent diabetes. Eur. J. Clin. Invest. *19* (1989) 518–526.
[22] Laws, A., M. L. Stefanick, G. M. Reaven: Insulin resistance and hypertriglyceridemia in non-diabetic relatives of patients with non-insulin dependent diabetes mellitus. J. Clin. Endocrinol. Metab. *69* (1989) 343–347.
[23] Lerner, D. J., W. B. Kannel: Patterns of coronary heart disease morbidity and mortality in the sexes. A 26 year follow-up of the Framingham population. Am. Heart J. *111* (1986) 383–390.
[24] Lillioja, S., D. M. Mott, B. V. Howard et al.: Impaired glucose tolerance is a disorder of insulin action: Longitudinal and cross-sectional studies in Pima Indians. N. Engl. J. Med. *318* (1988) 1217–1225.
[25] Manolio, T. A., P. J. Savage, G. L. Burke et al.: Association of fasting insulin with blood pressure and lipids in young adults: The Cardia study. Arteriosclerosis *10* (1990) 430–436.
[26] Mitchell, B. D., M. P. Stern, S. M. Haffner et al.: Risk factors for cardiovascular mortality in Mexican-Americans and non-Hispanic whites. Am. J. Epidemiol. *131* (1990) 423–433.
[27] Pollare, T., H. Lithell, C. Berne: Insulin resistance is a characteristic feature of primary hypertension independent of obesity. Metabolism *39* (1990) 167–174.
[28] Pyorala, K., M. Laakso, M. Uusitupa: Diabetes and atherosclerosis: An epidemiologic view. Diabetes Metab. Rev. *3* (1987) 463–524.

[29] Pyorala, K., E. Savolainen, S. Kaukola et al.: Plasma insulin as coronary heart disease risk factor; relationship to other risk factors and predictive value. The 9½ year follow-up of the Helsinki Policeman Study population. Acta Med. Scand. Suppl. 701 (1985) 38 – 52.

[30] Reaven, G. M.: Insulin resistance, hyperinsulinemia and hypertriglyceridemia in the etiology and clinical course of hypertension. Am. J. Med. *90* Suppl. 2 (1991) 7 – 12.

[31] Reaven, G. M.: Insulin resistance in non-insulin-dependent diabetes mellitus: does it exist and can it be measured? Am. J. Med. *74* (1983) 3 – 17.

[32] Reaven, G. M.: Insulin secretion and insulin action in non-insulin dependent diabetes mellitus: which defect is primary? Diabetes Care *7* Suppl. 1 (1984) 17 – 24.

[33] Reaven, G. M.: Role of insulin resistance in human disease. Diabetes *37* (1988) 1595 – 1607.

[34] Saad, M. F., S. Lillioja, B. L. Nyomba et al.: Racial differences in the relation between blood pressure and insulin resistance. N. Engl. J. Med. *324* (1991) 733 – 739.

[35] Shen, S.-C., S.-M. Shieh, M. M.-T. Fuh et al.: Resistance to insulin-stimulated glucose uptake in patients with hypertension. J. Clin. Endocrinol. Metab. *66* (1988) 580 – 583.

[36] Sicree, R., P. Zimmet, H. King et al.: The plasma insulin response amongst Nauruans: prediction of deterioration in glucose tolerance over six years. Diabetes *36* (1987) 179 – 186.

[37] Sievers, M. L.: Myocardial infarction among Southwestern American Indians. Ann. Intern. Med. *67* (1967) 800 – 807.

[38] Stout, R. W.: Insulin as a mitogenic factor: Role in the pathogenesis of cardiovascular disease. Am. J. Med. *30* Suppl. 2A (1991) 62 – 65.

[39] Swislocki, A. L. M., B. B. Hoffman, G. M. Reaven: Insulin resistance, glucose intolerance and hyperinsulinemia in patients with hypertension. Am. J. Hypertens. *2* (1989) 419 – 423.

[40] Voors, A. W., B. Radhakrishnamurthy, S. R. Srinivasan et al.: Plasma glucose level related to blood pressure in 272 children, ages 7 – 15 years sampled from a total biracial population. Am. J. Epidemiol. *113* (1981) 347 – 356.

[41] Welborn, T. A., K. Wearne: Coronary heart disease incidence and cardiovascular mortality in Busselton with reference to glucose and insulin concentration. Diabetes Care *2* (1979) 154 – 160.

[42] Zavaroni, T., E. Bonora, M. Pagliara et al.: Risk factors for coronary artery disease in healthy persons with hyperinsulinemia and normal glucose tolerance. N. Engl. J. Med. *320* (1989) 702 – 706.

[43] Zimmet, P.: Non-insulin-dependent (type II) diabetes mellitus: Does it really exist. Diabetic Medicine *60* (1989) 728 – 735.

Strategies for the treatment of hyperglycemia in Syndrome X

R. G. Josse

Introduction

In the past few years it has been increasingly recognized that a constellation of abnormalities exists that places individuals at increased risk for macrovascular disease, especially coronary artery disease. These abnormalities include: resistance to insulin stimulated glucose uptake, glucose intolerance, hyperinsulinemia, increased very low density lipoprotein triglyceride, decreased high density lipoprotein cholesterol and hypertension. Collectively these features have been designated Syndrome X [34]. An extensive body of experimental and clinical data has implicated insulin resistance as a key link between these diverse but interrelated variables. Current understanding suggests that the other changes are likely secondary to this basic abnormality [9, 10, 33, 34]. Over fifty years ago, Himsworth [14] first postulated that individuals with diabetes could be classified as either insulin sensitive or insulin insensitive, according to their glucose response to insulin administration. Since that time this concept has been validated and has now been incorporated into the classification of diabetes. More recent investigations using a variety of techniques including glucose clamp studies have demonstrated that resistance to insulin stimulated glucose uptake is present not only in those with non-insulin dependant diabetes mellitus (NIDDM) but also in individuals with glucose intolerance and in approximately 25% of non-obese people with normal oral glucose tolerance. Why subjects with IGT or normal people with insulin resistance do not develop frank hyperglycemia, revolves around the ability of the pancreatic beta cell to augment insulin secretion. The metabolic trade off is thus maintenance of normal or near normal glycemia at the expense of hyperinsulinemia. Superficially this may seem like a reasonable physiologic compromise. However a variety of epidemiologic, clinical and laboratory studies have shown that hyperinsulinemia is not necessarily a benign state [40].

At the tissue level it must be born in mind that the hyperglycemia consequent upon insulin resistance is due to different mechanisms in the basal as opposed to the post-absorptive state. This distinction, as we shall see later, has importance in terms of treatment options. In the fasting situation, increased hepatic glucose production is a key factor responsible for producing and maintaining the hyperglycemia. In the post-absorptive state however, despite hyperinsulinemia, it is a reduction in the efficacy of the oxidative and non-oxidative glucose disposal pathways principally in muscle that are responsible for the hyperglycemia [10]. Thus in developing treatment strategies it is important to direct our therapeutic interventions to reduce hepatic glucose production in order to lower hyperglycemia in the basal state, at the same time as attempting to increase oxidative and non-oxidative glucose disposal in the post-absorptive state. Moreover one must try and accomplish this metabolic improvement in intermediary metabolism by increasing insulin sensitivity and decreasing circulating insulin concentration.

Table 1: Therapeutic options to lower glycemia in NIDDM

1. ↓ Intestinal glucose absorption
   - Low glycemic index diets
   - Fibre
   - α-glucosidase inhibitors
2. ↑ Insulin secretion from β cell
   - Sulphonylureas
   - α_2 adrenergic blocking drugs
3. ↓ Hepatic glucose output
   - Insulin + Proinsulin
   - Glucagon inhibitors
   - Hydrazines
   - Inhibitors of fatty acid oxidation
4. ↑ Peripheral glucose uptake
   - Biguanides
   - Sulphonylureas
   - Ciglitazone
5. Insulin independant ↑ in glucose uptake – inhibitors of fatty acid oxidation
   - Nicotinic acid
   - Carnitine palmitoyl transferase inhibitors (Methyl palmoxirate)

Table 1 outlines some of the therapeutic options available to lower hyperglycemia. While agents such as sulphonylureas or alpha-2 adrenergic blocking drugs can increase pancreatic insulin secretion; and insulin and pro-insulin can decrease hepatic glucose output, and while both of these therapies may improve hyperglycemia they will not be considered further as they augment hyperinsulinemia.

Modulation of carbohydrate absorption

It is increasingly appreciated that delaying nutrient absorption is a useful therapeutic approach in the treatment of metabolic disease, especially diabetes. Methods by which this has been achieved include

1) "nibbling" (as opposed to "gorging") [24] (Fig. 1);
2) use of soluble fiber supplements and soluble fiber foods [5, 21] (Fig. 2);
3) alpha-glucosidase inhibition [7, 18, 31];
4) lowering the glycemic index of diets by appropriate food selection [6, 19, 23] (Fig. 3 – 5).

Theoretically slowing the rate of absorption would be accompanied by lower blood glucose and insulin responses, the latter being important also as a possible stimulus to hepatic lipogenesis and lipid synthesis in the arterial wall. These approaches could thus have important therapeutic implications for Syndrome X.

Soluble fiber

Consumption of both soluble fiber supplements (e.g. guar, pectin, locust bean gum) and fiber rich foods (e.g. barley, oats, legumes, beans, peas, and lentils) has been associated with improved blood glucose control in patients with diabetes [2, 22, 38] and lower blood lipids in normal [17, 25], diabetic[2, 38] and hyperlipidemic individuals [16, 29]. In keeping with the objective of controlling metabolic events by slowing the rate of absorption, soluble fiber and high fiber foods, such as legumes reduce the rate of glucose uptake in vivo [5] and slow carbohydrate digestion [16], glucose diffusion [12], and amino acid uptake in vitro (11]. Problems with the use of fiber have arisen from administration of ineffective, insoluble fiber types or, in the case of supplements, failure to allow for adequate mixing with the food. Although fiber has many positive beneficial attributes, a concern with the use of supplements, as opposed to high fiber foods is their effectiveness in the long term and the degree to which compliance can be maintained.

Low glycemic index foods

Direct ranking of foods (the glycemic index) by a physiological system according to the degree to which equicarbohydrate amounts raise the blood glucose has also been proposed as an indicator of a slowed absorption rate [16]. In this respect it has been demonstrated that the glycemic index (GI) is related to the rate of in vitro digestion (Fig. 6). It was hoped that this classification would encompass the many aspects of food which alter their absorption rates. These factors include the nature of the starch, amylose versus the more readily digested amylopectin; fiber; and the anti-nutrients, phytate, lectins, tanins and saponins

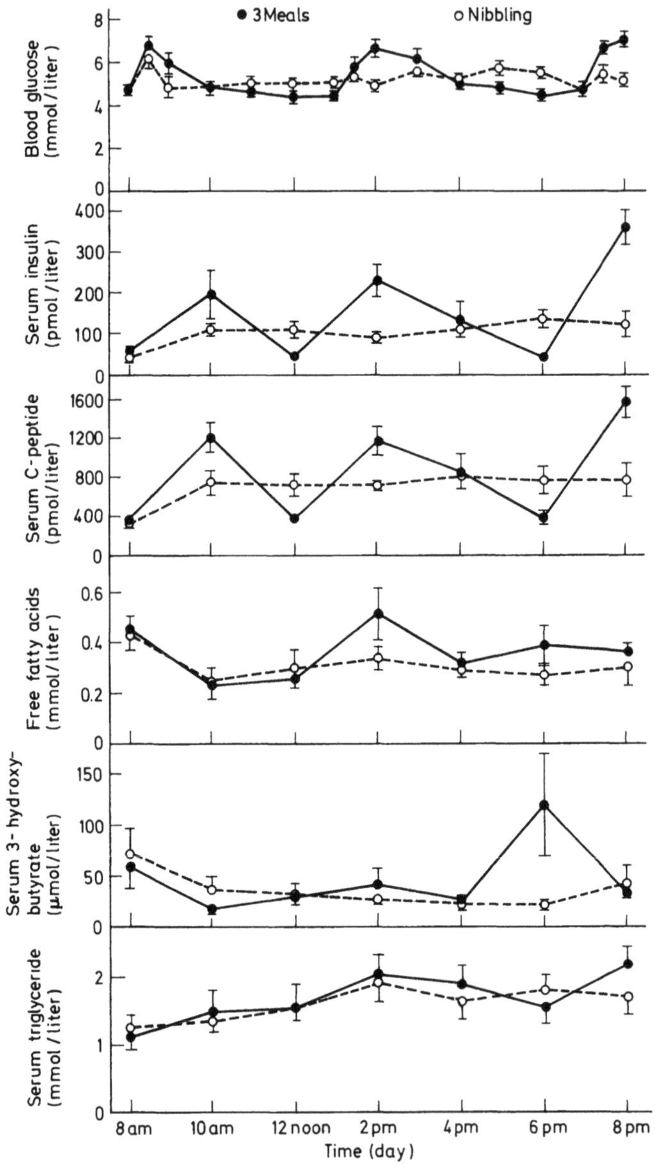

Fig. 1: Mean (± SE) blood glucose levels and serum concentrations of insulin, C-peptide, free fatty acids, 3-hydroxybutyrate, and triglyceride. Adapted from Jenkins, D. J. A. et al. [24].

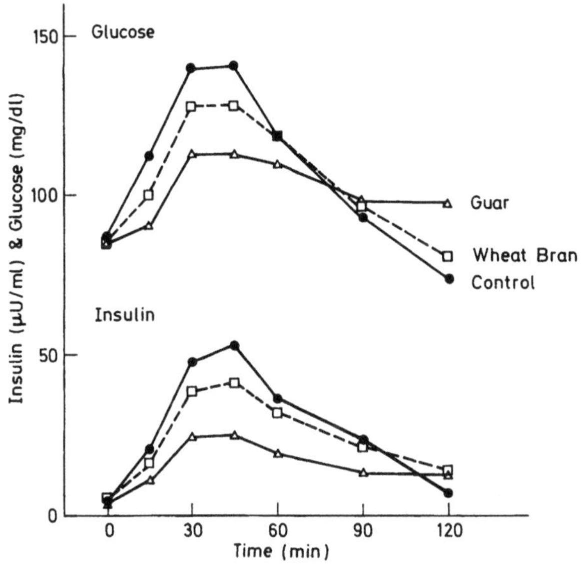

Fig. 2: Mean blood glucose and plasma insulin responses of healthy subjects after consuming 50 g glucose (control), 50 g glucose plus 14.5 g guar, or 50 g glucose plus 40 g wheat bran. Adapted from Jenkins, D. J. A. et al. [21].

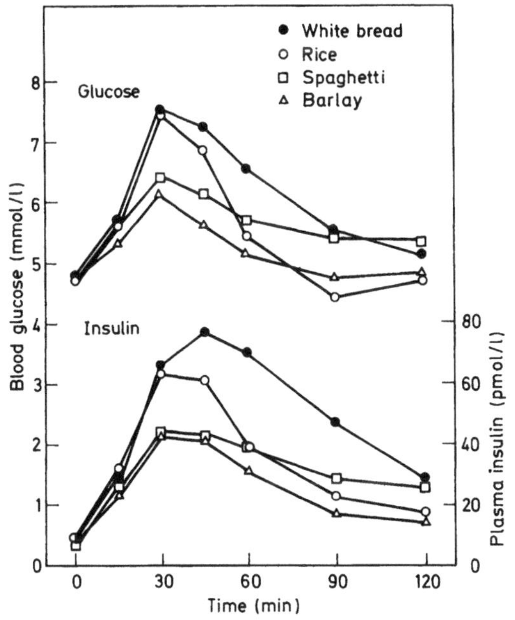

Fig. 3: Mean blood glucose and plasma insulin responses of 7 healthy subjects after consuming 50 g carbohydate portions of white bread, rice, spaghetti or barley to which were added 32 g cheddar cheese plus 100 g tomato. Adapted from Wolever, T. M. S., D. J. A. Jenkins, G. Collier et al.: Nutr. Res. *8* (1988) 573–581.

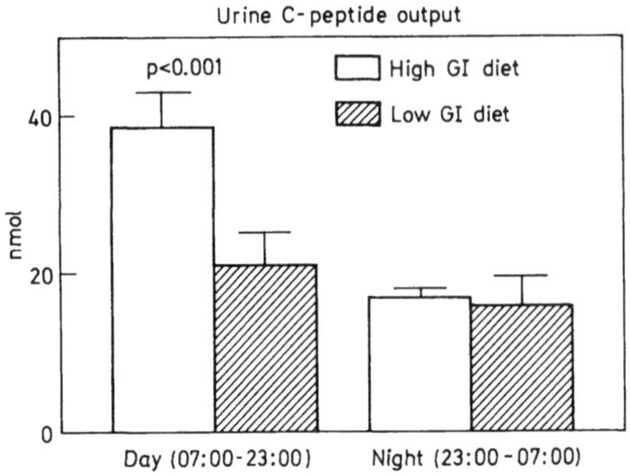

Fig. 4: Mean ± SEM urinary C-peptide excretion of 6 healthy subjects during the day and night after 2 weeks on metabolically controlled high or low glycaemic index (GI) diets. Each subject took each diet according to a randomized cross-over design. The nutrient composition of the low GI diet was identical to that of the high GI diet (60% energy as carbohydrate, 20% fat, 20% protein) but the starchy carbohydrate foods were different so that the diet GI was reduced by 40%. Adapted from Jenkins, D. J. A., T. M. S. Wolever, G. R. Collier et al.: Am. J. Clin. Nutr. *46* (1987) 968–975.

[41]. This concept is not new but more recent studies over the last decade have demonstrated that this principle has considerable promise. Reduced glucose profiles and urinary C-peptide excretion have been noted in normal volunteers, together with reduced total and LDL cholesterol and apo-B lipoprotein levels [16]. These changes have also been associated with lower serum fructosamine levels. Despite the fact that improvements in glucose tolerance with lower insulin responses mirrored by favorable changes in glycosylated hemoglobin can be achieved with low glycemic index diets, there is still controversy concerning the glycemic impact of a mixed meal based upon the calculated GI of the individual foods. Further exploration of the factors determining the glycemic responses to mixed meals will enhance the utility of existing tables. Nevertheless, the concept of selecting foods with slower rates of absorption on the basis of the glycemic index fits well with the overall principle of controlling metabolism by gut related mechanisms.

Enzyme inhibition

Another treatment strategy to utilize the metabolic benefits of a reduced rate of absorption has been the development and use of the alpha-glucosidase inhibitors. Early studies with kidney bean and wheat derived alpha-amylase inhibitors

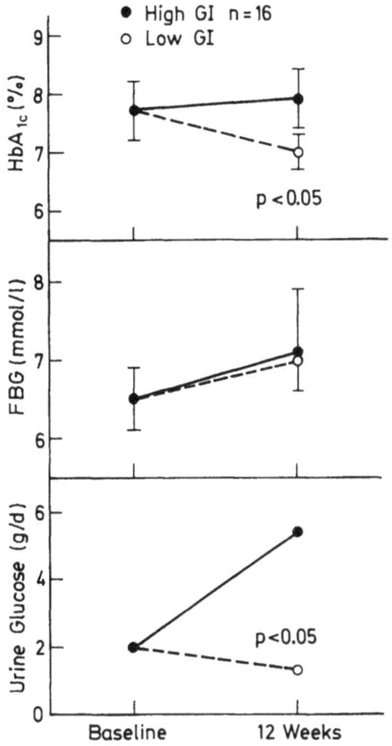

Fig. 5: Mean ± SEM glycosylated haemoglobin (HbA_{1c}), fasting blood glucose (FBG) and urinary glucose output of 16 patients with non-insulin dependent diabetes who took low and high glycaemic index (GI) diets on an outpatient basis according to a randomized cross-over design. The nutrient composition of the low GI diet was similar to that of the high GI diet, but the diet GI was reduced by 15%. Adapted from Brand, J. C., S. Colagiuri, S. Crossman et al. [6].

demonstrated that the rate of starch absorption could be reduced and postprandial glucose and insulin levels flattened [31]. The bacterially derived inhibitors (e.g. acarbose and miglitol) have a broader spectrum of activity with anti-amylolytic, anti-sucrase and anti-maltase activity [18]. Their use has been associated with reduced gut hormone responses (particularly of the potent incretin, gastric inhibitory polypeptide) [39] and flattened postprandial profiles of glucose and insulin [37, 42]. This is accompanied in the longer term by reduced glycosylated hemoglobin and serum VLDL triglyceride levels. New data concerning the beneficial effects of alpha-glucosidase inhibition will be covered elsewhere in this volume. In terms of meeting the goals of improving glycemia (and lipid profiles) without increasing insulin levels, these agents look promising.

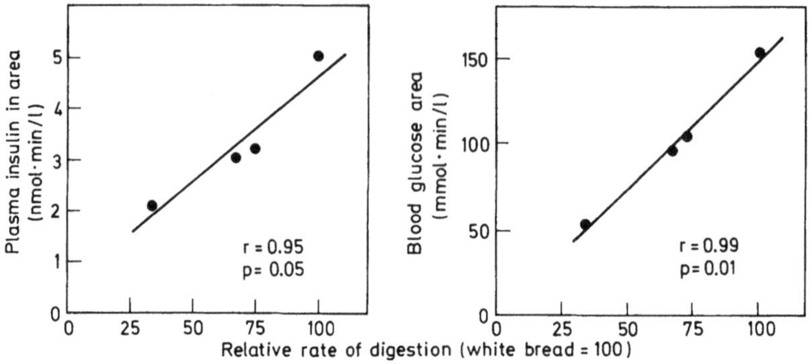

Fig. 6: Relationships between the mean incremental areas under the plasma insulin (left) and blood glucose (right) response curves of healthy subjects after consuming 50 g carbohydrate from white bread, rice, spaghetti and barley (plus cheese and tomato) and the rates of digestion of the same foods in vitro. The rate of digestion is the sum of the glucose, maltose and maltotriose released after 3 h digestion of each food expressed as a percent of that released from white bread. Adapted from Wolever, T. M. S., D. J. A. Jenkins, G. Collier et al.: Nutr. Res. *8* (1988) 573–581.

Meal frequency

Some twenty-five years ago, antedating the major attention given to fiber, enzyme inhibitors and glycemic index, there was much interest in the effect of altering the frequency of meals on the intermediary metabolism of normal, obese, hyperlipidemic and diabetic subjects. This concept of spreading the nutrient load throughout the day ("nibbling" vs "gorging"), results in lower cholesterol, phospholipid, and triglyceride levels as well as improved glucose tolerance. Studies from our own group have confirmed the hypocholesterolemic effect of nibbling and demonstrated reduction in apo-B lipoprotein levels [24]. With respect to carbohydrate metabolism, this concept had itself been anteceded by the Staub-Traugott phenomenon, where one carbohydrate meal was found to improve the response to the next in proportion to the time interval between the meals. The shorter the interval, the better the subsequent tolerance. We have also demonstrated that a 50 gm glucose load taken as a bolus drink produces a significantly greater insulin response area than is seen when the same amount of glucose is sipped at an even rate over 3.5 hours. Furthermore subsequent glucose disposal at 4 hours following a 5 gm glucose IVGTT was improved as judged by a 30% increase in glucose disappearance rate (i. e. a reduction in K_g at the end of the sipping, compared with the bolus experiment) [20]. Insulin levels during the IVGTTs were similar but over the preceding 4 hour period there had been an increase in urinary catecholamine excretion and reduced glucagon levels were also seen during the post sipping IVGTT. As further evidence of increased insulin sensitivity, branched chain amino acid levels were reduced despite similar insulin levels. Although in the clinical context this approach is impractical, the experimental paradigm may be seen as supporting the concept of slow absorption as a means of favourably influencing carbohydrate and lipid metabolism without augmenting insulin secretion.

Colonic effects

Factors which reduce the rate of carbohydrate absorption are also associated with a varying degree of carbohydrate delivery to the colon. In therapeutic terms this loss is not sufficient to account for the flatter blood glucose and endocrine responses [8]. Although some caloric loss may occur, the short chain fatty acids generated as a result of carbohydrate fermentation by colonic bacteria are absorbed, act as energy substrates and may have important metabolic effects [7, 8]. These short chain fatty acids (e.g. acetate, butyrate, and propionate) formed during bacterial fermentation may have mixed effects both favourable and unfavourable on glycemia, insulin sensitivity and lipid synthesis. Propionate, for example, can act as a gluconeogenetic substrate but can also inhibit cholesterol synthesis in the liver.

An impressive body of data is accumulating attesting to the metabolic benefits that can accrue to slowing the rate of nutrient absorption. The maneouvres that I have discussed, especially with respect to treatment of Syndrome X merit further exploration.

Enhancing peripheral glucose uptake

Biguanides

Biguanides in clinical usage for over thirty years have had a checkered career as oral agents for the treatment of type II diabetes. Phenformin due to its toxicity, principally lactic acidosis, is no longer used. The disubstituted biguanide metformin is an effective agent for the treatment of both obese and nonobese patients with NIDDM. However despite many years of clinical experience with this drug, its precise mechanism of action is still unknown. Theoretically this drug could improve glucose tolerance by decreasing intestinal glucose absorption, stimulating pancreatic insulin secretion, decreasing hepatic glucose output and increasing glucose uptake in peripheral tissues (principally muscle and fat). It has been claimed that metformin may have a modest anorectic and weight reducing action as well as decreasing intestinal glucose absorption [3]. As will be seen for many of the postulated actions of metformin, data is both inconsistent and contradictory. Perhaps the only issue on which there is general consensus is that metformin does not increase insulin secretion. If there is a modest effect on intestinal glucose absorption, it is quite insufficient to account for the hypoglycemic action of the drug.

Recent data in both animals and man implicate a role for reduced gluconeogenesis as a significant mechanism of action. Although still controversial it appears that permissive (albeit modest) concentrations of insulin are necessary for this effect to be manifest [3].

Implicit in the observation that metformin is ineffective in the absence of insulin (and does not increase insulin secretion) is the postulate that it potentiates insulin mediated glucose disposal. Glucose clamp studies are the traditional method for assessing glucose utilization. Most have shown that metformin can increase glucose disposal in peripheral tissues by 50% at high insulin infusion rates and by 25% at low insulin infusion rates. However the results from a recent study indicate that steady state plasma glucose and insulin concentrations were similar during the glucose clamps performed before and after initiation of metformin therapy. The ability of insulin to promote glucose uptake was assessed by measurement of the metabolic clearance rate of glucose and in this investigation there was no change in glucose uptake that was associated with metformin treatment. In addition, values for hepatic glucose production were indistinguishable from zero during the clamp studies. The authors have suggested that the fact that their patients had substantially higher plasma glucose concentrations than noted in other studies may perhaps explain why no significant change in insulin action with metformin treatment was noted [44]. Clearly further work is required to reconcile these differences.

Extensive study of the effect of metformin on insulin receptor binding does not suggest that this is an important mechanism of action. While metformin has been shown in many studies, though not all, to increase insulin binding to cells, this effect does not appear to be directly related to the subsequent metabolic and clinical effects of the drug [26]. Thus since the anti-hypoglycemic effect of metformin is often poorly correlated with insulin binding and there is no relationship between the antihypoglycemic effect and insulin concentration, the impression is evolving that its direct action may occur at a post-insulin binding level.

Specialized units, called glucose transporters, embedded in the cell membrane are responsible for mediating glucose transport. These transporters belong to a family of related transmembrane polypeptides, two isoforms of which designated GLUT-1 and GLUT-4, exist in insulin sensitive tissue. GLUT-1 is located predominately in the plasma membrane whereas GLUT-4 is primarily in a storage pool in intracellular membranes. Addition of insulin to adipocytes or skeletal muscle causes a migration of the intracellularly located GLUT-4 isoforms to the cell membrane. It is this insulin activated recruitment of glucose transporters which is thought to represent a primary action of insulin that stimulates glucose transport activity into the cell. In a muscle cell line, metformin has been shown to increase the number and activity of GLUT-4 transporters present in the plasma membrane. This effect is thus similar to the action of insulin, although in culture insulin is not required for metformin to induce this effect [26].

Thus although the precise mechanism(s) of action of metformin remains to be clarified, a plethora of clinical studies has shown both an improvement in carbohydrate and lipoprotein metabolism in type II diabetic patients which can be achieved without augmenting insulin secretion.

Metabolic inhibitors of key biochemical pathways

At steady state the blood glucose level is determined by the balance between glucose production and glucose utilization. In the basal state glucose production is primarily a function of the liver, accomplished by two mechanisms, glycogenolysis and gluconeogenesis. Glycogen stores are limited and when exhausted glucose availability will depend on gluconeogenesis. This in turn has two major components, true gluconeogenesis principally from amino acids (and to a much lesser extent from glycerol) and glucose reformation from lactate in the Cori cycle. Nearly thirty years ago Randle [32] described the glucose fatty acid cycle in which he proposed that increased free fatty acid oxidation, by influencing the redox state and by inhibiting several critical enzymes (especially pyruvate dehydrogenase), would restrain glucose oxidation. In addition to impairing glucose oxidation there is also a reduction in glucose storage (as glycogen) since in the process of free fatty acid oxidation there is inhibition of glycogen synthase [10]. Pharmacologic manipulation of various metabolic pathways can inhibit gluconeogenesis either directly through inhibition of regulatory steps in the gluconeogenic pathway itself or indirectly through prevention of fatty acid oxidation [1]. An alternative and as we will see an adjunctive manoeuvre is to limit substrate supply. However since intermediary metabolism is so intimately interrelated, pharmacologic tampering with key metabolic pathways is not without potential risk and significant toxicity. For example depending upon the locus of action, inhibitors of gluconeogenesis, particularly if they interfere with argininosuccinate production could interfere with the urea cycle and toxicity from hyperammonemia would occur. Likewise blockade of the removal of organic acids formed from carbohydrate metabolism, either because gluconeogenesis is inhibited or because fatty acid oxidation is ongoing could result in their accumulation resulting in major acid based disturbances. The same problem will of course apply to inhibition of gluconeogenesis through the Cori cycle which would result in lactic acidosis. Lastly as an extreme example, inhibition of glucose-6-phosphatase would be an extremely effective blocker, preventing both gluconeogenesis and glycogenolysis, but this is of course tantamount to creating type I glycogen storage disease. Nevertheless judicious administration of certain metabolic inhibitors has been studied in both animals and man with potentially promising results.

Inhibitors of carnitine acyltransferase which block the movement of fatty acids across the inner mitochondrial membrane (e.g. methylpalmoxirate or etomoxir) improve blood glucose levels in both diabetic animals and man [1, 4, 27, 28]. The downside with the use of these drugs is the accumulation of fatty acid in the circulation where they may be toxic while in the liver they would accumulate as triglycerides.

Further along the fatty acid oxidation pathway beyond translocation into the mitochondria, several hypoglycemic compounds have been described which inhibit beta oxidation. A well known example of such agents is hypoglycin (the active principal from the Jamaican ackee fruit). Although none of these agents has yet found clinical utility their mechanism of action is of interest. It appears that they decrease acetyl Co-A formation. This results in inhibition of pyruvate decarboxylase, a key enzyme in gluconeogenesis and at the same time the reduction in acetyl Co-A allows flux through pyruvate dehydrogenase.

An alternative metabolic approach is to limit the supply of fatty acid substrate. This is achieved by inhibition of lipolysis. Several agents have been used in man primarily to treat hyperlipidemias. Thus far the data in man is limited [1] but recent studies in diabetic rats have shown very encouraging results using phenylisopropyl adenosine (PIA) and nicotinic acid. Interfering with fatty acid metabolism at two different loci in diabetic rats can produce an even more significant effect. This has been demonstrated in a recent study where etomoxir and nicotinic acid were used together [35].

Many attempts have been made to capitalize on the pivotal interrelationship between glucose and fatty acid metabolism. A number of compounds look promising but problems with tissue specificity and toxic side effects have thus far limited their clinical utility. Nevertheless pharmacologic manipulation of lipolysis and hepatic fat oxidation offer another approach to moderate hyperglycemia, without altering insulin secretion.

Conclusion

The pivotal abnormality in Syndrome X is insulin resistance. This is accompanied by hyperinsulinemia, now recognized as a significant risk factor for atherosclerosis. Control of hyperglycemia has been traditionally through mechanisms which further raise insulin levels. This brief review has discussed some alternative treatment strategies to control hyperglycemia which do not raise insulin levels and at times are actually associated with reduction in insulin concentration. Whether utilization of these therapeutic options can in time achieve the goal of reducing macrovascular disease remains to be seen.

References

[1] Alberti, K. G. M. M., H. S. A. Sherratt, P. L. Selby: Metabolic inhibitors in the treatment of diabetes mellitus. In: W. Creutzfeldt, P. Lefèbvre (eds.): Diabetes Mellitus, Pathophysiology and Therapy, pp. 164 – 171. Springer-Verlag, Berlin – New York 1989.

[2] Anderson, J. W., K. Ward: Long term effects of high carbohydrate, high fibre diets on glucose and lipid metabolism: A preliminary report on patients with diabetes. Diabetes Care *1* (1978) 77 – 82.

[3] Bailey, C. J.: Metformin revisited: Its actions and indications for use. Diab. Med. *5* (1988) 315 – 320.

[4] Bailey, J. W., M. D. Jensen, J. M. Miles: Effects of intravenous methyl palmoxirate in the turnover and oxidation of fatty acids in conscious dogs. Metabolism *40* (4) (1991) 428 – 431.

[5] Blackburn, N. A., J. S. Redfern, H. Jarjis et al.: The mechanism of action of guar gum in improving glucose tolerance in man. Clin. Science *66* (1984) 329 – 336.

[6] Brand, J. C., S. Colagiuri, S. Crossman et al.: Low glycemic index foods improve long term glycemic control in NIDDM. Diabetes Care *14* (2) (1991) 95 – 101.

[7] Caspary, W. F.: Inhibitors influencing carbohydrate absorption. In: W. Creutzfeldt, P. Lefèbvre (eds.): Diabetes Mellitus, Pathophysiology and Therapy, pp. 172 – 191. Springer-Verlag, Berlin – New York 1989.

[8] Cummings, J. H.: Short chain fatty acids in the human colon. Gut *22* (1981) 763 – 779.

[9] DeFronzo, R. A., E. Ferrannini: Insulin Resistance: A multifaceted syndrome responsible for NIDDM, obesity, hypertension, dyslipidemia and atherosclerotic cardiovascular disease. Diabetes Care *14* (3) (1991) 173 – 195.

[10] DeFronzo, R. A.: The triumvirate: B cell, muscle, liver. A collusion responsible for NIDDM. Diabetes *37* (1988) 667 – 687.

[11] Eisenhaus, B., V. Sufke, R. Blume et al.: The influence of carbohydrate gelling agents on rat intestinal transport of monosaccharides and neutral amino acids in vitro. Clin. Sci. *59* (1980) 373 – 380.

[12] Edwards, C. A., N. A. Blackburn, L. Graigen et al.: Viscosity of food gums determined in vitro related to their hypoglycemic actions. Am. J. Clin. Nutr. *45* (1987) 72 – 77.

[13] Gérard, J., A. S. Luyckx, P. J. Lefèbvre: Improvement in metabolic control in insulin dependant diabetes treated with the alpha glucosidase inhibitor Acarbose for two months. Diabetologia *21* (1981) 446 – 457.

[14] Himsworth, H.: Diabetes Mellitus: A differentiation into insulin sensitive and insulin insensitive types. Lancet *1* (1936) 127 – 130.

[15] Jenkins, D. J. A., D. Cuff, T. M. S. Wolever et al.: Digestability of carbohydrate foods in an ileostomate: relationship to dietary fibre, in vitro digestibility and glycemic response. Am. J. Gastroenterol. *82* (1987) 709–717.

[16a] Jenkins, D. J. A., Ghafari, T. M. S. Wolever et al.: Relationship between the rate of digestion of foods and post-prandial glycaemia. Diabetologia *22* (1982) 450–455.

[16b] Jenkins, D. J. A., A. L. Jenkins, T. M. S. Wolever et al.: Aims of diet in diabetes management. In: W. Creutzfeldt, P. Lefèbvre (eds.): Diabetes Mellitus, Pathophysiology and Therapy, pp. 299–308. Springer-Verlag, Berlin–New York 1989.

[17] Jenkins, D. J. A., A. R. Leeds, M. A. Gassull et al.: The cholesterol lowering properties of guar and pectin. Cli. Sci. Mol. Med. *51* (1976) 8.

[18] Jenkins, D. J. A., R. H. Taylor, D. V. Goff et al.: Scope and specificity of Acarbose in slowing carbohydrate absorption in man. Diabetes *30* (1981) 951–954.

[19] Jenkins, D. J. A., T. M. S. Wolever, A. L. Jenkins et al.: The glycemic response to carbohydrate foods. Lancet *2* (1984) 388–391.

[20] Jenkins, D. J. A., T. M. S. Wolever, A. M. Ocana et al.: Metabolic effects of reducing rate of glucose ingestion by single bolus versus continuous sipping. Diabetes *39* (1990) 775–781.

[21] Jenkins, D. J. A., T. M. S. Wolever, A. R. Leeds et al.: Dietary fibres: fibre analogues and glucose tolerance: Importance of viscosity. Br. Med. J. *1* (1978) 1392–1394.

[22] Jenkins, D. J. A., T. M. S. Wolever, R. Nineham et al.: Guar crispbread in the diabetic diet. Br. Med. J. *2* (1978) 1744–1746.

[23] Jenkins, D. J. A., T. M. S. Wolever, R. H. Taylor et al.: Glycemic index of foods: a physiological basis for carbohydrate exchange. Am. J. Clin. Nutr. *34* (1981) 362–366.

[24] Jenkins, D. J. A., T. M. S. Wolever, V. Vuksan et al.: Nibbling versus gorging: Metabolic advantages of increased meal frequency. New. Eng. J. Med. *321* (1989) 929–934.

[25] Kay, R. M.: Dietary Fibre. J. Lipid Res. *23* (1982) 221–242.

[26] Klip, A., L. A. Leiter: Cellular mechanisms of action of metformin. Diabetes care *13* (6) (1990) 696–704.

[27] Mandarino, L., E. Tsalikian, S. Bartold et al.: Mechanism of hyperglycemia and response to treatment with an inhibitor of fatty acid oxidation in an patient with insulin resistance due to anti-insulin receptor antibodies. J. Clin. Endo. Metab. *59* (1984) 658–664.

[28] Martin, C., M. Odeon, R. Cohen et al.: Mechanisms of the glucose lowering effect of a carnitine palmitoyl transferase inhibitor in normal and diabetic rats. Metabolism *40* (4) (1991) 420–427.

[29] Miettinen, T. A., S. Tarpila: Effect of pectin on serum cholesterol fecal bile acids and biliary lipids in normolipidemic and hyperlipidemic individuals. Clin. Chim. Acta. *79* (1977) 471–474.

[30] National Diabetes Data Group: Report of the expert committee on glycosylated hemoglobin. Diabetes Care *7* (1984) 602–606.

[31] Puls, W., V. Kemp: Influence of an alpha-glucoside inhibitor (Bay d7781) on blood glucose, serum insulin and NEFA in starch loading tests in rats, dogs and man. Diabetologia *9* (1973) 97–101.

[32] Randle, P. J., P. B. Garland, C. N. Hales et al.: The glucose fatty acid cycle – its role in insulin sensitivity and the metabolic disturbances of diabetes mellitus. Lancet *1* (1963) 785 – 789.

[33] Reaven, G. M.: Insulin resistance, hyperinsulinemia, hypertriglyceridemia and hypertension: Parallels between human disease and rodent models. Diabetes Care *14* (3) (1991) 195 – 203.

[34] Reaven, G. M.: Role of insulin resistance in human disease. Diabetes *37* (1988) 1595 – 1607.

[35] Reaven, G. M., H. Chang, B. B. Hoffman: Additive hypoglycemic effects of drugs that modify free fatty acid metabolism by different mechanisms in rats with sterep-tozotocin-induced diabetes. Diabetes *37* (1988) 28 – 32.

[36] Reaven, G. M., H. Chang, H. Ho et al.: Lowering of plasma glucose in diabetic rats by antilipolytic agents. Am. J. Physiol. *254* (1988) 23 – 30.

[37] Samed, A. H. B., T. S. T. Willing, K. G. M. M. Alberti et al.: Effects of BAYm1099, a new alpha glucosidase inhibitor on acute metabolic responses and metabolic control in NIDDM over 1 month. Diabetes Care *2* (1988) 337 – 344.

[38] Smith, V., G. Holm: Effect of a modified guar gum preparation on glucose and lipid levels in diabetes and healthy volunteers. Atherosclerosis *45* (1982) 1 – 10.

[39] Solsch, V. R., R. Ebert, W. Creutzfeldt: Response of serum levels of gastric inhibitory polypeptide and insulin to sucrose ingestion during long-term application of Acarbose. Scan. J. Gastroenterol. *16* (1981) 629 – 632.

[40] Stout, R. W.: Insulin and Atheroma: 20 year perspective. Diabetes Care *13* (6) (1990) 631 – 654.

[41] Thorne, M. J., L. V. Thompson, D. J. A. Jenkins: Factors affecting starch digestibility and the glycemic response with special references to legumes. Am. J. Clin. Nutr. *38* (1983) 481 – 488.

[42] Walhon, R. J., G. A. Now, I. T. Sherif et al.: Improved metabolic profiles in insulin treated patients given an alpha-glucosidehydrolase inhibitor. Br. Med. J. *1* (1979) 220 – 221.

[43] Wolever, T. M. S.: Metabolic effects of continuous feeding. Metabolism (1990) 947 – 951.

[44] Wu, M. S., P. Johnston, W. H. H. Sheu et al.: Effect of metformin on carbohydrate and lipoprotein metabolism in NIDDM patients. Diabetes Care *13* (1) (1990) 1 – 8.

Treatment strategies of Syndrome X – hypertension and vascular complications

H. Lithell

Introduction

It seems likely that our lack of knowledge regarding the genesis of essential hypertension is partly responsible for the strategy for the treatment of hypertension during the 60's, 70's and 80's: drug treatment should be instituted when the blood pressure exceeded a certain cut-off level. This strategy was based on extremely good survival results in the first studies that were carried out using a placebo-treated control group [24]. Much of the effect noted in these studies could probably be ascribed to the inclusion of patients with severe hypertension who were at a very high risk of death from hemorrhagic stroke, aorta rupture, cardiac or renal insufficiency. However, already at that time a few voices were heard claiming that "we should adopt an attitude of scepticism and restraint in accepting drugs that lower blood pressure as even part of the answer of the management of hypertensive disease" [5]. In the following studies, patients with mild to moderate hypertension were also included and the cut-off point for definition of hypertension that should be treated with drugs was accordingly reduced first from 115 to 105 and then to 95 mm Hg. In all these studies the effect with regard to reduction of risk of stroke and other complications that are pressure-related turned out to be statistically significant and of the same magnitude as in the earlier studies. However, the effect on coronary heart disease was not statistically significant in most of the studies. A discussion started about the reasons.

The risk of coronary heart disease

It has been suggested that a severely pronounced blood pressure reduction may be responsible for part of the failure in reducing CHD events [2]. The blood pressure in the coronary arteries may become reduced below a critical perfusion pressure in patients who have signs of coronary artery disease or left ventricular hypertrophy [10]. On the other hand, thosc individuals in different studies who did not obtain an optimal blood pressure level but stayed with a treatment, diastolic pressure of $\geq 95-100$ mm Hg were also at a high risk [21]. However, these two patient groups represented only a minor part of the study populations. The majority of those suffering from a coronary heart disease complication should have belonged to the greater part of the population that had a blood pressure between 80 and 95 mm Hg.

In a series of meta-analyses [1, 8] it has become quite obvious that the results of this type of analysis are totally dependent on the trials included in the analysis. The trials included depend on the question asked. So, recently a large meta-analysis including results from 14 different prospective trials was published [1]. It reported that a reduction in CHD incidence by 14% was obtained at a blood pressure reduction of about 6 mm Hg. The expected CHD reduction was about 22%. In this analysis, studies including patients who had severe hypertension were also incorporated. One might argue that today we do not see any patients with severe hypertension and therefore the relevant analysis is the one carried out on the trials that included only patients with mild-to-moderate hypertension. Such an analysis has been done [8] and the average calculated net reduction in those trials was 8% (ns) compared with the expected 22 to 25%. However, if only trials in which drug treatment was used were included and not trials that also used non-pharmacological means, then the net reduction was only 3% (ns) [8]. In the same three meta-analyses the obtained reduction by about 40% with regard to risk for stroke corresponded well to the expected reduction of about 40%.

The risk for coronary heart disease is determined by factors such as blood pressure, lipoprotein concentration, thrombotic factors and smoking. The risk for coronary heart disease is linearly related to the blood pressure level. Therefore blood pressure is less important as a risk factor in patients with mild-to-moderate hypertension than in patients with more severe hypertension. The result of one of the meta-analyses [8] also indicates the possibility that the drug treatment itself, as it was carried out in those trials using primarily beta-blockers and diuretics, may in one way or the other counteract the beneficial effect of the blood pressure reduction.

It was not until recently that it was suggested that insulin resistance may be a common, underlying cause of hypertension, hyperlipidemia, impaired glucose tolerance and diabetes mellitus [16] in today's community explaining why many of these entities appear in one and the same patient [3]. The theory that the different clinical appearances of these phenomena are due to genetic factors predisposing to the development of hypertension, hyperlipidemia or diabetes mellitus [3] in the presence of insulin resistance has also been put forward.

Insulin sensitivity

It was as early as 1966 that the first publication appeared reporting higher insulin concentration in hypertensives than in normotensives [25]. Modan et al. [9] suggested hyperinsulinemia to be the common link between obesity, hypertension and impaired glucose tolerance. Ferrannini et al. in 1987 [4] clearly demonstrated that in a group of hypertensives the insulin sensitivity was lower than in a group of normotensives with similar body weight and body mass index. Shen et al. confirmed these observations in similar studies [17]. They also pointed out that hypertensives treated with beta-blockers and/or diuretics had still lower insulin sensitivity than those hypertensives who had been withdrawn from treatment [14]. This indicated that treatment with both beta-blockers and diuretics may have a worsening effect on insulin sensitivity.

We recently reported that a large group of previously untreated hypertensives recruited from an ongoing health survey had a reduction of insulin sensitivity by about 33% compared with a normotensive control group recruited from the same health survey [12]. When the hypertensive group was subdivided into a non-obese and an obese subgroup according to body mass index ($\geq$ 26 for women and $\geq$ 27 for men as cut-off points), it turned out that the non-obese subgroup was very similar to the control group with regard to average body weight and body mass index. In spite of this, insulin sensitivity was 20% lower in the hypertensives. In the obese hypertensive subgroup that made up 60% of the hypertensives, insulin sensitivity was reduced by 43%. This study therefore proves that in non-selected hypertensives in a Western community the hypertensive state per se is an insulin resistant state. However, the insulin sensitivity at a given level of blood pressure may vary considerably from normal values to very resistant values indicating that high blood pressure can certainly develop in the absence of insulin resistance as well [12].

Today a series of studies have demonstrated that treatment with selective beta-blockers [13, 15] as well as non-selective beta-blockers (to be published) as well as thiazide diuretics [11] impair insulin sensitivity by 15 – 30% (Fig. 1). In evaluations of insulin concentrations in the fasting state (Fig. 2) as well as after glucose injection, (using the i. v. glucose tolerance test), it turns out that the concentrations during active treatment are increased with these types of drugs with the exception for the early insulin increment (Fig. 3) above the fasting insulin value that seems to be relatively impaired.

During treatment with a calcium-channel blocker, diltiazem, there was no significant effect on insulin sensitivity, insulin concentrations or lipoprotein concentrations [13]. Similar findings using nifedipine in a slow-release form were reported by Sheu et al. [18].

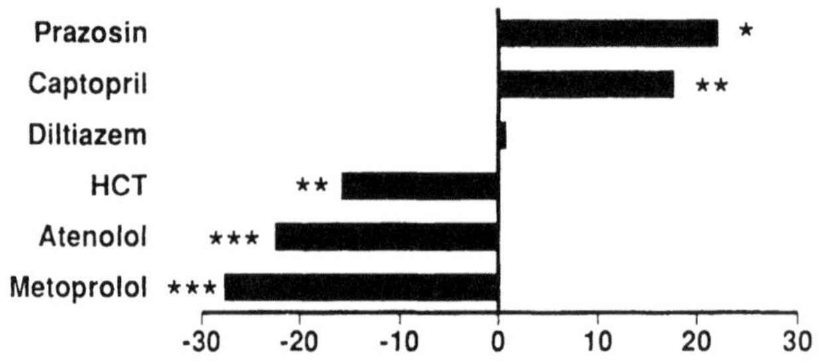

Fig. 1: Effects on insulin sensitivity during treatment with different antihypertensive drugs: change (%) of insulin sensitivity index [11, 13 – 15].

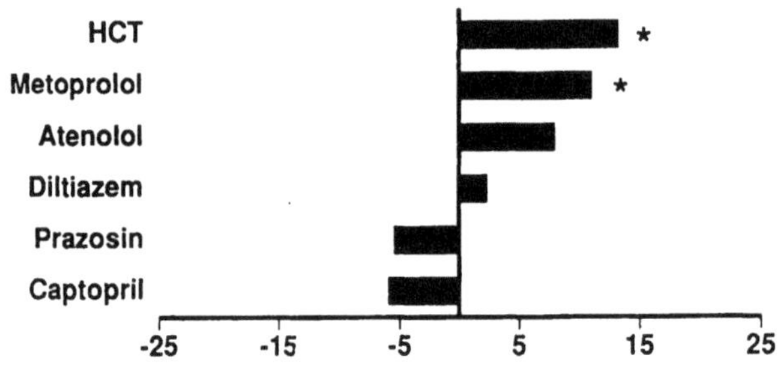

Fig. 2: Effects on fasting insulin concentration during treatment with different antihypertensive drugs [11, 13 – 15].

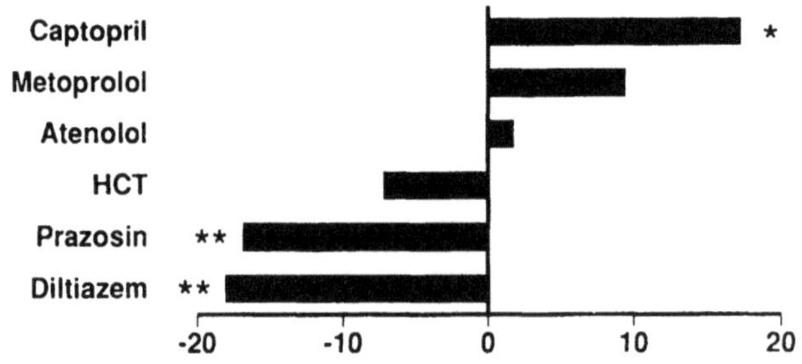

Fig. 3: Effects on insulin increment during treatment with different antihypertensive drugs [11, 13 – 15].

With the ACE-inhibitor captopril, an improvement in insulin sensitivity resulting in lower insulin concentrations during the IVGTT was reported [11]. The lipoprotein concentrations during that regimen were not affected.

We [14] and others [23] have reported that during prazosin treatment insulin sensitivity is improved, insulin concentrations and glucose concentrations are decreased and lipoprotein concentrations tend to change in a favourable way with decreased triglyceride concentrations and slightly elevated high density lipoprotein cholesterol concentrations.

Treatment of hypertension in the future

Since it is now recognized that several life-style factors that lead to an increase in body weight may considerably increase the risk of the development of hypertension, it is a desirable goal for the society to work for an improvement in dietary habits and physical exercise habits that would lead to a lower prevalence of obesity in the population. An increase of body weight also in late middle age increases the risk of the development of hypertension [19, 20]. However, not only is obesity a risk factor for hypertension, but hyperinsulinemia in itself is also associated with an increased risk for development of hypertension [19]. Better dietary and exercise habits not only help in preventing the development of obesity but also favourably influence insulin sensitivity. A lower prevalence of individuals with insulin resistance should be a result of an improvement in these life-style factors and consequently a lower prevalence of hypertension.

When hypertension is manifest it is now generally agreed upon and recommended that the initial treatment for those with mild-to-moderate hypertension should be a decrease in body weight in cases of obesity. This should be obtained by a change in dietary avoiding saturated fatty acids and increasing the intake of fibre-rich carbohydrates, monounsaturated fatty acids and polyunsaturated fatty acids, in particular those of the n-3 type. A lower fat intake, a substitution of fibre-rich carbohydrates for fats will lead to body-weight reduction. Such a prudent diet will in itself reduce the intake of salt. All these factors taken together may have a beneficial effect on the blood-pressure situation but most importantly, other risk factors of coronary heart disease are also changed in a fashion that should decrease the risk of coronary heart disease.

It is now recognized that the effect on the risk of stroke seems to be linearly related to the degree of blood-pressure reduction independent of how this is obtained. It seems reasonable to upgrade calcium-channel blockers and ACE-inhibitors, as was recently done by WHO/ISH [6] to first-line drugs for treatment of hypertension. It must be remembered though, that this was a decision based on an extrapolation of available data and that neither ACE-inhibitors, calcium-channel blockers or $alpha_1$ blockers have been tested in prospective trials with regard to the effect on stroke.

Considering the poor effect of risk reduction for coronary heart disease in patients with mild-to-moderate hypertension treated with drugs only, it seems reasonable to advocate the use of drugs with fewer effects on metabolic risk factors than beta-blockers and diuretics, at least in patients who have more profound deteriorations of e. g. glucose or lipoprotein metabolism. This should benefit these individuals. In prospective trials in which lowering of low density lipoprotein cholesterol or increasing high density lipoprotein cholesterol have been obtained by drugs or diet, such changes are accompanied by a significant decrease in the risk of coronary heart disease [7]. Consequently, every change in lipoprotein concentration must be regarded as if it were associated with a change in risk for coronary heart disease until the opposite has been proved. In addition, several studies have indicated that increased plasma insulin concentrations may in themselves constitute a risk for coronary heart disease. Therefore, the elevations of insulin concentration during antihypertensive treatment may also counteract the beneficial effect of the blood pressure reduction. In a prospective study of about 1800 middle-aged men it has been demonstrated that both fasting hyperinsulinemia as well as a low insulin increment were significant risk factors for development of diabetes [19a]. Furthermore, treatment with beta-blockers and/or diuretics was an independent risk factor for development of diabetes mellitus. This may be regarded as a confirmation that the induced metabolic effects by these types of drugs have clinical implications after long-term treatment.

Again, it must be emphazised that these are extrapolations and that we do not have prospective studies where the metabolic effects of the different used antihypertensive drugs have been evaluated prospectively with regard to their impact on risk for coronary heart disease. A more general recommendation of a change from beta-blockers and diuretics to ACE-inhibitors, calcium channel blockers and α_1-blockers must probably await results from further prospective trials. Today an individualized therapy should be recommended.

References

[1] Collins, R., R. Peto, S. MacMahon et al.: Blood pressure, stroke, and coronary heart disease. Part 2, short-term reductions in blood pressure: overview of randomized drug trials in their epedemiological context. Lancet *335* (1990) 827–838.

[2] Cruickshank, J. M., J. M. Thorp, F. J. Zacharias: Benefits and potential harm of lowering high blood pressure. Lancet *I* (1987) 581–584.

[3] DeFronzo, R. A., E. Ferrannini: Insulin resistance: a multifaceted syndrome responsible for NIDDM, obesity, hypertension, dyslipidemia, and atherosclerotic cardiovascular disease. Diab. Care *14* (1991) 173–194.

[4] Ferrannini, E., G. Buzzigoli, Bonadonna et al.: Insulin resistance in essential hypertension. N. Engl. J. Med. *317* (1987) 350–357.

[5] Goldring, W., H. Chasis: Antihypertensive drug therapy: an appraisal. In: F. J. Ingelfinger, A. S. Relman, M. Finland (eds.): Controversy in internal medicine, pp. 83–91. Philadelphia: W B Saunders Co, 1966.

[6] 1989 Guidelines for the management of mild hypertension: memorandum from a WHO/ISH meeting. J. Hypertens. *7* (1989) 689–693.

[7] Holme, I.: An analysis of randomized trials evaluating the effects of cholesterol reduction on total mortality and coronary heart disease incidence. Circulation *82* (1990) 1916–1924.

[8] Holme, I.: Medikamentell behandling av mild hypertension. En oversiktsanalyse av randomiserte forsök. Tidsskr. Nor. Laegeforen. *108* (English abstract) (1988) 1932–1936.

[9] Modan, M., H. Halkin, A. Almog et al.: Hyperinsulinemia: A link between hypertension, obesity and glucose intolerance. J. Clin. Invest. *75* (1985) 809–817.

[10] Pepi, M., M. Alimento, A. Maltagliati et al.: Cardiac hypertrophy in hypertension. Repolarization abnormalities elicited by rapid lowering of pressure. Hypertension *11* (1988) 84–91.

[11] Pollare, T., H. Lithell, C. Berne: A comparison of the effects of hydrochlorothiazide and captopril on glucose and lipid metabolism in patients with hypertension. N. Engl. J. Med. *321* (1989) 868–873.

[12] Pollare, T., H. Lithell, C. Berne: Insulin resistance is a characteristic feature of primary hypertension independent of obesity. Metabolism *39* (1990) 167–174.

[13] Pollare, T., H. Lithell, C. Mörlin et al.: Metabolic effects of diltiazem and atenolol: results from a randomized, double-blind study with parallel groups. J. Hypertens. *7* (1989) 551–559.

[14] Pollare, T., H. Lithell, I. Selinus et al.: Application of prazosin is associated with an increase of insulin sensitivity in obese patients with hypertension. Diabetologia *31* (1988) 415–420.

[15] Pollare, T., H. Lithell, I. Selinus et al.: Sensitivity to insulin during treatment with atenolol and metoprolol: a randomized, double blind study of effects on carbohydrate and lipoprotein metabolism in hypertensive patients. Br. Med. J. *298* (1989) 1152–1157.

[16] Reaven, G. M.: Role of insulin resistance in human disease. Diabetes *83* (1988) 609–612.

[17] Shen, R.-C., S.-M. Shieh, D. A. Fuh et al.: Resistance to insulin-stimilated glucose uptake in patients with hypertension. J. Clin. Endocrinol. Metab. *66* (1988) 580–583.

[18] Sheu, W. H.-H., A. L. M. Swislocki, B. Hoffman et al.: Comparison of the effects of atenolol and nifedipine on glucose, insulin, and lipid metabolism in patients with hypertension. Am. J. Hypertens. *4* (1991) 199–205.

[19] Skarfors, E. T., H. O. Lithell, I. Selinus: Risk factors for the development of hypertension: a 10-year longitudinal study in middle-aged men. J. Hypertens. *9* (1991) 217–223.

[19a] Skarfors, E. T., K. I. Selinus, H. O. Lithell: Risk factors for developing non-insulin-dependent diabetes a 10 year follow up of men in Uppsala. Br. Med. J. *303* (1991) 755 – 760.

[20] Stamler, R., J. Stamler, F. C. Gosch et al.: Primary prevention of hypertension by nutritional-hygienic means. Final report of a randomized, controlled trial. JAMA *262* (1989) 1801 – 1807.

[21] Strate, M., K. Thygesen, C. Ringsted et al.: Prognosis in treated hypertension. Acta Med. Scand. *219* (1986) 153 – 159.

[22] Swislocki, A. L. M., B. B. Hoffman, G. M. Reaven: Insulin resistance, glucose intolerance and hyperinsulinemia in patients with hypertension. Am. J. Hypertens. *2* (1989) 419 – 423.

[23] Swislocki, A. L. M., B. B. Hoffman, W. H.-H. Scheu et al.: Effects of prazosin treatment on carbohydrate and lipoprotein metabolism in patients with hypertension. Am. J. Med. *86* (1989) 14 – 18.

[24] Veterans Administration Cooperative Study Group on Antihypertensive Agents. Effects of treatment on morbidity in hypertension. Results in patients with diastolic blood pressures averaging 115 through 129 mm Hg. JAMA *202* (1967) 116 – 122.

[25] Welborn, T. A., A. Breckenridge, A. H. Rubinstein et al.: Serum insulin in essential hypertension and in peripheral vascular disease. Lancet *I* (1966) 1336 – 1337.

Lipid metabolism: metabolic consequences of moderate hypertriglyceridemia

G. L. Vega

Introduction

Moderate hypertriglyceridemia, defined as plasma triglyceride levels between 250 mg/dl and 500 mg/dl (3.39 – 5.65 mmoles/L), can be either primary or secondary [1]. *Primary moderate hypertriglyceridemia* is defined as a rise in plasma triglyceride resulting from a genetic defect in triglyceride metabolism, whereas *secondary moderate hypertriglyceridemia* is a rise in plasma triglycerides resulting from another metabolic abnormality, such as diabetes mellitus or obesity. Moderate hypertriglyceridemia is not associated with the presence of chylomicrons. All of the increase in triglycerides occur in very low density lipoproteins (VLDL).

High triglyceride levels have been implicated from epidemiologic studies as a risk factor for coronary heart disease (CHD) [2]. Further, a number of alterations of the plasma lipoproteins have been reported as a consequence of high blood triglycerides, and these alterations may be atherogenic. For example, small, dense low density lipoproteins (LDL) occur frequently with hypertriglyceridemia, and epidemiologic data suggest that their presence may be atherogenic [3]. Dense LDL apparently are prone to oxidation [4] which may be atherogenic, and they have been reported to have a low affinity for the LDL receptors [5]. Hypertriglyceridemia also is associated with abnormalities in VLDL [6 – 8] and high density lipoproteins (HDL) [9]. An inverse correlation between triglyceride levels and HDL-cholesterol concentrations has been demonstrated [10], and low HDL-cholesterol levels are an independent risk factor for CHD [11].

In this review we shall consider the connection between moderate hypertriglyceridemia and the metabolism of plasma lipoproteins containing hepatic apolipoprotein B; the effect of drugs that lower plasma triglycerides also will be examined.

Metabolism of lipoproteins containing hepatic apolipoprotein B (Lp B-100)

The liver secretes lipoproteins containing one apolipoprotein B-100 per lipoprotein particle; newly secreted lipoproteins of this type can be called "nascent" LpB-100 (Fig. 1). The core of these particles is enriched with triglycerides, and

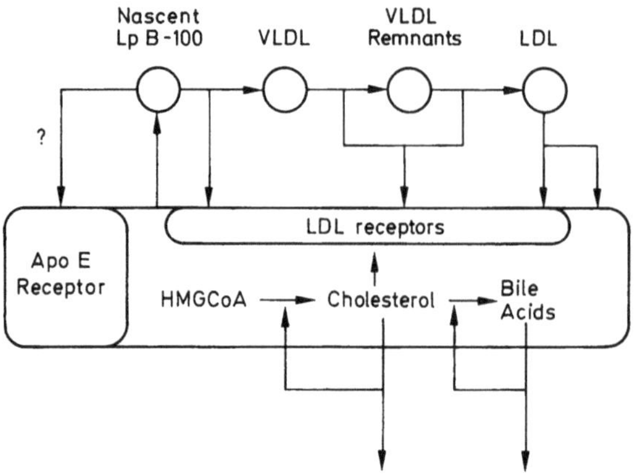

Fig. 1: Metabolic pathways for lipoproteins containing hepatic apolipoprotein B (Lp B-100). The liver secretes triglyceride-rich lipoproteins ("Nascent") which are precursors of plasma VLDL, and LDL. Each of these lipoproteins undergoes triglyceride hydrolysis; in the process they are enriched in cholesteryl esters. VLDL and VLDL remnants (including IDL), have two metabolic fates: (1) they can be converted to LDL, or (2) they can be removed from circulation by LDL receptors. The latter regulate levels of Lp B-100 particles in plasma.

the surface has a high content of unesterified cholesterol, phospholipid, and apolipoproteins. Nascent LpB-100 are secreted into the space of Disse [12], and thereafter, enter the systemic circulation. As the particles circulate, their triglyceride is hydrolyzed by lipoprotein lipase [13], and after removal of some triglycerides, LpB-100 have three metabolic fates: (a) direct removal by a receptor-mediated pathway, (b) conversion to plasma VLDL or (c) direct conversion to LDL. The details of these processes have not been completely elucidated. In plasma, most of the VLDL can undergo further catabolism; triglycerides continue to be hydrolyzed by lipoprotein lipase and hepatic triglyceride lipase; free cholesterol is esterified by lecithin-cholesteryl-acyl transferase (LCAT), and the core of the lipoprotein exchanges triglyceride for cholesteryl esters from other lipoproteins through the action of cholesterol ester transfer protein (CETP) [14]. In this process, VLDL remnants, including intermediate density lipoproteins (IDL), are formed; remnant particles are enriched in cholesterol esters, and partially depleted of triglycerides. Remnant particles can either be removed directly by a receptor-mediated pathway in the liver, or they can be converted to LDL [15, 16]. The latter in turn, has two metabolic fates: (a) a receptor-mediated clearance, and (b) a receptor-independent removal.

LpB-100 lipoproteins clearly vary in their affinities for the LDL receptor; at each step of their catabolism a fraction of the lipoproteins is removed through the receptor-mediated pathway, and the remainder is gradually converted to smaller lipoproteins. Factors promoting the direct uptake of LpB-100 particles include: (a) the content and/or conformation of apolipoprotein (apo) E on the surface of LpB-100 particles (apo E is another hepatic apolipoprotein that can bind to the LDL receptor), (b) the content of apolipoprotein C-III, which may interfere with the binding of LpB-100 particles to the LDL receptor, and (c) the activity of hepatic triglyceride lipase, an enzyme located on the surface of hepatocytes, which seemingly facilitates the conversion of VLDL remnants and IDL to LDL [15, 16].

One function of the LDL receptor is to remove LpB-100 particles from plasma when hepatic cholesterol biosynthesis is not sufficient to maintain intracellular cholesterol balance [17]. Once LpB-100 particles bind to the receptor, they are internalized and degraded within lysosomes by hydrolases and esterases. The LDL receptor dissociates from the ligands before any degradation of the lipoproteins takes place, and it is recycled to the surface of hepatocytes [17]. Thus, the number of receptors available on the surface of hepatocytes for binding LpB-100 particles are determined not only by the rate of synthesis, but also by the rate of recycling of the receptor. Synthesis of receptors, in turn, is regulated by factors that respond to intracellular cholesterol concentrations.

Repletion of intracellular cholesterol triggers a series of reactions that also lead to the suppression of receptor biosynthesis, hence to its decreased activity and reduced uptake of LpB-100 particles [17]. Within the hepatocyte (Fig. 1) cholesterol regulates its own synthesis by modulating the activity of 3-hydroxy-3-methylglutaryl coenzyme A (HMGCoA) reductase. This enzyme is rate limiting in the biosynthesis of cholesterol; it catalyzes the conversion of HMGCoA to mevalonate. Finally, excess cholesterol can be secreted directly into bile or be converted into bile acids. The rate limiting enzyme in bile acid synthesis is cholesterol-7-alpha-hydroxylase.

Recently, a protein with structural similarities to the LDL receptor has been identified [18]. It was designated the LDL-receptor-related protein (LRP), and in Figure 1 it is postulated to be the *apo E receptor* for reasons detailed below. LRP also is located on the surface of hepatocytes. One of its functions may be to remove plasma lipoproteins of intestinal origin which have acquired apo E, the protein that mediates binding of intestinal lipoproteins to this receptor. Unlike the LDL receptor, the apo E receptor seemingly is not regulated by the cholesterol content of liver cells. Since nascent LpB-100 particles may be secreted with apo E, and/or acquire the apolipoprotein after secretion, these particles also could be removed by the apo E receptor. If LRP is not the true apo E receptor, it is likely that another protein, yet to be identified serves this purpose.

Metabolism of Lp B-100 lipoproteins during moderate hypertriglyceridemia

Tracer kinetics have been instrumental in defining the changes in the lipoprotein metabolism in patients with hypertriglyceridemia [1922]. Two methods have been employed: (a) radioactive precursors of plasma triglycerides, and (b) radioactive tracers for apolipoprotein B-100 [19 – 23]. The methods require injection of tracers, collection of blood at selected time points after injection, and determination of fraction of injected dose remaining in either plasma VLDL-triglyceride or apo B-100 in VLDL, IDL, and LDL [20]. The data are analyzed by multicompartmental analysis, and fractional catabolic rates (pools/day) as well as transport rates (mg/kg-day) are estimated. Kinetic data suggests that there are at least two kinetic species of plasma VLDL. One type of VLDL undergoes rapid hydrolysis of triglyceride and formation of remnants, and the other is catabolized much more slowly [20]. Normally, most plasma VLDL consists of Lp-B-100 particles that are rapidly degraded to IDL and LDL. However, kinetic studies suggest that catabolism of VLDL particles does do not account for all of plasma LDL. In our view, plasma LDL can also be derived from direct catabolism of "nascent" Lp B-100 lipoproteins which bypasses VLDL (Fig. 1).

Hypertriglyceridemia usually is associated with a prolonged residence time of VLDL, VLDL remnants and IDL in circulation. This delayed clearance may lead to changes in the physicochemical properties of these triglyceride-rich lipoproteins; for example, they become enriched in cholesteryl esters. Also, Gianturco et al. [6 – 8] have shown that "hypertriglyceridemic" VLDL are more rapidly taken up by LDL receptors in fibroblast culture, and likewise, some triglyceride-rich lipoproteins are recognized as modified lipoproteins by macrophages. VLDL from normolipidemic subjects are not taken up by LDL receptors, and the uptake of "hypertriglyceridemic" VLDL may reflect a change in the conformation of apo E on the surface of VLDL particles. The mechanism for uptake of "hypertriglyceridemic" VLDL by scavenger receptors on macrophages are not well understood. Many patients also have increased conversion of VLDL to LDL, possibly due to a decreased direct removal of VLDL remnants and IDL; this may lead to an increase in LDL-apo B levels.

LDL of hypertriglyceridemic patients is polydisperse (heterogeneous in size), and at least two subfractions have been isolated which differ in physicochemical properties [21, 25]. Both of these subfractions are rapidly removed from circulation as is typical of the whole LDL fraction in hypertriglyceridemic patients [25 – 27]. The predominant species of LDL in hypertriglyceridemia tends to be small, and dense [28]. Some workers suggest that this type of LDL confers a high risk for atheroclerotic disease [29].

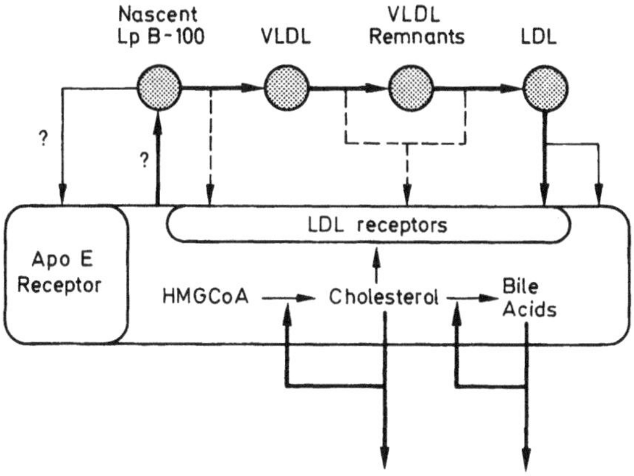

Fig. 2: Metabolism of Lp B-100 particles in moderate hypertriglyceridemia. Three causes of moderate hypertriglyceridemia can be defined: (1) hepatic secretion of triglyceride-enriched Lp B-100 particles, (2) increased secretion in the number of Lp B-100 particles carrying a normal content of triglycerides, and (3) a lipolytic defect in combination with either (1) or (2). The consequences of these alterations are two-fold: (1) change in physicochemical and biological properties of Lp B-100 particles, and (2) an abnormally high rate of removal of LDL from circulation. The latter may occur, despite normal levels of LDL cholesterol.

Figure 2 summarizes our current understanding of the metabolism of Lp B-100 particles during moderate hypertriglyceridemia. The liver may secrete a normal number of particles that are enriched in triglyceride, or it may secrete an increased number of particles each having a normal content of triglyceride. With the former, total apo B levels are not increased. The latter may lead to hypertriglyceridemia, but in addition serum levels of apolipoprotein B-100 are increased. A third mechanism that pertains is an abnormality in catabolism of triglyceride-rich lipoproteins which results in a slow processing of "nascent" lipoproteins, VLDL, and VLDL remnants. In most patients with hypertriglyceridemia, there is a marked alteration in the metabolism of VLDL, and VLDL remnants, leading to a rapid clearance of LDL. The high rate of clearance of LDL may reflect increased availability of LDL receptors for LDL clearance since VLDL and its remnants, in some patients, may have a low affinity for the LDL receptor.

Some patients with moderate hypertriglyceridemia have an increased synthesis of cholesterol and/or bile acid [30, 31]. These observations have been confirmed in liver biopsies of patients with moderate hypertriglyceridemia; these tests showed increased activity of HMGCoA reductase and cholesterol-7-alpha-hydroxylase, the rate limiting enzymes for synthesis of cholesterol and bile acids, respectively [32, 33]. The increase in hepatic cholesterol synthesis and bile acid synthesis may occur more frequently in patients secreting a normal number of Lp B-100 particles that are enriched in triglyceride, and less frequently in patients who secrete an increased particle number of normal composition.

Metabolism of Lp B-100 lipoproteins during secondary moderate hypertriglyceridemia

Two disorders in which moderate hypertriglyceridemia may occur are obesity and non-insulin-dependent diabetes mellitus (NIDDM). Each will be considered briefly in turn.

Obesity

Obese patients apparently have an increased secretion of hepatic Lp B-100 particles having a normal content of triglyceride [22, 34 – 35]. The degree of hypertriglyceridemia, however, in obese patients will depend on the individual's lipolytic capacity. Likewise, the lipoprotein pattern of an obese subject will depend on the capacity to catabolize Lp B-100 particles at the various sites noted in Figure 1. A large fraction of obese patients do not have hypertriglyceridemia, despite the increased secretion of Lp B-100 particles by the liver, because they have efficient catabolic pathways; i. e. receptor number, and lipolysis.

Non-insulin-dependent diabetes mellitus (NIDDM)

Two metabolic abnormalities may cause an increase in plasma triglyceride levels in patients with NIDDM. A relative deficiency of peripheral insulin activity apparently reduces the synthesis of lipoprotein lipase, and it may stimulate secretion of Lp B-100 particles enriched in triglycerides [36 – 38]. A number of factors may contribute to this alteration of hepatic triglyceride secretion; these are (a) increased influx of fatty acids into the liver, (b) increased plasma glucose, (c) hyperinsulinemia, and (d) hyperglucagonemia.

Alterations in the metabolism of Lp B-100 lipoproteins have been reported in NIDDM patients that are similar to those noted with obesity [39]. It may well be that some of these patients have an increased secretion of triglyceride-enriched Lp B-100 lipoproteins, and that they have an altered metabolism of VLDL and remnants, leading to an increased conversion of VLDL to LDL, shown in Figure 2. However, more detailed studies are needed to confirm these mechanisms. Most of the effects of NIDDM on Lp B-100 metabolism may be reversed in the early stages either by weight reduction or specific hypoglycemic therapy.

Drug management of moderate hypertriglyceridemia

Diet modification is the first line of therapy for management of moderate hypertriglyceridemia. The first step is to modify dietary factors that alter the metabolism of triglycerides; thus, excess ingestion of carbohydrates and alcohol should be eliminated. Weight reduction in obese subjects and in NIDDM patients, is indicated, but this does not always result in normalization of the metabolism of Lp B-100 lipoproteins. A number of drugs are effective in curtailing the abnormalities in the metabolism of the lipoproteins. Management may differ depending on the cause of the hypertriglyceridemia.

Management of increased secretion of triglyceride-enriched Lp B-100 lipoproteins and of decreased lipolysis of VLDL-triglyceride

Several fibric acids – clofibrate, gemfibrozil, bezafibrate, and fenofibrate – appear to inhibit the synthesis of triglycerides in the liver as shown in animals models; if this mechanism pertains in humans, this class of drugs should reduce hepatic secretion rates of triglyceride without affecting the normal secretion rate of apo B-100. In other words, these drugs may reduce the content of triglyceride in VLDL. Additionally, fibric acids, particularly gemfibrozil, enhance lipolysis of plasma VLDL, which tends to normalize the metabolism and chemical composition of LDL [40]. Fibric acids are effective in reducing levels of plasma triglyceride and are generally recommended in cases of severe hypertriglyceridemia, which predisposes to pancreatitis.

Management of increased secretion in the number of Lp B-100 lipoproteins

Two drugs may be effective in the management of hypertriglyceridemia resulting from increased number of Lp-B-100 particles secreted into plasma. These are nicotinic acid, and competitive inhibitors of 3-hydroxy-3-methylglutaryl coenzyme (HMGCoA) reductase.

Nicotinic acid is a potent triglyceride-lowering drug which curtails hepatic secretion of Lp B-100 particles [41, 42]. As a result, this drug lowers plasma cholesterol and apo B-100 levels [42]. However, nicotinic acid is not well tolerated by patients with gastrointestinal disorders, or a history of gout, and uricemia; the drug also may result in hepatotoxicity. In NIDDM patients, poor glycemic control has been noted [43]. More recently, an analogue of nicotinic acid – acipimox – has been introduced. This drug may not have the same side effects as nicotinic acid in causing flushing, rashes, or poor glycemic control, but neither is it as potent for lipid lowering.

HMGCoA reductase inhibitors have been used extensively in the management of hypercholesterolemia [44], but they also may have a place in management of hypertriglyceridemia [45, 46]. These drugs inhibit cholesterol biosynthesis, which in turn causes an increase in the number of LDL receptors on the surface of liver cells (Fig. 1). The cholesterol-lowering effect in plasma results from an increased removal of Lp B-100 particles; i. e., the drug causes a reduction in the number of Lp B-100 particles in circulation [44]. Compared to gemfibrozil, HMGCoA reductase inhibitors have proven superior in lowering the number of Lp B-100 particles in patients having moderate hypertriglyceridemia, borderline high cholesterol and elevated serum apo B-100 [46].

In patients with moderate hypertriglyceridemia caused by a lipolytic defect in combination with increased hepatic secretion of Lp B-100 particles, two drugs may be needed [44]. Combination of an HMGCoA reductase inhibitor with gemfibrozil would be useful. However, carefull monitoring of the patient may be necessary since this combination has been reported to cause severe myosytis [47].

Bile acid sequestrants are another class of drugs that induce an increase in receptor number and a reduction in the number of Lp B-100 particles in circulation [48]. However, these drugs generally should not be used in patients with hypertriglyceridemia because they cause increases in hepatic secretion of triglyceride [49, 50].

Use of hypolipidemic agents in the management of moderate hypertriglyceridemia in NIDDM

Patients with NIDDM have additional metabolic complications which warrant careful consideration in the selection of hypolipidemic agents. The causes of moderate hypertriglyceridemia in NIDDM may result from a combination of increased secretion of triglyceride-enriched Lp B-100 lipoproteins, and poor lipolysis of plasma VLDL-triglyceride. If these mechanisms pertain, it would seem reasonable to first test the effectiveness of nicotinic acid. However, recent studies indicate that this drug usually worsens hyperglycemia in NIDDM patients [43]. Another drug that is being tested in Europe is acipimox, and preliminary studies suggest that this compound may have hypolipidemic effects without side effects. Fibric acid derivatives, such as gemfibrozil, may be indicated in cases of severe hypertriglyceridemia; they do not appear to cause deterioration of glycemic control, but they may increase lithogenicity of bile. Finally, HMGCoA reductase inhibitors have been tested in NIDDM with hypercholesterolemia [51, 52]. This class of drugs do not affect glycemic control, which may be a benefit for their use.

Conclusion

Moderate hypertriglyceridemia causes a number of alterations in the metabolism of hepatic Lp B lipoproteins. Three types of abnormalities in the metabolism of Lp B lipoproteins are found in patients with hypertriglyceridemia: (1) increased secretion of Lp B particle number, (2) normal secretion of Lp B particles that are enriched in triglyceride content, and (3) a combination of either of these with decreased lipolytic capacity. The choice of drugs for the management of the dyslipidemia may depend on the clinical presentation of the patient. For example, a patient with elevated plasma triglyceride with normal levels of plasma cholesterol may benefit from treatment with a fibric acid derivative, whereas a hypertriglyceridemic subject with borderline high cholesterol and elevated serum apo B-100 may require either nicotinic acid or a first line treatment of the increased plasma cholesterol and serum apo B with competitive inhibitors of HMGCoA reductase.

Acknowledgements

This work was supported by the Veterans Administration, National Institutes of Health grants HL-29252 and M01-R00633, the Southwestern Medical Foundation, and the Moss Heart Foundation of Dallas, Texas. The author acknowledges the valuable discussions of this manuscript with Professor Scott M. Grundy.

References

[1] Consensus Development Conference 1984. Treatment of hypertriglyceridemia. JAMA *251* (1984) 1196–1200.

[2] Carlson, L. A., L. E. Bottiger: Ischaemic heart-disease in relation to fasting values of plasma triglycerides and cholesterol: Stockholm prospective study. Lancet *1* (1972) 865–868.

[3] Austin, M. A., J. L. Breslow, C. H. Hennekens et al.: Low-density lipoprotein subclass patterns and risk of myocardial infarction. JAMA *260* (1988) 1917–1921.

[4] de Graaf, J., H. L. M. Hak-Lemmers, M. P. C. Hectors et al.: Enhanced susceptibility to in vitro oxidation of the dense low density lipoprotein subfraction in healthy subjects. Arteriosclerosis and Thrombosis *11* (1991) 298–306.

[5] Kleinman, Y., S. Eisenberg, Y. Oschry et al.: Defective metabolism of hypertriglyceridemic lipoprotein in cultured human skin fibroblasts. Normalization with bezafibrate. J. Clin. Invest. *75* (1985) 1796–1803.

[6] Gianturco, S., A. U. Sr. Gotto, R. L. Jackson et al.: Control of 3-Hydroxy-3-Methylglutaryl-CoA reductase activity in cultured human fibroblasts by very low density lipoproteins of subjects with hypertriglyceridemia. J. Clin. Invest. *61* (1978) 320–328.

[7] Gianturco, S. H., G. J. Packard, J. Shepherd et al.: Abnormal suppression of 3-hydroxy-3-methylglutaryl-CoA reductase activity in cultured human fibroblasts by hypertriglyceridemia very low density lipoprotein subclasses. Lipids *15* (1980) 456–463.

[8] Gianturco, S. H., S. G. Eskin, L. T. Navarow et al.: Abnormal effects of hypertriglycerolemia very low-density lipoproteins in 3-hydroxy-3-methylglutaryl-CoA reductase activity and viability of cultured bovine aortic endothelial cells. Biochem. Biophys. Acta *618* (1980) 143–152.

[9] Deckelbaum, R. J., E. Granot, R. Oschry et al.: Plasma triglyceride determines structure-composition in low and high density lipoproteins. Arterisclerosis *4* (1984) 225–231.

[10] Nikkila, E. A.: HDL in relation to the metabolism of triglyceride rich lipoproteins. In: N. E. Miller, G. J. Miller (eds.): Clinical and metabolic aspects of high-density lipoproteins. Elsevier Science Publishers, Amsterdam 1984.

[11] Miller, N. E.: Associations of high-density lipoprotein subclasses and apolipoproteins with ischemic heart disease and coronary atherosclerosis. Am. Heart. J. *113* (1987) 589–597.

[12] Williams, K. J., R. W. Brocia, K. Petrie et al.: Lipoprotein lipase modulates net apolipoprotein-B output by HepG2 cells. Circulation *82* (III) (1990) 283a.

[13] Havel, R. J.: Metabolism of lipids in chylomicrons and very low density lipoproteins. Section 5. In: Handbook of physiology, pp. 499–471, 1970.

[14] Tall, A. R.: Plasma lipid transfer proteins. J. Lipid Res. *27* (1986) 361–367.

[15] Havel, R. J.: The formation of LDL: mechanisms and regulation. J. Lipid Res. *25* (1984) 1570–1577.

[16] Goldberg, I. J., N. A. Le, J. R. Paterniti, Jr. et al.: Lipoprotein metabolism during acute inhibition of hepatic triglyceride lipase in the cynomolgus monkey. J. Clin. Invest. *70* (1982) 1184–1192.

[17] Goldstein, J. L., M. S. Brown: Progress in understanding the LDL receptor and HMG CoA reductase, two membrane proteins that regulate the plasma cholesterol. J. Lipid Res. *25* (1984) 1450–1461.

[18] Beisiegel, U., W. Weber, G. Ihrke et al.: The LDL-receptor-related protein, LRP, is an apolipoprotein E-binding protein. Nature *341* (1989) 162–164.

[19] Janus, E. D., A. Nicoll, R. Wootton et al.: Quantitative studies of very low density lipoprotein in normal controls and primary hyperlipidemic states and the role of direct secretion of low density lipoprotein in heterozygous familial hypercholesterolemia. Eur. J. Clin. Invest. *10* (1980) 149–159.

[20] Packard, C. J., A. Munro, A. R. Lorimer et al.: Metabolism of apolipoprotein B in large triglyceride-rich very low density lipoproteins of normal and hypertriglyceridemic subjects. J. Clin. Invest. *74* (1984) 2178–2192.

[21] Fisher, W. R.: Apoprotein B kinetics in man: concepts and modeling. In: M. Berman, S. M. Grundy, B. V. Howard (eds.): Lipoprotein and modeling, pp. 43–66. Academic Press, New York 1982.

[22] Grundy, S. M., H. Y. Mok, L. Zech et al.: Transport of very low density lipoprotein triglycerides in varying degrees of obesity and hypertriglyceridemia. J. Clin. Invest. *63* (1979) 1274–1283.

[23] Beltz, W. F., Y. A. Kesaniemi, N. H. Miller et al.: Studies on the metabolism of apolipoprotein B in hypertriglyceridemic subjects using simultaneous administration of tritiated leucine and radioiodinated very low density lipoprotein. J. Lipid Res. *31* (1990) 361–374.

[24] Grundy, S. M., G. L. Vega: What is beta-VLDL?. In: M. Berman, S. M. Grundy, B. V. Howard (eds.): Lipoprotein Kinetics and Modeling, pp. 208–216. Academic Press, New York 1982.

[25] Vega, G. L., S. M. Grundy: Kinetic heterogeneity of low density lipoproteins in primary hypertriglyceridemia. Arteriosclerosis *6* (1986) 395–406.

[26] Vega, G. L., S. M. Grundy: Influence of Lovastatin therapy on the metabolism of low density lipoproteins in mixed hyperlipidemia. J. Intern. Med. (1991) (In press).

[27] Vega, G. L., W. Beltz, S. M. Grundy: Low density lipoprotein metabolism in hypertriglyceridemic and normolipidemic patient with coronary heart disease. J. Lipid Res. *26* (1985) 115–126.

[28] Miettinen, T. A.: Faecal fat, bile acid excretion, and body height in familial hypercholesterolaemia and hypertriglyceridemia. Scand. J. Clin. Invest. *30* (1972) 85–88.

[29] Austin, M. A., M. C. King, K. M. Vranizan et al.: Atherogenic lipoprotein phenotype: a proposed genetic marker for coronary heart disease risk. Circulation *82* (1990) 495–506.

[30] Beil, U., S. M. Grundy, J. R. Crouse et al.: Triglyceride and cholesterol metabolism in primary hypertriglyceridemia. Arteriosclerosis *2* (1982) 44–57.

[31] Angelin, B., K. S. Hershon, J. D. Brunzell: Bile acid metabolism in hereditary forms of hypertriglyceridemia: Evidence for an increased synthesis rate in monogenic familial hypertriglyceridemia. Proc. Natl. Acad. Sci. USA *84* (1987) 5434–5438.

[32] Ahlberg, J., B. Angelin, I. Bjorkhem et al.: Hepatic cholesterol metabolism in normo and hyperlipidemic patients with cholesterol gallstones. J.Lipid Res. *20* (1979) 107–115.

[33] Nicolau, G., S. Shefer, G. Salen et al.: Determination of hepatic cholesterol 7-a-hydroxylase activity in man. J. Lipid Res. *15* (1974) 146–151.

[34] Kesaniemi, Y. A., W. F. Beltz, S. M. Grundy: Comparisons of metabolism of apolipoprotein B in normal subjects, obese patients, and patients with coronary heart disease. J. Clin. Invest. *76* (1985) 586–595.

[35] Egusa, G., W. F. Beltz, S. M. Grundy et al.: Influence of obesity on the metabolism of apolipoprotein B in man. J. Clin. Invest. *76* (1985) 596–603.

[36] Abrams, J. J., H. Ginsberg, S. M. Grundy: Metabolism of cholesterol and plasma triglycerides in nonketotic diabetes mellitus. Diabetes *31* (1982) 903–910.

[37] Taskinen, M. R., W. F. Beltz, I. Harper et al.: Effects of NIDDM on very-low-density lipoprotein triglyceride and apolipoprotein B metabolism. Studies before and after sulfonylurea therapy. Diabetes *35* (1986) 1268–1277.

[38] Dunn, F. L., P. Raskin, D. W. Bilheimer et al.: The effect of diabetic control on very low-density lipoprotein-triglyceride metabolism in patients with type II diabetes mellitus and marked hypertriglyceridemia. Metabolism *33* (1984) 117–123.

[39] Kissebah, A. H., S. Alfarsi, P. W. Adams et al.: The metabolic fate of plasma lipoproteins in normal subjects and in patients with insulin resistance and endogenous hypertriglyceridemia. Diabetologia *12* (1976) 501–509.

[40] Vega, G. L., S. M. Grundy: Gemfibrozil therapy in primary hypertriglyceridemia associated with coronary heart disease. Effects on metabolism of low-density lipoproteins. JAMA *253* (1985) 2398–2403.
[41] Grundy, S. M., H. Y. I. Mok, L. Zech et al.: Influence of nicotinic acid on metabolism of cholesterol and triglycerides in man. J. Lipid. Res. *22* (1981) 24–36.
[42] Langer, T., R. I. Levy: The effect of nicotinic acid on turnover of low density lipoproteins Type II hyperlipoproteinemia. In: K. F. Gey, L. A. Carlson (eds.): Metabolic Effect of Nicotinic Acid and Its Derivatives, p. 641. Huber and Bern, New York 1971.
[43] Garg, A., S. M. Grundy: Nicotonic acid as therapy for dyslipidemia in non-insulin-dependent diabetes mellitus. JAMA *264* (1990) 723–726.
[44] Grundy, S. M.: HMG-CoA reductase inhibitors for treatment of hypercholesterolemia. N. Engl. J. Med. *319* (1988) 24–33.
[45] Vega, G. L., S. M. Grundy: Management of primary mixed hyperlipidemia with lovastatin. Arch. Int. Med. *150* (1990) 1313–1319.
[46] Vega, G. L., S. M. Grundy: Primary hypertriglyceridemia with borderline high cholesterol and elevated apolipoprotein B concentrations. JAMA *264* (1990) 2759–2763.
[47] East, C., P. A. Alivizatos, S. M. Grundy et al.: Rhabdomyolysis in patients receiving lovastatin after cardiac transplantation [letter]. N. Engl. J. Med. *318* (1988) 47–48.
[48] Packard, C. J., J. Shepherd: The hepatobiliary axis and lipoprotein metabolism: effects of bile acid sequestrants and ileal bypass surgery. J. Lipid Res. *23* (1982) 1081–1098.
[49] Grundy, S. M., E. H. Ahrens, Jr., G. Salen: Interruption of the enterohepatic circulation of bile acids in man: comparative effects of cholestyramine and ileal exclusion on cholesterol metabolism. J. Lab. Clin. Med. *78* (1971) 94–121.

Update on the treatment of NIDDM

P. J. Lefèbvre, A. J. Scheen

Introduction

Non-insulin-dependent diabetes mellitus (NIDDM or type II diabetes) is a frequent disorder. Its prevalence in most countries is at least 2%, but detection campaigns have shown that for every case identified there is at least one which is not diagnosed, a finding that we have recently confirmed in Belgium [28]. In some populations such as the Pima Indians in Arizona or the inhabitants of some Pacific islands like Nauru, the prevalence of NIDDM can reach 25 – 30%. It has long been recognized that drugs represent only part of the management of NIDDM and that other interventions such as education of the patient, modifications of diet and promotion of physical activity, when feasible, are useful therapeutic tools. Two concepts have more recently emerged: (a) the therapeutic approach must be tailored to the needs and specifics of each patient and must take into consideration parameters such as life expectancy and quality of life; (b) NIDDM is often part of a larger syndrome that may include obesity, hypertension, hypertriglyceridemia, or hyperuricemia; when this is the case it is no longer permitted to treat separately every component of the syndrome. The best example in this respect is the recently recognized fact that several treatments of hypertension indeed reduce insulin sensitivity and, consequently, render more difficult the control of the accompanying diabetes [36].

The various aspects of the management of NIDDM have been taken into consideration by the European NIDDM Policy Group which recently summarized the primary objectives of treatment as being: relief of symptoms, improvement of quality of life, prevention of acute and long-term complications, reduction of mortality and treatment of accompanying disorders.

Non-pharmacological approach to NIDDM

Diet

a) Caloric content

Most patients with NIDDM present overweight or frank obesity and it is well recognized today that these features represent a major factor of insulin resistance. Consequently, reduction of weight excess comes to the front line in the management of NIDDM. A dietary interview (ideally by a dietician) is needed to evaluate the daily caloric intake of the patient, to know his food habits (nibbling versus gorging for instance) and to get information about his/her food preferences, or even addictions. Together with the informations about his/her type of physical activities (see below), the dietary interview will be the ground on which the caloric content of the prescribed diet will be calculated. When extreme caloric restriction are indicated and when rapid weight loss seems desirable, a very low calorie diet (VLCD) or protein-sparing modified fast (PSMF) may be considered.

b) Macronutrients

The ideal distribution of the daily caloric intake into carbohydrates, lipids and proteins in NIDDM is still a matter of discussion. The European Consensus recommended that carbohydrates provide 50 – 60% of total energy, proteins no more than 15% of total energy and total fat some 30 – 35% of total energy. It has been recently recognized that 60% of carbohydrates, even avoiding sugars, may favor the dyslipidemia of diabetes. Consequently, Reaven [51] recently advocated the "Stanford diet" in which carbohydrates, proteins and lipids provide 45%, 15% and 40% respectively of the daily energy intake, for type II diabetes.

Carbohydrates are recommended to be predominantly complex and high in soluble dietary fibers; food with a low glycemic index [33] are to be preferred, although moderate intake of simple sugars such as sucrose does not seem to be detrimental [61].

Proteins should not exceed the requirements since high protein intake seems to be harmful to kidney function. Whatever the daily lipid allowance (30, 35 or 40% of daily total energy), there is a general agreement that ⅓ should be polyunsaturated, ⅓ monounsaturated and ⅓ saturated.

c) Dietary fibers

Numerous studies recently reviewed by Horwitz [29] have shown that in addition to certain types of soluble fibers, especially guar and pectin may result in a significant reduction of postprandial glucose and insulin levels in patients with NIDDM. Tables of food fiber content are available to aid in making dietary recommendations [3, 14].

d) Fish oils

There is some evidence that fish oils or derived omega-3 fatty acids may play some role in preventing atherosclerotic vascular disease by reducing plasma triglyceride and lipoprotein levels [4]. However there is some indication that, in

NIDDM, the decrease in plasma triglyceride is counterbalanced by adverse effects on blood glucose or LDL cholesterol [25, 39, 67]. At present, it is not recommended to favor omega-3 fatty acid systematic supplementation in patients with NIDDM [4].

e) Magnesium

As recently reviewed [41], low plasma and erythrocyte magnesium levels are frequently found in patients with NIDDM. It has been suggested that low intracellular magnesium levels result from both increased urinary losses and insulin resistance. Furthermore, there are some indications that a reduced intracellular magnesium content might contribute to the impaired insulin response and action that are seen in NIDDM. Recent observations suggest that chronic magnesium supplementation can contribute to an improvement in both islet B-cell response [42] and insulin action [43] in NIDDM.

Physical activity

Recent clinical investigations have clarified the mechanisms by which exercise may help in controlling excessive blood glucose levels [7]. Furthermore, there is good evidence that regular exercise has a positive influence on various cardiovascular risk factors which worsen the prognosis in type II diabetic patients [1]. However, in a few patients exercise may be harmful and therefore should not be prescribed.

a) Metabolic effects of training

Regular exercise improves insulin sensitivity and, as a consequence, may help improving glucose tolerance [27]. Such effect is result in part from enzymatic adaptations in skeletal muscles (considered to be responsible for the improvement of maximal oxygen uptake or $\mathring{V}O_{2max}$) and in part from a decrease in body weight, body fat, and maybe also fat cell size. Such effects are beneficial in type II diabetics since they enhance work capacity, enrich quality of life and potentially may help to reduce the dosage (or even need) for insulin or oral hypoglycemic agents.

b) Physical training and cardiovascular disease in NIDDM

As analyzed by Kemmer and Berger [34], and when measured by such objective criteria as mortality rate, the incidence of coronary heart disease, or the concurrence of coronary risk factors, there is little doubt concerning the overall beneficial effect of chronic physical activity. In several prospective studies, physical training has been shown to reduce the plasma concentrations of triglycerides and cholesterol and to increase HDL-cholesterol which is associated with a decreased risk of coronary heart disease. In trained subjects with normal glucose tolerance, plasma insulin levels are particularly low and a physical training program has been shown to lower plasma insulin concentrations in non-diabetic patients. Recently, hyperinsulinemia has been implicated as a coronary risk factor. Thus, training by improving insulin sensitivity and lowering plasma insulin levels may contribute to a reduction in coronary risk. Finally, physical training can help to reduce body weight and hypertension and may even prevent or at least minimize the development of atherosclerosis.

c) Prescription of exercise in patients with NIDDM

It is generally agreed that the intensity and duration of physical exercise should be adjusted to the general health and physical training of the patient [58]. As with the diet, the program of exercise should also consider the interests of the patient. Before prescribing an exercise programme, the physician should analyze with the patient the amount of physical activity spent in everyday life conditions. Encouraging walking, using staircases instead of elevators, etc., are simple means to increase the daily caloric expenditure. The use of a cheap podometer may help in proving to the patient that he/she indeed has little activity. Simply recommending progressive increase in the number of steps to at least 5000 – 6000 per day would correspond to a significant increase in physical activity. Before prescribing a program of more intense exercise, performing a detailed medical evaluation, including cardiovascular examination (pulse, blood pressure, ECG at rest and during exercise, chest X-ray, eye fundus examination) is mandatory.

The amount of exercise recommended should always start at low work doses, and gradually increase to higher work loads. Regular medical supervision and reevaluation are also mandatory. Practice of sport involving particular hazards, i. e. deep diving, parachute, etc., should not be recommended for patients at risk of hypoglycemia.

Drug therapy of NIDDM

Drug therapy of NIDDM should be considered when diet, education and increased physical activity have failed to achieve the individual treatment goals.

Sulfonylureas

As recently reviewed by Melander et al. [37], "although controversies remain as to the usefulness of sulfonylureas most evidence is in favor of their use in many if not most patients with non-insulin-dependent diabetes mellitus". We consider sulfonylureas as the first-line drug treatment in NIDDM patients who are not grossly obese. The main pharmacological effect of sulfonylureas is to stimulate insulin release, but extrapancreatic effects of these drugs are likely to exist [19, 38] including a reduction of the hepatic clearance of insulin [2, 23, 54, 56]. Rate of onset and duration of action of the various drugs available are important parameters to consider [19]. Rapid onset drugs are interesting because they reduce the delay in acute insulin release and consequently reduce the elevation and duration of postprandial hyperglycemia. Long duration of action drugs increase the risk of delayed hypoglycemia and, probably desensitization to sulfonylureas. Another reason for recommending rapid onset-short duration of action sulfonylureas is to attempt to minimize chronic hyperinsulinemia suspected to be a major risk factor for atherosclerosis [15, 47]. A useful analysis of which sulfonylurea to choose and how it should be used can be found in the already mentioned review [37]. The major acute risk of sulfonylurea is hypoglycemia, a risk which is markedly increased in the elderly and in the presence of renal insufficiency. Sulfonylurea-induced hypoglycemia can result from interaction with numerous drugs including alcohol, aspirin, sulfonamides, phenylbutazone, dicoumarol, clofibrate, monoamine oxidase inhibitors, tricyclic antidepressive, etc.

Biguanides

Due to the risk of lactic acidosis, two biguanide compounds widely used in the treatment of NIDDM, namely phenyl-ethyl biguanide or phenformin and butyl-biguanide or buformin, have been banned in most countries. The only remaining compound, metformin or dimethylbiguanide, is presently still not available in several countries including the USA. It is widely used in Europe. The mode of action of metformin is still a matter of discussion [5, 32, 59]. It may include reduced glucose absorption by the gut, increased peripheral glucose uptake, and reduced liver glucose output. As others do, we consider metformin a first line drug treatment for the obese NIDDM patient. Metformin should be ingested with the meal and the maximal daily dose is 3 × 500 mg or 2 × 850 mg. Interestingly metformin improves blood glucose control despite decreasing plasma insulin levels. It favors weight loss. Metformin contraindications include renal insufficiency and major liver or cardiovascular disease. Kidney function and plasma lactate levels must be regularly checked.

Acarbose and other α-glucosidase inhibitors

Acarbose and related compounds such as miglitol delay the intraluminal production of monosaccharides, particularly glucose, by competitively inhibiting the α-glucosidases associated with the brush-border membrane of the small intestine. These enzymes are responsible for the digestion of complex polysaccharides and sucrose [11 and 12]. As reviewed by Clissold and Edwards [10], several non-comparative multicenter clinical studies and many placebo-controlled studies performed in patients with NIDDM have shown that acarbose reduces postprandial blood glucose peaks and postprandial plasma insulin levels, improves the indices of blood glucose stability and lowers HbA_{1c} levels in the majority of studies in which this parameter has been adequately investigated. When present this last effect lies between −0.5 to −3.0%. Innerfield and Connif [31] have recently presented in an abstract form, the preliminary results of a multicenter, double-blind, placebo-controlled study on the long-term efficacy and safety of acarbose in the treatment of 212 patients with NIDDM treated by diet alone: 107 patients were randomized to placebo and 105 to acarbose (50 to 300 mg t. i. d. for 24 weeks). Treatment started after a 6 week run-in period and was followed by a 6 week wash-out period. Acarbose was superior to placebo in all variables studied, the effect being due to an improvement in patients treated by diet + acarbose, a deterioration in those treated by diet + placebo, or both. The resulting effects: all in favor of acarbose were −0.59% HbA_{1c}, −15.6 mg/dl for fasting food glucose, −59.8 mg/dl on 60 min postprandial blood glucose, −50.4 mg/dl on 120 min postprandial blood glucose and −55 mg/dl in maximum blood glucose levels.

As emphasized by Toeller [63], it is extremely important in acarbose treatment that diabetic patients follow the dietary guidelines which advise the intake of complex carbohydrates instead of simple sugars.

Combined oral therapy

Once the target of treatment has been defined for a given patient, one is often confronted with considering combining diet with more than one drug to attain, or attempt to attain, the target.

a) Sulfonylureas and biguanides

This approach has been considered for more than 30 years. As we have seen, sulfonylureas are preferred as first-line drugs in non-obese patients and metformin is considered as the treatment of choice in obese NIDDM patients, not controlled by diet alone. In patients with sulfonylurea failure, the addition of metformin may provide satisfactory control for several years while the addition of a sulfonylurea to an initial metformin treatment is less often used [26]. When using such combination, the well-known contraindications of both types of drugs (see above) have to be taken into consideration. As discussed by Hermann [26], this type of oral combination therapy as a primary drug treatment has not been assessed yet, and more data is needed to evaluate the full clinical potential and the combined mechanism of action of the association sulfonylureas plus biguanides.

b) Sulfonylureas and acarbose

As reviewed by Clissold and Edwards [10], several placebo-controlled studies have demonstrated an improvement in diabetes control in NIDDM patients treated simultaneously by a sulfonylurea compound and acarbose. For instance, in the study performed by Uttenthal et al. [66], 17 NIDDM patients, poorly controlled by diet and sulfonylureas, were treated for 20 – 52 weeks with acarbose (3×100 mg daily): acarbose reduced integrated postprandial responses of glucose to $58 \pm 10\%$ ($p < 0.0001$), insulin to $61 \pm 10\%$ ($p < 0.01$) and GIP to $45 \pm 8\%$ ($p < 0.001$) of control values; the effect of acarbose remained approximately constant throughout the trial period; values returned to pretreatment levels within 2 days of stopping treatment. In another study performed by Gérard et al. [21], a single dose of 5 mg glibenclamide was administered in 6 NIDDM patients immediately before a standardized breakfast; the patients were studied twice in a random order after having been treated for one week with a placebo or with acarbose (3×100 mg daily). Acarbose induced a significant improvement in blood glucose profile (AUC: -18%; $p < 0.05$) together with a significant diminution in plasma insulin levels (AUC: -15%; $p < 0.005$). Interestingly acarbose had no significant effect on the pharmacokinetics of glibenclamide.

The interest in combining acarbose and sulfonylureas was also shown by Reaven et al. [50], who demonstrated significant reductions in fasting and postprandial blood glucose, HbA_{1c} and plasma triglyceride levels in 12 patients with NIDDM poorly controlled by diet plus sulfonylureas drugs.

c) Biguanides and acarbose

We are not aware of any controlled study investigating the effects of the combined therapy biguanides plus acarbose probably because of the fear of adding the gastrointestinal effects of these two types of drugs. If such combination is envisaged, it should probably be taken into consideration that, as demonstrated in healthy subjects, acarbose significantly modifies the pharmacokinetics of metformin [53].

Other oral drugs

a) Fenfluramine and dexfenfluramine

Fenfluramine and its dextro-stereo-isomer, dexfenfluramine, are widely used drugs in the pharmacological treatment of obesity [24]. Fenfluramine has been shown to improve the glycemic control in NIDDM patients, independently of the effects of the drug on food intake and body weight [67]. This effect was attributed to an increase in insulin sensitivity, an effect confirmed more recently in sulfonylurea-treated NIDDM patients [45]. Using the euglycemic hyperinsulincemic glucose clamp technique performed at three insulin levels and combined with 3-^{3}H-glucose turnover measurements, a recent study showed that a one-week treatment with dexfenfluramine induced better glucose control and improved insulin-induced glucose disposal in diet-treated obese patients with NIDDM, independent of any significant weight reduction [54].

b) Quinine derivatives

Recent studies have indicated that hydroxychloroquine at doses of 600 mg/day improves blood glucose control in patients with NIDDM refractory to sulfonylureas [49). Further studies are needed to confirm the long-term safety and usefulness of hydroxychloroquine or chloroquine [48, 62] in NIDDM.

Insulin therapy of NIDDM

When diet and the various drugs available, either alone or in combination, have failed in attaining the therapeutic goal in a given NIDDM patient, it is usual practice to declare the patient "insulin-requiring" and to initiate insulin therapy. It is beyond the scope of the present paper to review the rationale of the use of insulin in NIDDM or its modalities; the reader is referred to recent reviews on this topic [16, 18, 65]. We will briefly consider hereafter the potential interest of combining insulin and various oral antidiabetic drugs in this type of patients.

Insulin plus sulfonylureas

Several reviews on the interesting aspects of combination therapy in NIDDM patients have been published most recently [6, 22, 35, 57]. Several recent, well-designed and controlled studies have clearly shown that some patients can indeed benefit from this combination therapy. Most of the studies investigating the mechanism of action have shown that the beneficial effects (improved blood glucose control, reduction in HbA_{1c} levels and reduction in the daily insulin requirements) are mainly due to stimulation of residual insulin secretion with minimal or no effect on insulin sensitivity [9]. However, some studies have suggested that an additional effect of the sulfonylureas reducing the insulin metabolic clearance rate should also be taken into consideration [57].

Insulin plus biguanides

We have seen that biguanides, today metformin only, improve diabetes control despite reducing circulating insulin levels in the obese NIDDM patient [59].

Several studies have shown that metformin improves both peripheral [30, 40, 46] and hepatic [32, 46] insulin sensitivity in type II diabetic patients. However, to our knowledge and surprisingly, no studies gave definite data clearly showing the advantages of the combination of insulin and biguanides during a chronic treatment in obese type II diabetic patients.

Insulin plus acarbose

In many studies performed in type I (IDDM) patients, the dose of insulin had to be decreased under acarbose treatment [10]. Such is also the case in NIDDM patients. Out of the 32 patients studied by Gérard et al. [20], 10 had residual insulin secretion. Better metabolic control was obtained despite a small but significant reduction in insulin requirements. Addition of acarbose to insulin should be considered in insulin-requiring NIDDM patients when an excessive rise in blood glucose postprandially cannot easily be controlled by rapid acting pre-meal insulin.

Treatment of associated disorders

As said in the Introduction, NIDDM is often associated with other disorders and care should be taken not to use drugs that may render the treatment of diabetes itself more difficult or even more dangerous.

Obesity

Any dietary or behavioural treatment that may favor weight loss is welcome in the obese NIDDM patient. Significant weight loss will often permit reduction of the dose of the antidiabetic oral agents or of insulin. The pharmacological treatment of obesity comprises drugs that should not be used for diabetic or any other patients, like amphetaminc and drugs that may help in also improving diabetes control [8]. Such are the cases of metformin, dexfenfluramine [54] or acarbose [60].

Hypertension

As reviewed most recently by DeFronzo and Ferrannini [13] and by Reaven [51], new information indicates that resistance to insulin action on glucose metabolism in peripheral tissues is a common underlying mechanism in hypertension and diabetes. As reviewed by Lithell [36], the effects of antihypertensive agents have recently been evaluated on insulin sensitivity and lipoprotein metabolism. It has been shown that both β-blockers and thiazide diuretics worsen insulin resistance and deteriorate lipoprotein metabolism. In contrast, other antihypertensive agents like angiotensin-converting enzyme (ACE) inhibitors, Ca^{++}-channel blockers and α-blockers are neutral or improve these factors. The improvement of insulin sensitivity by ACE inhibitors has recently been confirmed in NIDDM patients by Torlone et al. [64]. Obviously, these factors must be taken into consideration when a decision is to be made regarding the choice of an antihypertensive agent in a patient with NIDDM.

Hyperlipidemia

Type II diabetes is a major risk factor for coronary heart disease, and the lipoprotein abnormalities that frequently occur with NIDDM probably contribute to this increased risk. For most NIDDM patients, lipid-lowering drugs should be considered only if a combination of diet, exercise and hypoglycemic therapy tried for 3 – 6 months fails to achieve desirable plasma lipid levels. As recently pointed out [17], the therapeutic target for cholesterol lowering in NIDDM should include both VLDL and LDL cholesterol(non-HDL-cholesterol) rather than LDL-cholesterol alone. To minimize the risk of coronary heart disease in NIDDM, the guidelines given by the National Cholesterol Education Program for the general population should probably be adapted for the diabetic population: Garg and Grundy [17] proposed that a minimum goal of therapy for non-HDL cholesterol be < 4.1 mM and the ideal goal be 3.4 mM. Particular emphasis should be given to weight reduction and in some NIDDM patients monounsaturated fatty acids may be a better replacement for saturated fatty acids than carbohydrates [17]. To obtain a substantial reduction of cholesterol levels, drug therapy may be required in many patients. As suggested by Garg and Grundy [17], HMG CoA reductase inhibitors (lovastatin, simvastatin, pravastatin) may be the drugs of choice for NIDDM patients with elevated LDL cholesterol and borderline hypertriglyceridemia, whereas fibric acid derivatives (fenofibrate, bezafibrate and gemfibrozil) appear preferable for NIDDM patients with severe hypertriglyceridemia. Finally, some studies have shown that a reduction in serum lipid parameters could improve blood glucose control in type II diabetic patients, probably via an increased insulin sensitivity [44].

Conclusions

The management of non-insulin-dependent diabetes mellitus or NIDDM requires education of the patient, modifications of diet and, when feasible, promotion of physical activity. It is only when such an integrated approach fails that drug therapy should be considered. Dietary therapy of NIDDM includes caloric restriction, when necessary, and appropriate distribution of the caloric intake into carbohydrates, lipids and proteins. Supplementation of diet with soluble fibers and checking of magnesium status are recommended. Systematic supplementation with fish oils or with derived omega-3 fatty acid is not recommended. Regular physical exercise can be useful providing that it is well accepted and flexible, and that contraindications are respected. Oral drug therapy for NIDDM includes: sulfonylurea derivatives, first line drug treatment in the patients who are not grossly obese, metformin, to be used first in obese patients, and α-glucosidase inhibitors, mainly to reduce postprandial blood glucose excursions. These three types of drugs can be used alone or in combination of two by two. Insulin therapy may be required to achieve control in some patients. In several instances, insulin therapy can be combined with sulfonylureas, essentially when residual insulin secretion is present, with metformin or with α-glucosidase inhibitors. The treatment of associated disorders like obesity, hypertension or hyperlipidemia requires particular attention in order not to render the treatment of diabetes itself more difficult or most dangerous. Whatever the treatment chosen, the approach must be tailored to the needs and possibilities of each patient and parameters such as life expectancy and quality of life must be systematically taken into consideration.

Acknowledgments

We acknowledge the expert secretarial help of E. Vaessen-Petit. This paper has been originally published under the title "Management of non-insulin-dependent diabetes" in a Supplement to DRUGS entitled: "Alpha-Glucosidase Inhibitors: A New Therapeutic Option in Diabetes Mellitus" ADIS Intl. Ltd, Auckland, New Zealand. We thank ADIS Intl. Ltd for permission to reproduce it in this volume.

References

[1] A. D. A. Position Statement: Diabetes mellitus and exercise. Diabetes Care *13* (1990) 804 – 805.

[2] Almer, L. O., E. Johansson, A. Melander et al.: Influence of sulfonylureas on the secretion, disposal and effect of insulin. Europ. J. Clin. Pharmacol. *22* (1982) 27 – 32.

[3] Anderson, J. W., S. K. Bridges: Dietary fiber content of selected foods. Am. J. Clin. Nutr. *47* (1988) 440–447.

[4] Axelrod, L.: Omega-3 fatty acids in diabetes mellitus. Gift from the sea? Diabetes *38* (1989) 539–543.

[5] Bailey, C. J.: Metformin revisited: its actions and indications for use. Diab. Med. *5* (1988) 315–320.

[6] Bailey, T. S., N. H. E. Mezitis: Combination therapy with insulin and sulfonylureas for type II diabetes. Diabetes Care *13* (1990) 687–695.

[7] Berger, M., P. Christacopoulos, J. Wahren (eds.): Diabetes and exercise. Hans Huber Publ., Bern–Stuttgart–Vienna 1982.

[8] Carpenter, M. A., H. J. Bodansky: Drug treatment of obesity in type II diabetes mellitus. Diab. Med. *7* (1990) 99–104.

[9] Castillo, M., A. J. Scheen, G. Paolisso et al.: The addition of glipizide to insulin therapy in type II diabetic patients with secondary failure to sulfonylureas is useful only in the presence of significant residual insulin secretion. Acta Endocrinol. (Copenh.) *116* (1987) 364–372.

[10] Clissold, S. P., C. Edwards: Acarbose. A preliminary review of its pharmacodynamic and pharmacokinetics properties, and therapeutic potential. Drugs *35* (1988) 214–243.

[11] Creutzfeldt, W. (ed.): Proc. First Internat. Symposium on acarbose, Excerpta Medica, Amsterdam 1982.

[12] Creutzfeldt, W. (ed.): Proc. Second Internat. Symposium on acarbose, Springer Verlag, Berlin 1988.

[13] DeFronzo, R. A., E. Ferrannini: Insulin resistance: A multifaceted syndrome responsible for NIDDM, obesity, hypertension, dyslipidemia, and atherosclerotic cardiovascular disease. Diabetes Care *14* (1991) 173–194.

[14] Del Tomma, E., A. Clementi, M. Maracelli et al.: Food fiber choices for diabetic diets. Am. J. Clin. Nutr. *47* (1988) 243–246.

[15] Ducimetière, P., E. Eschwège, L. Papoz et al.: Relationship of plasma insulin levels to the incidence of myocardial infarction and coronary heart disease mortality in a middle-aged population. Diabetologia *19* (1980) 205–210.

[16] Galloway, J. A.: Treatment of NIDDM with insulin agonists or substitutes. Diabetes Care *13* (1990) 1209–1239.

[17] Garg, A., S. M. Grundy: Management of dyslipidemia in NIDDM. Diabetes Care *13* (1990) 153–169.

[18] Genuth, S.: Insulin use in NIDDM. Diabetes Care *13* (1990) 1240–1264.

[19] Gerich, J. E.: Oral hypoglycemic agents. N. Engl. J. Med. *321* (1989) 1231–1245.

[20] Gérard, J., A. S. Luyckx, P. J. Lefèbvre: Improvement of metabolic control in insulin dependent diabetics treated with the α-glucosidase inhibitor acarbose for two months. Diabetologia *21* (1981) 446–451.

[21] Gérard, J., P. J. Lefèbvre, A. S. Luyckx: Glibenclamide pharmacokinetics in acarbose-treated type II diabetics. Eur. J. Clin. Pharmacol. *27* (1984) 233–236.

[22] Groop, L. C., P.-H. Groop, S. Stenman: Combined insulin-sulfonylurea therapy in treatment of NIDDM. Diabetes Care *13* (Suppl. 3) (1990) 47–52.

[23] Groop, L. C., P.-H. Groop, S. Stenman et al.: Comparison of pharmacokinetics, metabolic effects and mechanisms of action of glyburide and glipizide during long-term treatment. Diabetes Care *10* (1987) 671 – 678.
[24] Guy-Grand, B., M. Apfelbaum, G. Crepaldi et al.: International trial of long-term dexfenfluramine in obesity. Lancet *2* (1989) 1142 – 1145.
[25] Hendra, T. J., M. E. Britton, D. R. Roper et al.: Effects of fish oil supplements in NIDDM subjects. Controlled study. Diabetes Care *13* (1990) 821 – 829.
[26] Hermann, L. S.: Biguanides and sulfonylureas as combination therapy in NIDDM. Diabetes Care *13* (Suppl. 3) (1990) 37 – 41.
[27] Horton, E. S.: Exercise and physical training: effects on insulin sensitivity and glucose metabolism. Diab. Metab. Reviews *2* (1986) 1 – 17.
[28] Hortulanus-Beck, D., P. J. Lefèbvre, M. F. Jeanjean: Le diabète dans la province belge de Luxembourg: fréquence, importance de l'épreuve de surcharge glucosée orale et d'une glycémie à jeun discrètement accrue. Diab. Metab. (Paris) *16* (1990) 311 – 317.
[29] Horwitz, D. L.: Dietary adjuncts: efficacy and inadequacy. In: C. J. Bailey, P. R. Flatt (eds.): New antidiabetic drugs, pp. 53 – 63. Smith-Gordon, London and Nishimura, Japan 1990.
[30] Hother-Nielsen, O., O. Schmitz, P. H. Andersen et al.: Metformin improves peripheral but not hepatic insulin action in obese patients with type II diabetes. Acta Endocrinol. (Copenh.) *120* (1989) 257 – 265.
[31] Innerfield, R. J., R. F. Coniff: A multi-center, double-blind, placebo-controlled study of the long-term efficacy and safety of acarbose (BAY g 5421) in the Rx of obese patients with NIDDM Rxed by diet alone. Diabetes *39* (Suppl. 1) (1990) 211A, Abstract 829.
[32] Jackson, R. A., M. I. Hawa, J. B. Jaspan et al.: Mechanism of metformin action in non-insulin-dependent diabetes. Diabetes *36* (1987) 632 – 640.
[33] Jenkins, D. J. A., A. L. Jenkins, T. M. S. Wolever et al.: Aims of diet in diabetes management. In: W. Creutzfeldt, P. Lefèbvre (eds.): Diabetes mellitus: pathophysiology and therapy, pp. 299 – 308. Springer Verlag, Berlin – Heidelberg – New York – London – Paris – Tokyo 1989.
[34] Kemmer, F. W., M. Berger: Therapy and better quality of life: the dichotomous role of exercise in diabetes mellitus. Diab. Metab. Reviews *2* (1986) 62 – 68.
[35] Lebovitz, H. E., R. M. Pasmantier: Combination insulin-sulfonylurea therapy. Diabetes Care *13* (1990) 667 – 675.
[36] Lithel, H. O. L.: Effect of antihypertensive drugs on insulin, glucose and lipid metabolism. Diabetes Care *14* (1991) 203 – 209.
[37] Melander, A., H. E. Lebovitz, O. K. Faber: Sulfonylureas. Why, which, and how? Diabetes Care *13* (Suppl. 3) (1990) 18 – 25.
[38] Melander, A., P.-O. Bitzen, O. Faber: Sulphonylurea antidiabetic drugs. An update of their clinical pharmacology and rational therapeutic use. Drugs *37* (1989) 58 – 72.
[39] Mori, T. A., R. Vandongen, J. R. L. Masarei: Fish oil-induced changes in apolipoproteins in IDDM subjects. Diabetes Care *13* (1990) 725 – 732.
[40] Nosadini, R., A. Avogaro, R. Trevisan et al.: Effect of metformin on insulin-stimulated glucose turnover and insulin binding to receptors in type II diabetes. Diabetes Care *10* (1987) 62 – 67.

[41] Paolisso, G., A. Scheen, F. D'Onofrio et al.: Magnesium and glucose homeostasis. Diabetologia *33* (1990) 511 – 514.

[42] Paolisso, G., N. Passariello, G. Pizza et al.: Dietary magnesium supplements response to glucose and arginine in elderly non-insulin dependent diabetic subjects. Acta Endocrinol. (Copenh.) *21* (1989) 16 – 20.

[43] Paolisso, G., S. Sgambato, G. Pizza et al.: Improved insulin response and action by chronic magnesium administration in aged NIDDM subjects. Diabetes Care *12* (1989) 265 – 269.

[44] Paolisso, G., S. Sgambato, S. Deriu et al.: Simvastatin reduces plasmalipid levels and improves insulin action in elderly, non-insulin-dependent diabetics. Eur. J. Clin. Pharmacol. *40* (1991) 27 – 31.

[45] Pestell, R. G., P. A. Crock, G. M. Ward et al.: Fenfluramine increases insulin action in patients with NIDDM. Diabetes Care *12* (1989) 252 – 258.

[46] Prager, R., G. Schernthaner, H. Graf: Effect of metformin on peripheral insulin sensitivity in non insulin dependent diabetes mellitus. Diab. Metab. (Paris) *12* (1986) 346 – 350.

[47] Pyörälä, K.: Relationship of glucose tolerance and plasma insulin to the incidence of coronary heart disease: results from two population studies in Finland. Diabetes Care *2* (1979) 131 – 141.

[48] Quatraro, A., G. Consoli, A. Ceriello et al.: Is there a role for chloroquine treatment in diabetes? A three case report (letter). Lancet *4* (1988) 666 – 667.

[49] Quatraro, A., G. Consoli, M. Magno et al.: Hydroxychloroquine in decompensated, treatment-refractory noninsulin-dependent diabetes mellitus. A new job for an old drug? Ann. Intern. Med. *112* (1990) 678 – 681.

[50] Reaven, G. M., C. K. Lardinois, M. S. Greenfield et al.: Effect of acarbose on carbohydrate and lipid metabolism in NIDDM patients poorly controlled by sulfonylureas. Diabetes Care *13* (Suppl. 3) (1990) 32 – 36.

[51] Reaven, G. M.: Insulin resistance, hyperinsulinemia, hypertriglyceridemia, and hypertension: parallels between human disease and rodent models. Diabetes Care *14* (1991) 195 – 202.

[52] Reaven, G. M.: Personal communication 1990.

[53] Scheen, A. J., A. C. F. A. de Magalhaes, T. Salvatore et al.: Modifications de la pharmacocinétique de la metformine après inhibition des alpha-glucosidases intestinales par l'Acarbose chez le sujet sain. Diab. Metab. (Paris) *15* (Suppl. XIV), (1989), résumé n° 53.

[54] Scheen, A. J., G. Paolisso, T. Salvatore et al.: Improvement of insulin-induced glucose disposal in obese patients with NIDDM after 1-wk treatment with d-fenfluramine. Diabetes Care *14* (1991) 325 – 332.

[55] Scheen, A. J., M. J. Castillo, P. J. Lefèbvre: Decreased or increased insulin metabolism after glipizide in type II diabetes? Diabetes Care *11* (1988) 687 – 689.

[56] Scheen, A. J., P. J. Lefèbvre, A. S. Luyckx: Glipizide increases plasma insulin but not C-peptide level after a standardized breakfast in type II diabetic patients. Eur. J. Clin. Pharmacol. *26* (1984) 471 – 474.

[57] Scheen, A. J., P. J. Lefèbvre: Insulin versus insulin plus sulfonylureas in type II diabetic patients with secondary failure to sulfonylureas. Diab. Res. Clin. Pract. *6* (1989) 33 – 43.

[58] Schneider, S. H., N. B. Ruderman: Technical review: Exercise and NIDDM. Diabetes Care *13* (1990) 785 – 789.

[59] Shäfer, G.: Biguanides. A review of history, pharmacodynamics and therapy. Diab. Metab. (Paris) *9* (1983) 148 – 163.

[60] Sjöström, L., T. William-Olsson: Relapse-reducing effects of acarbose after weight reduction in severely obese subjects. In: W. Creutzfeldt (ed.): Proceedings of the Second International Symposium on Acarbose, pp. 137. Springer Verlag, Berlin – Heidelberg – New York – London – Paris – Tokyo 1988.

[61] Slama, G.: L'alimentation des diabétiques. In: G. Tchobroutsky, G. Slama, R. Assan, P. Freychet (eds.): Traité de Diabétologie, pp. 657 – 678. Editions Pradel, Paris 1990.

[62] Smith, G. D., T. A. Amos, R. Mahler et al.: Effect of chloroquine on insulin and glucose homeostasis in normal subjects and in patients with non-insulin-dependent diabetes mellitus. Br. Med. J. (Clin. Res.) *294* (1987) 465 – 467.

[63] Toeller, M.: Modulation of intestinal glucose absorption: postponement of glucose absorption by α-glucosidase inhibitors. In: C. E. Mogensen, E. Standl (eds.): Pharmacology of diabetes, pp. 93 – 112. De Gruyter, Berlin – New York 1991.

[64] Torlone, E., A. M. Rambotti, G. Perriello et al.: ACE-inhibition increases hepatic and extrahepatic sensitivity to insulin in patients with type II (non-insulin-dependent) diabetes mellitus and arterial hypertension. Diabetologia *34* (1991) 119 – 125.

[65] Turner, R. C., R. R. Holman: Insulin use in NIDDM. Rationale based on pathophysiology of disease. Diabetes Care *13* (1990) 1011 – 1020.

[66] Uttenthal, L. O., O. O. Ukponmwan, M. Ghiglione et al.: Long-term effects of acarbose treatment on postprandial glucose, pancreatic and gut hormones responses and fasting serum lipids in non-insulin-dependent diabetics on sulphonylureas. In: W. Creutzfeldt (ed.): Proceedings of the Second International Symposium on Acarbose, pp. 133. Springer Verlag, Berlin – Heidelberg – New York – London – Paris – Tokyo 1988.

[67] Verdy, M., L. Charboneau, I. Verdy: Fenfluramine in the treatment of non-insulin dependent diabetics: hypoglycemic versus anorectic effect. Int. J. Obes. 7 (1983) 289 – 297.

[68] Vessby, B., M. Boberg: Dietary supplementation with n-3 fatty acids may impair glucose homeostasis in patients with non-insulin-dependent diabetes mellitus. J. Intern. Med. *228* (1990) 165 – 171.

Hyperinsulinemia and macrovascular complications in NIDDM

E. Standl, H. U. Janka, H. Stiegler, H. Mehnert

Introduction

Coronary, cerebral and peripheral vascular disease represent the major macrovascular complications of patients with NIDDM in the Western World, irrespective of the subtype of diabetes, and largely determine the prognosis of these patients. More than 50% of all NIDDM patients die from cardiac disease and another 25% from stroke, as evidenced by a number of epidemiological studies [16].

In our still ongoing Schwabing Study on Macrovascular Disease in Diabetes mellitus, a more than fourfold increase of peripheral artery disease was found in diabetics compared to non-diabetics, and a doubling of signs for coronary and carotid artery disease [23]. Similar results have also been generated by the Framingham Study [10] or the MR FIT experience [21]. Furthermore, the outcome of macrovascular disease seems to be much poorer in diabetics, as indicated by a greatly reduced survival rate after myocardial infarction [20] or after a stroke [15]. Hence, it is not surprising that the death toll due to macrovascular disease is considerable among patients with NIDDM and amounts to a reduction of life expectancy of about one decade for patients with onset of diabetes between the ages of 40 and 49, and the loss of life is also more pronounced in older age groups [16]. It is, however, surprising that during the 1970's and 1980's, a large body of evidence has been accumulated that this excess of macrovascular disease in patients with NIDDM appears to be somehow associated with insulin and the degree of insulinemia present in the blood of these patients [9, 22, 25, 30, 31].

The metabolic syndrome – a concept

In 1991, an intriguing way of looking at the issue of hyperinsulinemia as related to the risk of macrovascular disease in NIDDM is within the framework of the hyperinsulinemia/insulin resistance syndrome, which is perhaps best described as the "metabolic" syndrome and is also called Syndrome X by others [11, 18, 28]. Whatever the appropriate name, the concept suggests a cluster of risks associated with insulin resistance and consisting of hyperinsulinemia, hypertension, dyslipoproteinemia and NIDDM. Insulin resistence has moved to the top of the list, been incriminated as the secret killer [5], and put into perspective with NIDDM and macrovascular disease, not only crossectionally, but also longitudinally, over time. Insulin resistance appears to be a life sentence in prone individuals. It is yet unknown when it starts, but it can be detected in predisposed subjects inspite of normal body weight and perfectly normal glucose tolerance [2]. It seems to be aggravated by upper body or central obesity and a sedentary life style, hyperinsulinemia is a consequence of insulin resistance with a link to dyslipidemia and perhaps in a vicious circle with hypertension (Fig. 1). Finally, after 10, 20,

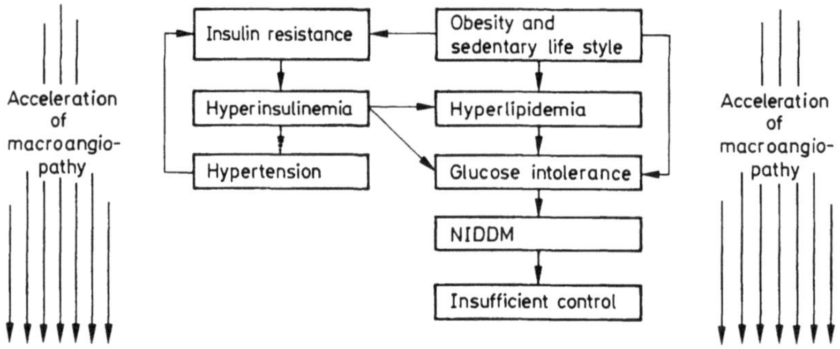

Fig. 1: The hyperinsulinemia/insulin resistance syndrom in the context with NIDDM and macrovascular disease.

30 years, glucose intolerance and NIDDM may develop. The syndrome, however, has already been operating and exerting its detrimental effects in terms of accelerating macroangiopathy, long before NIDDM emerges [28].

Evidence compatible with the existence of the metabolic syndrome

For the time being, a number of findings seem to support the concept of the metabolic syndrome as depicted in Figure 1, although the situation is still far from being settled and may be different in different ethnical groups. The following points pertain mainly to white westernized populations:

a) Insulin resistant, hyperinsulinemic, yet normal glucose tolerant, non-obese subjects exhibit statistically significant higher triglycerides, lower HDL cholesterol, and both higher systolic and diastolic blood pressure values, referring to an early networking of the risky syndrome [34].

b) Insulin resistant, hyperinsulinemic, but otherwise perfectly normal offspring of two NIDDM parents develop subsequent NIDDM almost ten times more often compared to matched controls. In other words: Hyperinsulinemia precedes the onset of NIDDM [14].
c) Even in the absence of NIDDM, the metabolic syndrome as represented by hyperinsulinemia, hypertension, hypertriglyceridemia strongly predicts the risk of cardiovascular death at a later time, although with a variable power of the single factor at different time points, as assessed by multivariate analysis in the large population based studies in Helsinki, Busselton, and Paris [3, 4, 17, 33].
d) At the time point of clinical diagnosis of NIDDM, there is already excessive macrovascular disease, e.g. in terms of coronary heart disease, both in men and women and compared to matched controls in Finland [32], and in addition in terms of peripheral and carotid artery disease, as seen in the context of the NIDDM Program for General Practitioners in the Greater Munich Area [27].
e) Furthermore, at the time point of clinical diagnosis of NIDDM, also the other key players of the metabolic syndrome seem to be in full action. Eighty per cent of all recently diagnosed NIDDM patients seen in the above mentioned NIDDM Program for GPs in the Greater Munich Area exhibited in addition hypertension, another 80% hypertriglyceridemia, 50% hyperinsulinemia and with a striking interdependence between these variables [27].
f) In the Schwabing Study on Macrovascular Disease in Diabetes mellitus, again a similar risk profile clustering of hypertension, hypertriglyceridemia, obesity etc. was observed in relation to fasting C-peptide levels on the one hand, and in the subgroup of the insulin treated NIDDM patients with the size of the daily insulin dose on the other [25].
g) That this syndrome predicts to a large extent the macrovascular risk in NIDDM has been established by several large scale population studies of NIDDM patients, e.g. the Paris Prospective Study, the Diabetes Intervention Study, one study in Oxford, and the Schwabing Study [3, 4, 6, 7, 8, 22, 25, 26].
h) In view of the discussion about proinsulinemia and its split products in NIDDM, the finding in the Schwabing Study was even more interesting that, in the subgroup of the insulin treated NIDDM patients, the size of the daily insulin dose (which cannot be confounded by the issue of proinsulin) was among the most significant prospective determinants of risk – in conjunction with triglycerides and blood pressure – for major vascular complications, i.e. cardiovascular death, myocardial infarction, stroke etc., as well as for newly occurring leg artery disease within 5 years of follow up [9, 22, 25].

So, various ingredients of the metabolic syndrome cluster predict macrovascular risk in various studies, whereby it should be pointed out that triglycerides are probably not a risk as such, but rather indicate an atherogenic lipid profile with low HDL-cholesterol, active VLDL-remnants etc., and facilitated by poor blood glucose control. As far as triglycerides as cardiovascular risk markers are concerned, the situation might be different between diabetics and clearly non-diabetics. In addition it should be emphasized that in diabetics systolic hypertension, not only diastolic hypertension, represent a major predictor of cardiovascular risk. Finally, one point must explicitly be stated: although enormous progress has been made in defining a series of parameters associated with, anticipatory of, or predicting macrovascular disease in diabetic patients during recent years, we are not (yet) entitled to speak of risk factors in a true sense as proven by intervention, i. e. that a lower macrovascular complication rate would have been established after elimination of a given factor.

Potential links between hyperinsulinemia and macrovascular disease

Besides hyperinsulinemia being part of the risky syndrome in association with lipid and blood pressure disorders, we are still more or less ignorant as to if and how insulin by itself might exert its effects on the cells of the arterial vessel wall, i. e., endothelial cells and smooth muscle cells, although several working hypotheses have been put forward [24, 30, 31]. There is probably no direct effect of insulin on endothelial cells of large arteries, whereas smooth muscle cells apparently become stimulated by insulin to proliferate, migrate, incorporate lipids, and generate fibrous tissue. Insulin may release the growth factor IGF 1 and play a role in the regulation of the plasminogen activator inhibitor PAI 1, thereby inhibiting fibrinolysis. Also macrophages, the precursors of foam cells in early atheroma, seem to be under the regulation of insulin.

Perhaps a new clue, how many features of the metabolic syndrome might be interrelated, seems to come from studies of the so-called waist-to-hip ratio or – more precisely – of the intraabdominal fat mass. Astounding associations of the waist-to-hip ratio with all the factors of the entire metabolic syndrome, with blood pressure, triglycerides, HDL-cholesterol, insulin, and diabetes have been found [13], and there has been further evidence, also experimentally, that the mass of the mesenteric fat tissue assessed by CAT scan determines the amount of FFA flowing through the portal vein to the liver, higher concentrations putting the so called Randle mechanism into action, inducing a higher hepatic glucose output and some kind of a central insulin resistance. Just to close the circle, there are already old data that a high waist-to-hip ratio is strongly associated with cardiac mortality, independently of the BMI [12].

Other risk markers of macrovascular disease in NIDDM

Undoubtedly, beyond the likely impact of the metabolic syndrome, macrovascular disease in NIDDM is also associated with other risk parameters, in particular age, smoking, hypercholesterolemia, (micro-)albuminuria, and clotting abnormalities [25, 26]. On the other hand, diabetes mellitus by itself, especially if uncontrolled, affects a number of risk variables like triglyceridemia, cholesterolemia, kidney and clotting function. In this respect, NIDDM seems to act by aggravating preexisting background risk in a given general population. Hence, it is not surprising that very recent evidence of the Schwabing Study even suggests a strong predictive power of the initial HbA_1 value for cardiovascular death during a 9 year follow up. Conversely, other key players of the metabolic syndrome like hypertension and dyslipoproteinemia apparently facilitate the manifestation of (micro-)albuminuria or hemostasiological and hemorheological disturbances, besides the manifestation of NIDDM [27]. So, it seems literally impossible to conceive and successfully perform a single factor intervention for the prevention of macrovascular disease in NIDDM.

Distinct characteristics of macroangiopathy in NIDDM

Although morphologically atherosclerotic disease in NIDDM is practically indistinguishably from that in nondiabetics ("not-yet-diabetics?"), which – in the light of the above chapter – is probably not by mere chance, there are, however, distinct characteristics of macroangiopathy in NIDDM [26, 19]. The strong male preponderance of atherosclerotic disease seen in nondiabetic populations is virtually abolished, if not reversed, and female patients with NIDDM are at the same risk as their male counterparts [8, 10, 23]. Furthermore, besides being more frequent and severe, the atherosclerotic process appears to be more diffuse and shows a pronounced predilection for more peripheral arterial segments, i. e. medium and small arteries. This phenomenon holds true for all major targets of macrovascular complications in NIDDM, in particular for the cerebrovascular, coronary, and peripheral vascular bed [26, 29], and probably contributes to the low grade symptomatology of macroangiopathy in diabetes.

Another feature is the frequent coexistence with neuropathy, both sensory-motor and autonomic neuropathy, which leads to a disordered regulation of local blood flow and masking of symptoms inspite of the presence of critical tissue ischemia. Autonomic neuropathy seems also be associated with mediasclerosis of the Mönckeberg type [1, 26]. Unlike the patchy calcification of the vessel intima within the framework of atherosclerosis in non-diabetics, Mönckeberg sclerosis is characterized by a linear dystrophic calcification of the tunica media and subsequent smooth muscle atrophy and collagen fibre proliferation. The pathologic significance of these metaplastic changes, however, is still unclear as they do not appear to contribute to arterial occlusion, yet are accompanied by occlusive disease in almost every other case. At any rate, due to the decreased function of vasoconstriction, blood flow through shunt vessels seems to be favoured so that the actual tissue blood supply falls short.

Practical consequences

a) In view of their high risk, it seems advisable to screen all subjects with a pre-NIDDM state for all the pertinent cardiovascular risk parameters and for emerging macrovascular disease on a regular basis. For practical purposes, pre-NIDDM states could be defined by clinical criteria, such as first degree relationship with a NIDDM patient, essential hypertension, dyslipidemia, gestational diabetes mellitus.
b) The same recommendations should be applied to all patients with ouvert NIDDM.

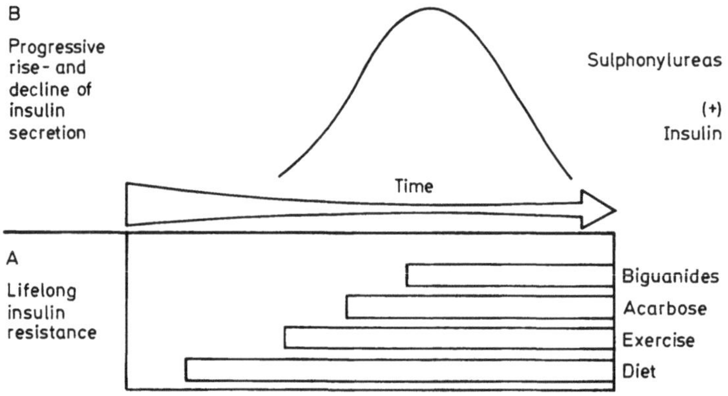

Fig. 2: Pathogenetically targeted treatment of NIDDM.

c) Any treatment in those subjects should be designed not to stimulate insulin resistance and booster the metabolic syndrome further, but rather to decrease insulin resistance and insulinemia. This principle seems to be of importance both in the treatment of diseases like hypertension or cardiac insufficiency, and in particular in the blood glucose lowering therapy of NIDDM patients. As far as the latter point is concerned, Figure 2 suggests a new and more pathogenetically oriented approach: Priority should be given to the reduction of insulin resistance and insulinemia by means of nutrition, physical exercise,

α-glucosidase inhibition with acarbose, or the use of the biguanide metformin (if applicable). Only when insulin secretion gradually declines – and this may be different from population to population and even from patient to patient – sulfonylurea and – later on – insulin treatment should be implemented and insulinemia be kept as low as possible, provided the individual goal for glycemia is secured.

References

[1] Edmonds, M. E., N. Morrison, J. W. Laws: Medical arterial calcification and diabetic micropathy. Br. Med. J. *284* (1982) 928–930.

[2] Eriksson, J., A. Franssila-Kallunki, A. Ekstrand et al.: Early metabolic defects in persons at increased risk for non-insulin-dependent diabetes mellitus. N. Engl. J. Med. *321* (1989) 337–343.

[3] Eschwege, E., J. L. Richard, N. Thibult et al.: Coronary heart disease mortality in relation with diabetes, blood glucose and plasma insulin levels. The Paris Prospective Study, ten years later. Horm. Metab. Res. Suppl. *15* (1985) 41–46.

[4] Fontbonne, A., E. Eschwege, F. Cambien et al.: Hypertriglyceridemia as a risk factor of coronary heart disease mortality in subjects with impaired glucose tolerance or diabetes: results from the 11-year follow up of the Paris Prospective Study. Diabetologia *32* (1989) 300–304.

[5] Foster, D. W.: Insulin resistance, a secret killer? N. Engl. J. Med. *320* (1989) 733–734.

[6] Hanefeld, M.: Relationship between insulin and coronary heart disease. In: E. Standl (ed.): Perspectives of the hyperinsulinemia/insulin resistance syndrome in NIDDM, pp. 70–73. MMV, Munich 1990.

[7] Hockaday, T. D. R., D. Phil: Serum insulin concentrations and anticipatory factors of cardiomyopathy in NIDDM. Diab. Metab. *13* (1987) 354–358.

[8] Janka, H. U.: Five year incidence of major macrovascular complications in diabetes mellitus. Horm. Metab. Res. (Suppl.) *15* (1985) 15–19.

[9] Janka, H. U., A. G. Ziegler, E. Standl et al.: Daily insulin dose as a predictor of macrovascular complications in diabetes mellitus. Diab. Metab. *13* (1987) 359–364.

[10] Kannel, E. B., D. L. Mc Gee: Diabetes and glucose tolerance as risk factors for cardiovascular disease: The Framingham Study. Diabetes Care *2* (1979) 120–126.

[11] Kaplan, N. M.: The deadly quartet: upper-body obesity, glucose intolerance, hypertriglyceridemia, and hypertension. Arch. Intern. Med. *149* (1989) 1514–1520.

[12] Lapidus, L., C. Bengtsson, B. Larsson et al.: Distribution of adipose tissue and risk of cardiovascular disease and death: a 12 year follow up of participants in the population study of women in Gothenburg, Sweden. Br. Med. J. *289* (1984) 1257–1261.

[13] Mc Keigue, P. M., B. Shah, M. G. Marmot: Rclation of central obesity and insulin resistance with high diabetes prevalence and cardiovascular risk in South Asians. Lancet *337* (1991) 382–386.

[14] Martin, B. C., J. H. Warram, A. S. Krolewski et al.: Slow glucose removal rate and hyperinsulinemia are predictors of the risk of type II diabetes. Diabetologia *33* (1990) Suppl. A 80.

[15] Olsson, T., M. Viitanen, K. Asplund et al.: Prognosis after stroke in diabetic patients. A controlled prospective study. Diabetologia *33* (1990) 244 – 249.

[16] Panzram, G.: Mortality and survival in type II (non-insulin-dependent) diabetes mellitus. Diabetologia *30* (1987) 123 – 131.

[17] Pyörälä, K., E. Savolainen, S. Komkola et al.: Plasma insulin as coronary heart risk factor: relationship to other risk factors and predictive value during 9.5 years follow-up of the Helsinki Policemen Study population. Acta Med. Scand. *701* (Suppl. 1) (1985) 38 – 52.

[18] Reaven, G. M.: Role of insulin resistance in human disease. Diabetes *37* (1988) 1595 – 1607.

[19] Rudermann, N. B., C. Haudenschild: Diabetes as an atherogenic factor. Progr. Cardiovasc. Dis. *26* (1984) 373 – 412.

[20] Smith, J. W.: Survival rate after myocardial infarction in diabetic patients. Am. J. Cardiol. *54* (1984) 718 – 721.

[21] Stamler, J., D. Wentworth, J. Neaton: Diabetes and risk of coronary, cardiovascular, and all cause mortality. Findings of 356000 men screened by the multiple risk factor intervention trial. Circulation *70* (1984) 11 – 16.

[22] Standl, E., H. U. Janka: High serum insulin concentrations in relation to other cardiovascular risk factors in macrovascular disease of type II diabetics. Horm. Metabol. Res. (Suppl.) *15* (1985) 46 – 51.

[23] Standl, E.: Die Angiopathien des Typ II-diabetes. Verh. Dtsch. Ges. Inn. Med. *92* (1986) 579 – 586.

[24] Standl, E., P. Vague: Hyperinsulinemia as a possible risk factor of macrovascular disease in diabetes mellitus. Diab. Metab. *13* (1987) 277 – 394.

[25] Standl, E., H. Stiegler, H. U. Janka et al.: Risk profile of macrovascular disease in diabetes mellitus. Diab. Metab. *14* (1988) 505 – 511.

[26] Standl, E., H. Stiegler, H. U. Janka et al.: Cerebral and peripheral vascular disease. In: C. E. Mogensen, E. Standl (eds.): Prevention and Treatment of Diabetic Late Complications, pp. 169 – 198. de Gruyter, Berlin – New York 1989.

[27] Standl, E., H. Stiegler, R. Roth et al.: On the impact of hypertension on the prognosis of NIDDM. Results of the Schwabing GP-Program. Diab. Metab. *15* (1989) 352 – 358.

[28] Standl, E. (ed.): Perspectives of the hyperinsulinemia/insulin resistance syndrome in NIDDM, pp. 1 – 111. MMW, Munich 1990.

[29] Steinke, W., S. Al-Deeb, M. Hennerici: Prävalenz extrakranieller Gefäßprozesse und Risikoprofil bei Patienten mit peripherer und koronarer Arteriopathie. Vasa *16* (1987) 283 – 290.

[30] Stout, R. W.: Insulin and atheroma – an update. Lancet *I* (1987) 1077 – 1079.

[31] Stout, R. W.: Insulin and atheroma. 20-yr. perspective. Diabetes Care *13* (1990) 613 – 655.

[32] Uusitupa, M., L. Niskanen, O. Siitonen et al.: Hyperinsulinemia and hypertension in patients with newly diagnosed non-insulin-dependent diabetes. Diab. Metab. *13* (1987) 369 – 374.

[33] Welborn, T. A., K. Wearne: Coronary heart disease incidence and cardiovascular mortality in Busselton with reference to glucose and insulin concentration. Diabetes Care 2 (1979) 154 – 160.

[34] Zavaroni, I., S. Mazza, L. Luchetti et al.: High plasma insulin and triglyceride concentrations and blood pressure in offspring of people with impaired glucose tolerance. Diab. Medicine 7 (1990) 494 – 498.

II Quality of life in diabetes mellitus

Diabetes and quality of life: some current issues in definition and research

S. H. Croog

Introduction

It is being increasingly recognized that quality of life is an important outcome variable that should be examined in the conduct of clinical trials for the evaluation of medical interventions. In the case of diabetes and its treatment, quality of life considerations have special importance. One evidence of this recognition is the number of recent publications on diabetes which have begun to center on quality of life and on psychosocial factors related to the illness [1, 11, 17, 21, 28]. Another is the effort to develop instruments and measures which can be used for studies of the diabetic patient in particular, with reference to quality of life issues [3, 6, 7]. The importance of these considerations was underlined a few years ago by a National Conference on Diabetes at the National Institutes of Health which concluded that social, emotional, and psychological factors can be as strongly associated with treatment outcomes as are bio-medical factors [13].

However, despite these efforts in the field of diabetes studies and despite the developing attention to quality of life issues in the medical and health care literature as a whole, in many ways this whole emphasis is relatively new. The focus is subject to continuing discussion, refinement, and controversy. At this point in the development of this area of systematic research, it will be useful to review some of the principal issues and problems that are now facing researchers carrying out work on quality of life and diabetes. This paper presents a brief overview of some of these tasks and issues in the field.

Quality of life in relation to diabetes – focus of interest in several principal ways

As an outcome variable

First, quality of life of the diabetic patient has been examined as a dependent variable in studies to assess the effects of treatment. The evaluation of these types of outcomes of treatment has special importance in diabetes. If the impact of therapy is unacceptable to the patient in terms of his or her quality of life, the patient will not comply with the therapeutic regimen or may comply only partially [8, 16, 18]. In carrying out the therapeutic regimen in terms of adherence to blood glucose monitoring, diet, medications, exercise, and to life style modifications, the intensity of the motivation and drive of the diabetic patient can be of critical importance to health and survival [29].

As an independent variable and as a mediating variable

Quality of life has been studied also as an independent variable in diabetes, and it functions as a mediating variable as well insofar as lifestyle of the patient can influence the course of diabetes itself. For example, as Cox et al. [4] have shown, external stressors as part of the quality of life of the patient can influence the metabolism of glucose and thus have an impact on the course of the disease. This may be through direct influence as in the effects of stress on blood glucose levels. Or quality of life factors can have indirect mediating effects such as through their influence on diet and exercise. These factors can be seen, for example, when work responsibilities impede the patient's ability to attend to all the tasks of keeping to a complicated regimen day after day [4, 9, 10, 12].

Assessment of progress and prognosis in treatment: as a descriptor

The impact of having diabetes itself can have pervasive and complex effects on the life and functioning of the patient, as shown by measures of anxiety, depression, cognitive performance, interpersonal relations, and perspectives on one's personal future [23, 26]. The Medical Outcomes Study followed over 800 diabetes patients for two years, tracking substantial impairment in their physical, emotional, social, and role functioning [27]. Use of the construct, quality of life, can assist as one means of providing a systematic descriptive focus on the course of the illness in many of its biochemical, physical, social and psychological aspects.

As an element in clinical decision making

Another important use of quality of life considerations has been in decision-making about treatment options. Which course of therapy or which treatment regimen is best for this particular patient, given considerations of such factors as disease type and severity, age, sex, socioeconomic status, ethnic and cultural background? In diabetes as well as in the case of many other illnesses, such as cancer or heart disease, the predictable consequences for the quality of life of the patient may be important factors in determining which treatment course to follow.

Defining and employing the construct in research

What is the construct?

During the past few years there have been continuing debates in regard to the utility of quality of life as a construct in health-related research. Among the severest critics, some hold that the concept is too ambiguous, too corrupted by colloquial use, that it is only a faddish rubric for describing a concern with social and psychological variables, and that the whole approach really represents nothing new. Many partisans maintain, on the other hand, that the quality of life approach is clearly important and promising, and that virtually every clinical trial evaluating a therapy should include quality of life measures.

At the core of many of the problems in carrying out research in this area is the state of conceptualization of the construct [14, 19, 20]. At present there is high ambiguity and wide variability in regard to conceptualization and definition. In fact, one of the remarkable features of this field is the tremendous volume of writing concerning the topic without specification of the core construct which is being discussed. If we review the substantial literature, we see numerous ways in which quality of life has been treated analytically without adequate specification or definition.

First, in a great many publications using the construct, it is never explicitly defined. Many empirical studies characterized by their authors as assessing quality of life focus on reporting data from such measures as return to work, freedom from angina, depression, anxiety, lists of a series of symptoms, and a whole range of psychosocial variable indicators. With the absence of a definition in these reports, the implication is that the construct is presumably defined by what the measures assess. Thus, at best it is an emergent definition, dependent on measures which act as "indicators" of quality of life.

A second widely used procedure is the specification of the dimensions of the construct while omitting discussion of what the construct is in itself. Commonly, in such an approach the authors indicate that the 'construct contains the following dimensions' – or they state that to assess quality of life certain essential areas should be measured, such as functional capacity, physical health, emotional status, well-being, etc. In these writings there is no statement which clearly delineates the core concept of which the components or dimensions are a part. Does specifying the dimensions to be measured really tell us about the phenomenon itself?

A third prominent method is definition by analogy. Here the reader is informed that quality of life is in a general way equivalent to such constructs as health or health status, functional capacity, well-being, life satisfaction, or happiness. One is presumably interchangeable with another, according to this orientation.

In a fourth approach the authors make a systematic effort to define the construct. However, among the many articles and books focusing on quality of life, such efforts at definition are relatively rare, and the results are often divergent definitions [2, 15, 22, 24, 25].

Despite the major ambiguities and problems of definition in the literature, it seems important to have at least a common general framework to guide research on diabetes and quality of life. At this point we can draw together many of the common themes in the research. A definition can be based on the developing agreement on specification of the relevant dimensions for study. I have already mentioned some of the areas which are often cited as components of quality of life.

Defining the construct as rubric

The format of the definition outlined here is modeled on the dictionary format used in definition of another complex construct, "personality". That definition focuses on the totality of elements which comprise personality. This approach to quality of life is similarly framed in broad terms to provide a general rubric within which researchers can work, and it is based on a common ground of elements which are already in use. The rubric or umbrella approach in this definition is similar, of course, to that which is commonly seen also in research-oriented approaches to studies of "health", "mental health", "culture", "intelligence" and other constructs which are analogous in many ways to "quality of life" in their scope.

Following are some principal elements in a working definition for discussion.

Health-related quality of life: the totality of characteristics of the way of life of an individual or group with particular reference to (a) the areas of physical health, emotional health, cognitive function, social role performance, well-being and/or life satisfaction and (b) the objective conditions of existence, including living conditions, and environmental stressors. Thus, this broad working definition centers on "quality of life" as characterized as a way of life of individuals or groups. It emphasizes the totality of traits which describe that way of life, then includes a series of specific health related areas to be measured, including in particular, both subjective and objective indicators.

What are the specific components to be measured in the context of this broad concept of quality of life? In 1988, a Workshop on Quality of Life and Cardiovascular Disease was sponsored by the National Heart, Lung and Blood Institute and Bowman Gray School of Medicine. As one product of the meetings some specific parameters for measurement were outlined. This listing drew upon a developing congruence among researchers in regard to core elements of the construct which should be measured. Table 1 shows the major dimensions and sub-dimensions for assessment as suggested at those meetings.

Table 1: Some suggested areas for review in the clinical interview with hypertensive patients

Physical status	
	Symptoms
	Sleep and rest
	Sexual functioning
Functional status	
	Physical activity
Emotional status	
	Anxiety
	Depression
	Irritability and anger
	Stress
	Spiritual well-being
Cognitive function	
	Attention and concentration
	Clarity of thinking
	Psychomotor functioning
Performance of social roles	
	Family membership roles (spouse, parent, sibling, etc.)
	Work performance
	Household management
	Community activities
General well-being	
	Life satisfaction
	Energy and vitality

The various major dimensions relevant for measurement provide at least a partial snapshot of the totality, assuming that no individual research program can ever capture the whole of quality of life.

In regard to measures of the objective conditions which are part of quality of life, one can note with reference to living conditions such elements as, for example:

(a) type of residence (private home, nursing home, hospital, etc.)
(b) number of persons per room
(c) level of quality of residence (the range can be from slum conditions to luxurious structures)

In regard to environmental stressors, one can note, for example:

a) level of air pollution
b) level of noise
c) level of sanitation and water purity
d) measures of threat of crime and attack

These areas for measurement can be applicable cross-culturally, relevant in some way in all societies. However, depending on the goals and orientation of the clinical trial, the relevance of some may be more primary than others. In a study of quality of life in a western industrialized society, for example, level of sanitation and water purity may not be as directly pertinent to the goals of the research as in a study set in a Brazilian slum or a set of villages in Ethiopia.

Thus, this description of the construct is designed as a working definition to draw together the various themes already in the literature – through describing health-related quality of life as the totality of health-related characteristics of the way of life of an individual or group – then specifying particular primary elements which are relevant for consideration. It refers to subjective and objective measures. Like many constructs, it is built on other constructs which are themselves diffuse in many ways. For example, if we think of health-related quality of life, what is health? How are the various other sub-dimensions to be defined, such as the components of emotional status or well-being?

Using the construct in this way as a broad rubric for research permits flexibility in research design at the present stage of development of the field. In a research program, defining the relevant areas of health-related quality of life can be done depending on the specific goals of the study. Everything in the construct does not have equal priority or relevance in every study as a rigid format. Thus, if one is studying a large population of free-living diabetic patients in a clinical trial testing a medication, one can specify the areas of quality of life which are relevant to this particular purpose. If one is studying the quality of life of cardiac patients in nursing homes, one would center on somewhat different sets of relevant elements for measure, including the characteristics of the nursing home environment, rehabilitation facilities, use of wheelchairs, etc.

Prominent issues and concerns

I would now like to turn to consideration of some other principal issues and challenges relating to quality of life assessment in clinical trials.

Validity and reliability

A first set of concerns centers on the basic issues of validity and reliability of measures. At present, there are numerous instruments which are being used to measure the construct. In his comprehensive review Hollandsworth lists 83 prominent instruments used from 1980 to 1985 [14]. The areas of quality of life which are commonly measured vary greatly in their degree of complexity and diffuseness. For example, the assessment of physical functioning, while difficult in many ways, is of a different, somewhat more concrete order than assessment of such areas as morale, social participation, and sexual functioning. Not surprisingly the precision and quality of available instruments reflects this range in the difficulty of measurement.

At present, in the array of available instruments, some have been validated with large populations in repeated studies and we know a good deal about their reliability. Others have passed through the process of validity and reliability testing – but this has taken place within the limited context of a single study or a small set of studies, often with small numbers of patients. Hence the question of their validity and reliability when used with other study populations remains to be demonstrated.

In quality of life studies is the instrument still measuring what it is supposed to measure when it is employed with populations differing by social class, by ethnic origins, by cultural background, or by sex? Determination of psychometric properties of instruments requires large investment of effort, time, and budget – and for many instruments used in quality of life studies, the special requirements of rigorous instrument development and testing have not been met.

Impact of methods on validity of assessments

Complicating the determination of the reliability and validity of instruments for assessing quality of life is the fact that patient responses on some areas of life can be strongly affected by how the data are collected, by whom, and in what circumstance. The importance of the selection of data collection procedure is often not sufficiently recognized in studies of sensitive and subtle areas of quality of life. All too routinely, researchers hand out questionnaires to patients, do telephone interviews, or rely on physician's assessments or the judgements of other health care workers about the patient. However, the source of the information is a critical factor in assessing quality of life, and numerous studies have shown differences depending on who provided the data. In the case of diabetes, it would seem essential to rely on the patient's perception.

Objective versus subjective measures

Another set of discussions regarding measures deals with the use of objective measures versus subjective measures. The issue involves the relative merit of reporting on the patient's subjective perceptions of his condition – the patient's reporting of symptoms of depression or anxiety, reporting on life satisfaction or feeling of vitality – versus those which can be measured objectively, that is, whether or not the patient has returned to work after illness, whether he or she can climb a flight of stairs, or the patient's income level. In general, critics are suspicious of subjective measures, viewing them as "soft", and unreliable.

It appears that neither objective nor subjective measures alone are sufficient in adequately documenting quality of life. One cannot assume that in knowing about one area – the objective – one is also informed about the other, the subjective. In response to a common criticism of quality of life assessments that they are based too much on subjective measures, one obvious solution in research in clinical trials has been to use both subjective and objective indicators.

Specific and generic measures

Another current set of discussions in regard to quality of life assessment, centers on the relative merit of using specific, focused measures versus using those that are generic and applicable to broad populations. Among the different approaches, one can select measures specific to the disease one is studying, such as hypertension, heart disease, diabetes, or arthritis, or measures that are population-specific, such as those for elderly females or middle-aged black males. However, such instruments are not usually applicable beyond the groups for which they are specifically focused. Broad categories of measures – generic measures – are designed for use across diverse populations. Examples are the Rand General Well-Being Index, the Sickness Impact Profile, the McMaster Health Index, or the Nottingham Health Profile.

Because much work has been done in refining and testing generic instruments relevant to quality-of-life measurements, they have advantages in use as far as reliability and validity are concerned. A disadvantage of generic instruments is that they often contain questions that are irrelevant or inappropriate when applied to the specific illness groups with which the clinician is concerned. Quality of life studies often use conglomerate generic and specific indices along with questions from various sources, shaping them for the operational needs at hand. This condition leads, of course, to noncomparability between studies.

Aggregate score versus profile score

A continuing set of discussions concerns the optimum method to characterize the quality of life of either individuals or groups – whether through use of a single aggregate score or through use of a profile score, one which characterizes separately each of the dimensions being measured. For some limited purposes a single score may be useful and economical in making comparisons between groups. However, given the complex multidimensional nature of the construct, a single, aggregate score cannot adequately characterize the nature of quality of life.

The profile score has the advantage of reviewing separate relevant areas, each of which may constitute a separate, clinically relevant domain [5]. One advantage of the profile score is that one can at some later time construct an aggregate score, if desirable, provided that the weighting and measurement conditions are met.

The press toward parsimony in measurement: short forms and quality of life

Recently there has been special interest in preparation of "short forms" to measure quality of life. This reflects a need for refining and reducing instruments to the most basic elements which can still enable collection of valid data. There are many pressures underlying the demand for measures that are brief, easily administered, and easily scored. For example, federal and pharmaceutical sponsors of clinical trials increasingly wish to include quality of life in their studies. At the same time, they seek the most economical way in terms of patient time, personnel time, and monetary cost. They look as well for minimal intrusion on the clinical, biomedical parts of the clinical trial. Numerous short forms have become available over recent years, and numerous researchers are working to produce new ones.

However, a danger in the use of short forms lies in reductionism, in measurement of complex areas in overly condensed or superficial ways that generally will not fulfill goals of obtaining valid and reliable assessment. In the field of tests and measurements, assessment of complex quality of life phenomena requires a sufficient number of scale items for each dimension in order to ensure satisfactory reliability and validity. A short form usually aims to measure complex dimensions of quality of life with only one or several questions for each, a procedure that may preclude scientifically sound assessments. The problem currently is inherently a difficult one to solve, for if each relevant dimension of quality of life is to be measured in a valid way, the conceptual and statistical requirements tend to militate against a short form. The result of all this is a fundamental dilemma – the need for valid and reliable measures which will assess difficult and complex areas of emotion, symptoms, and morale, for example, but which will do so at minimal costs in time and money.

Responsiveness of measures and clinical meaning

An important problem is the question of the responsiveness of instruments or measures – and their clinical meaning. The selection of measures for use in clinical trials typically involves consideration of their responsiveness – an important issue for those studies which evaluate and compare the effects of one treatment versus another upon the dependent variables, quality of life measures. The issue is whether the measures are sufficiently sensitive or responsive in order to detect significant changes between treatments.

Considering quality of life measures, there are complex and controversial questions as to what constitutes clinically significant differences between treatments in a clinical trial. Significant differences can be demonstrated statistically between treatment groups, but the degree to which they are clinically meaningful is another matter. Small differences in scores on psychometric tests, given study populations that are large enough, can be shown to be statistically meaningful, but they may not be clinically meaningful. Further, because of the great costs in time, funds, and effort, thus far quality of life studies involved in testing treatments have rarely been replicated, and the pursuit of clinical meanings cannot be carried far.

Given this problem, to what extent should conclusions based on one or several studies of quality of life be used in making clinical decisions about whether to give a patient one drug rather than another – or to recommend one type of surgery over a drug treatment, as in Parkinson's disease or diseases of the eye? As quality of life studies grow in number, using the kinds of measures available to us today, researchers have a continuing responsibility to maintain a cautious approach to the translation of research results from a clinical trial into patient care and the framing of health care policy.

In conclusion

As a disease of great complexity, diabetes presents both special challenges and problems in terms of understanding its many intermeshing biologic, metabolic, and psychosocial aspects. For example, with the development of new therapies, and new psychosocial interventions and educational methods in the treatment of diabetes, what are the effects of such innovations on quality of life of the patient? What are their effects on compliance with the medical regimen and their further influences on quality of life? Questions on the effects of psychosocial factors on metabolic processes in the diabetic can be matched by counterpart questions concerning the effects of diabetes on quality of life of the patient, including cognitive function, mood, behavior, and performance of social roles.

As outlined here, there are substantial issues and problems which are outstanding in regard to conceptualization of quality of life, ensuring the quality of measures used to assess it, and building a knowledge base founded on comparable studies which meet high scientific standards. However, it is also evident we are on a new threshold for quality of life research, considering the development of new measures and techniques in the behavioral sciences and the increasing collaboration of the biomedical and behavioral science professions. We can now move more efficiently toward answering core questions in these difficult and important areas in the study of diabetes.

References

[1] Bernbaum, M., S. G. Albert, P. N. Duckro: Psychological problems in patients with visual impairments due to diabetic retinopathy. Diabetes Care *11* (1988) 551 – 557.

[2] Calman, K. C.: Quality of life in cancer patients – an hypothesis. J. Med. Ethics *10* (1984) 124 – 127.

[3] Carey, M. P., R. S. Jorgensen, R. S. Weinstock et al.: Reliability and validity of the appraisal of diabetes scale. J. Behavioral Med. *14* (1991) 43 – 51.

[4] Cox, D. J., A. B. Taylor, B. Nowacek et al.: The relationship between psychological stress and insulin-dependent diabetic blood glucose control: preliminary investigations. Health Psychology *3*(1984) 63 – 75.

[5] Croog, S. H., S. Levine, M. A. Testa et al.: The effects of antihypertensive therapy on quality of life. N. Engl. J. Med. *314* (1986) 1657 – 1664.

[6] DCCT Research Group: Reliability and validity of a diabetes quality-of-life measure for the diabetes control and complications trial (DCCT). Diabetes Care *11* (1988) 725 – 732.

[7] Dunn, S. M., H. H. Smartt, L. J. Beeney et al.: Measurement of emotional adjustment in diabetic patients: validity and reliability of ATT39. Diabetes Care *9* (1986) 480 – 489.

[8] Glasgow, R. E.: Compliance to diabetes regimens. Conceptualization, complexity, and determinants. In: J. A. Cramer, B. Spilker (eds.): Patient compliance and medical practice and clinical trials, pp. 209 – 223. Raven Press – New York 1991.

[9] Goetsch, V. L.: Stress and blood glucose in diabetes mellitus: a review and methodological commentary. Annals of Behav. Med. *11* (1989) 102 – 107.

[10] Gonder-Frederick, L. A., W. R. Carter, D. J. Cox et al.: Environmental stress and blood glucose change in insulin-dependent diabetes mellitus. Health Psychology *9* (1990) 503 – 515.

[11] Greenfield, S., S. H. Kaplan, J. E. Ware et al.: Patients' participation in medical care: effects on blood sugar control and quality of life in diabetes. J. Gen. Internal Med. *3* (1988) 448 – 457.

[12] Halford, W. K., S. Cuddihy, R. H. Mortimer: Psychological stress and blood glucose regulation in Type I diabetic patients. Health Psychology *9* (1990) 516 – 528.

[13] Hamburg, B. A., L. E. Lipsett, G. E. Inoff et al.: Behavioral and psychosocial issues in diabetes: proceedings of the National Conference, Washington, DC, U. S. Gov't Printing Office, 1979, NIH Publ. no. 80-1993.

[14] Hollandsworth, J. G.: Evaluating the impact of medical treatment on the quality of life: a 5-year update. Soc. Sci. Med. *26* (1988) 425 – 434.

[15] Hornquist, J. O.: The concept of quality of life. Scand. J. Soc. Med. *10* (1982) 57 – 61.

[16] Jacobson, A. M.: Current status of psychosocial research in diabetes. Diabetes Care *9* (1986) 546 – 548.

[17] Kaplan, R. M., S. L. Hartwell, D. K. Wilson et al.: Effects of diet and exercise interventions on control and quality of life in non-insulin dependent diabetes mellitus. J. Gen. Internal Med. *2* (1987) 220 – 228.
[18] Karam, J. H.: Diabetes mellitus, hypoglycemia, and lipoprotein disorders. In: S. A. Schroeder, M. A. Krupp, L. M. Tierney et al. (eds.): Current medical diagnosis and treatment, pp. 852 – 875. Appleton and Lange, Norwalk, Connecticut 1991.
[19] Levine, S., S. H. Croog: What constitutes quality of life? A conceptualization of the dimensions of life quality in healthy populations and patients with cardiovascular disease. In: N. K. Wenger, M. E. Mattson, C. D. Furberg et al. (eds.): Assessment of quality of life in clinical trials of cardiovascular therapies, pp. 46 – 58. LeJacq, New York 1984.
[20] Najman, J. M., S. Levine: Evaluating the impact of medical care and technology on the quality of life: a review and critique. Soc. Sci. Med. *15F* (1981) 107 – 115.
[21] O'Connor, P. J., A. M. Jacobson: Functional states measurement in elderly diabetic patients. Clinics in Geriatric Med. *6* (1990) 865 – 882.
[22] Patrick, D. L., M. Danis, L. I. Southerland et al.: Quality of life following intensive care. J. Gen. Intern. Med. *3* (1988) 218 – 223.
[23] Ryan, C., A. Vega, C. Longstreet et al.: Neuropsychological changes in adolescents with insulin-dependent diabetes. J. Consulting and Clinical Psychol. *52* (1984) 335 – 342.
[24] Schipper, H., J. Clinch, V. Powell: Definitions and conceptual issues. In: B. Spilker (ed.): Quality of life assessments in clinical trials, pp. 16. Raven Press, New York 1990.
[25] Shumaker, S. A., R. T. Anderson, S. M. Czajkowski: Psychological tests and scales. In: B. Spilker (ed.): Quality of life assessments in clinical trials, pp. 96. Raven Press, New York 1990.
[26] Skenazy, J. A., E. D. Bigler: Psychological adjustment and neuropsychological performance in diabetic patients. J. Clinical Psychol. *41* (1985) 391 – 396.
[27] Stewart, A. L., S. Greenfield, R. D. Hays et al.: Functional status and well-being of patients with chronic conditions. Results from the Medical Outcome Study. JAMA *269* (1989) 907 – 913.
[28] Tun, P. A., D. M. Nathan, L. C. Perlmuter: Cognitive and affective disorders in elderly diabetics. Clinics in Geriatric Med. *6* (1990) 731 – 746.
[29] Wing, R. R., L. H. Epstein, M. P. Nowalk et al.: Behavioral self-regulation in the treatment of patients with diabetes mellitus. Psychological Bulletin *99* (1987) 78 – 89.

Quality of life in patients with type II diabetes mellitus*

S. Waadt, G. Duran, M. Waadt, P. Herschbach, F. Strian

Introduction

Maintenance of quality of life is one of the chief goals in the treatment of diabetes mellitus. There are at least two reasons for this:

1. Diabetes mellitus is a chronic disease that cannot be cured; at best it can be compensated for in order to prevent the physical complaints that result from acute and late complications.

2. Low quality of life and psychological problems are generally thought to affect adversely metabolic control both directly, by means of hormonal stress reactions, and indirectly, through poor compliance.

The twofold target, compensation for the metabolic disorder *and* prevention of a reduction in the quality of life, is accepted not only for type I patients but also for the older, type II patients despite their shorter life expectancy and their less complex treatment regimen.

In an effort to achieve optimal compensation of diabetes, treatment concepts have greatly been changed in the past 20 years. With the concept of self-treatment and self-monitoring, responsibility for physical well-being relies no longer on the physician alone, but also on the patient, who is expected to cooperate. To enable the patient to perform the self-treatment, follow the dietary regimen, take hypoglycemic medication and do urine or blood glucose self-monitoring, many treatment centers now have patient education programs. Although the diabetes education programs have usually been successful in reducing Hb_1 levels and the number of late complications [9, 10, 39], a large percentage of patients still make mistakes within the regimen and are unable to achieve acceptable metabolic control [14, 29, 54]. For example, Watkins et al. [52] studied adherence to the diabetes regimen in 162 insulin-treated type II diabetics and found that 75% of the patients made dietary mistakes. This is true also for non-insulin-dependent diabetics (NIDDM). Although their treatment regimen is less complex and there are fewer restrictions on the temporal aspects of their dietary regimen [3, 47] physicians often wrongly attribute non-compliance to a lack of motivation and an unwillingness to adhere to the doctor's advice. House et al. [25] enquired 90

* Supported by the Robert-Bosch-Stiftung

type II diabetics and 50 physicians about the reasons for failure in adhering to the dietary regimen. 80% of the physicians cited motivational problems as a major reason for non-compliance; that is, they blamed the patients for not doing as advised. Only 10% thought that information deficiency was the reason for lack of compliance. On the other hand, only 34% of the diabetics indicated poor motivation as the reason for non-compliance, 38% cited barriers from the social environment and 26% physical complaints as the major reasons.

But what kind of deal do we ask the patients to make? In exchange for maintaining their quality of life through optimal metabolic control and prevention of late complications some time far in the future, they are asked to follow a regimen that is both complex and quite stressful. They must have the attitude that good health is the only important thing or at least the most important thing in life. To follow the regimen, patients have to change their daily habits in nearly all areas of life and have to cope with many types of difficulties. We want the patients to do this despite the fact that acute signs of poor metabolic control are often not perceived and that no real reassurance can be given that self-control will in fact prevent late complications [37, 41] or even lead to good metabolic control. On the other hand, there is evidence that poor physical health has a negative impact on the emotional well-being and that a high level of quality of life is associated with the absence of physical complaints [6, 28, 43]. We can describe the relationship between psychosocial factors and diabetes mellitus as a model of interaction: Psychosocial problems arise from diabetes and its treatment demands. These problems can restrain proper compliance and non-compliance can lead to stressful, acute and late complications. Consequently, if we want to hold the first goal high and optimize the patient's quality of life through prevention of late complications, we first have to understand which psychological, social, physical and environmental barriers detain the patients in adhering to treatment.

Psychosocial factors predictive of compliance and metabolic control

A vast number of variables which probably affect compliance and well-being have been studied. Sackett and Haynes [46] reviewed 246 publications and found 250 variables associated with compliance. As a first strategy to bring order into these variables, several studies used the usual personality questionnaires to determine a typical personality pattern for diabetic patients generally or for non-compliers. These efforts failed because of highly inconsistent results [16]. Due to the vast number of possible factors, a definite variable pattern characterizing the non-complier could not be demonstrated [23].

More recently some investigators have looked for correlations between psychological or psychiatric symptomatology and diabetes. They have found that patients with diabetes score significantly higher on clinical measures of depression and anxiety than non-diabetic, chronically ill patients [36, 43]. Wing et al. [56] compared 32 obese patients with type II diabetes and their obese, non-diabetic spouses on the Beck Depression Inventory [4]. The patients with diabetes had a significantly higher mean score and rated more items positively than their spouses.

One of the few remaining variables still considered to be associated with personality is the "locus of control", the expectation about the efficacy of ones own actions. A person with an internal locus of control believes that his or her own planning and action is effective and that responsibility for consequences lies within the self. Whereas, a person with an external locus of control thinks other people or a higher power are responsible for what happens to them. But the results proved to be inconsistent even with this well defined psychological construct. E. g. Alonga [1] found that the non-compliant subjects in a study of 50 obese, non-insulin-dependent diabetic patients showed mainly an external locus of control in respect to health behavior. However Anderson et al. [2] found that on the scores for affective and behavioral dimensions, the clinicians' desire for control was positively related to the patients satisfaction. Williams et al. [53] summarized some further conflicting findings on "locus of control".

An overview of personality-related studies shows that, in the more recent studies, the results are generally interpreted much more carefully than in the earlier ones. The personality patterns are not necessarily claimed to be invariant, following or producing the chronic disease. The authors take into account the interdependence of physical disease and psychological well-being, for example depression can follow symptoms and knowledge of poor metabolic control as well as trigger non-compliance and other processes [34] leading to physical health problems.

Much more encouraging than studies about non-specific personality patterns are surveys that look for more specifically disease-related variables. For instance, Jenny [29] studied 246 adult diabetic patients and found that young age, long duration of disease, poor metabolic control and highly complex instructions were positively associated with regimen adherence. Accordingly, non-insulin-dependent patients showed less stress and less adherence behavior than insulin treated patients, but had better metabolic control [12]. Introceptive awareness and symptom perception are also strongly related to adherence behavior and well being [18, 27]. E. g. the quality of adherence behavior may partly depend on the psychological characteristics of the long-term-complications. Pauli et al. [40] found that patients with mild neuropathy had fewer physical and psychological complaints than those with severe neuropathy or without any neuropathy.

Furthermore, within personality-near concepts, the most consistent results came from surveys that dealt with aspects of personality that are specific to disease and treatment. The most promising variable is a specific group of control beliefs, the "health beliefs". These are attitudes concerning perceived severity of illness, complexity and perceived efficacy of treatment regimen and expectancies about one's own responsibilities for health and well-being. Hopper and Schechtman [24] investigated 161 low income, black female, type II diabetic patients. The variables that were positively related to non-compliance and poor metabolic control were: a lack of belief in control over health and efficacy of treatment, a belief that diabetes is less serious than other illnesses that are curable and low level of satisfaction with the clinic. In a study of 46 female NIDDM patients by Hampson, Glasgow and Toobert [22], beliefs about the helpfulness of treatment and about the seriousness of the illness were most accurate in predicting self-care behavior. Conflicting results were reported by Davis et al. [12]. These investigators compared non-insulin-treated, type II patients with insulin-treated, type I and type II patients. The non-insulin-treated patients rated their treatment regimen less complex than the other groups did and they experienced less risk of complications. But at the same time they rated the treatment benefits lower than the insulin-treated patients did. They faced fewer barriers to adherence, reported fewer metabolic-control problems and fewer social problems. They also had better HbA_1 scores than the other groups.

A number of studies showed that social environment, social support and impact of the disease on social life were important predictors of treatment adherence and metabolic control. Hopper & Schechtman [24] related a reported lack of social support to poor adherence and poor metabolic control. In a study of 127 type II diabetic patients Glasgow and Toobert [17] showed that family support for the performance of diabetes self-care behavior is highly predictive of regimen adherence. Connell et al. [7] asked 77 NIDDM retirement community residents over the age of 60 about regime adherence and metabolic control symptoms. The residents who reported frequent symptoms of poor metabolic control recognized that their social relationships had been disrupted by their health status. But they also reported that a great deal of social support was available to them, perhaps because of the structure of the community in which they lived.

Another important social variable is the doctor-patient relationship. Many studies have shown that appropriate emphasis, understanding and a clearly structured, open style of communication are a prerequisite for a well established doctor-patient relationship [15]. Especially differences in treatment targets often lead to difficulties [38]. But health care professionals are not always responsible for poor relationships. Linn et al. [35] compared 75 male diabetic patients with 75 matched nondiabetic patients on a measured of self-assessed health. The patients in both groups who viewed their health as poor reported more symptoms and were less satisfied with the doctor-patient relationship. However, the physicians' rating of actual health status did not confirm the patients' self-assessment.

As supported by extensive summary studies, psychosocial variables in general are very important in understanding adherence to self-care behavior and metabolic control. Wilson et al. [55] investigated self-care adherence (diet, medication, glucose testing and exercise) in 184 NIDDM and found that 18–24% of the discrepancy was explained by psychosocial variables (health beliefs, social support). Demers et al. [13] gave 19 type II patients a short questionnaire about stress resulting from life events or life changes in the past year. Despite the small number of subjects, the correlation between stress and HbA_1 scores (r = .65) and fasting blood glucose levels (r = .49) were highly significant. Davis et al. [11] predicted the mortality rate in a follow up study of 343 NIDDM who were examined in 1981/1982 and 1985/1986. The variables most closely associated with mortality were age, social impact of diabetes, renal function (the only physical health index that correlated), complexity of dietary regimen and a history of smoking. These variables were more closely associated to the mortality than HbA_1 scores, hospitalization rate or frequency of heart attacks. In particular, the variable "social impact of diabetes" could well explain the mortality rate.

Furthermore, the best indications of compliance are a cluster of highly specific variables concerning perception and interpretation of the illness, the treatment and the impact of diabetes on psychosocial variables and lifestyle. Patients who view their illness as severe, who believe that they will benefit from the regimen and who rate the impact of treatment demands and of the illness on their daily life as low, will probably be more compliant than patients with other attitudes. A more complex regimen, short disease duration, few acute or long-term complications and older age can make adherence more difficult. And of course discontent with the source of care and a poor doctor-patient relationship will hinder the adherence to the regimen.

Day-to-day stress related to diabetes mellitus as a barrier to adherence

Although modern investigation strategies usually involve highly specific variables that are mainly as concrete as desired, one major problem remains beyond the poor consistency of the results: disagreements about how the correlations should be interpreted. Quality of life and metabolic state can be seen both as a dependent as well as an independent variable. Up until now, no consistent theory has been available about the possible interdependences of these variables. The study by Davis et al. [11] cited earlier showed the risk of mortality by measuring the impact of diabetes on the patient's social life. The results of in depth interviews of 10 NIDDM (34] showed life stress prior to diagnosis and depression prior to disease as relevant factors that influence current adherence. Connell demonstrates a particular example in her research strategy [6, 7]. 77 NIDDM patients were interviewed about their treatment adherence, their overall morale and their good or poor metabolic control symptoms. In the first study, "low level of morale" was used to predict poor adherence and poor metabolic control. In the second study, performed on the same population, "low level of morale" was examined as a function of adherence, metabolic control and psychosocial impact of diabetes mellitus.

To avoid these dilemmas, we used a strictly subject-related concept. Patients with diabetes were simply questioned about their experiences with diabetes and treatment demands. With such a concept we hoped to identify in clearly defined situations, concrete problems with diabetes and treatment demands. These problems could then be taken as stimuli in developing suitable interventions, with the goal of reducing the specific subjective diabetes related-stress and, as a result, improving the quality of life. Improved treatment adherence and metabolic control can be a desired side effect of such interventions if the intervention strategies take into consideration the special psychobiological interdependences detected mostly by clinical analysis.

We recorded "day-to-day causes of stress" in patients with diabetes mellitus on a questionnaire developed in three steps [51]. First we interviewed two diabetic patients and their spouses in depth about living with diabetes. At the same time we also collected possible problems from the literature and from diabetes care professionals (psychologists, physicians and diabetes counsellors). From this first screening pool we developed a semi-standardized interview consisting of open-ended, standardized question about 7 aspects of living with diabetes mellitus: work, leisure, treatment demands, physical well being, social contacts, psychosocial well being and family. Next we interviewed 76 patients (46 type I with a different disease duration, 14 type II insulin-treated, 17 type II non-insulin-treated). They verified the standardized questions as relevant and pointed out problems not yet on our list. In a third step, we had diabetes care professionals rate this new item pool for clinical relevance. The final version of the questionnaire consisted of 90 stressful situations specific to diabetes. We also developed a short form with 45 items that can be answered in 10 minutes, but it was not used in the study reported here [51].

The subjects rated both the relevance of the stress and its severity (5 point scale: from no burden to a very heavy burden). We gave the questionnaire to 617 patients, (392 with type I diabetes, 215 with type II diabetes and 10 not classified), both inpatients and outpatients from several different treatment centers in Germany. A factor analysis with all patients revealed 10 stress clusters in 10 scales. The Cronbach alpha scores indicating the homogeneity of the scales varied between a = .69 and a = .89 [51]. The following is a description of "day-to-day stresses" in 207 patients with type II diabetes, 90 on insulin and 117 not receiving

DPD	no problem	hardly a/a very heavy burden				
	0	1	2	3	4	5
14. I'm no longer able tó perform certain tasks	□	□	□	□	□	□
35. It's a heavy burden that I have to talk about diabetes when eating out	□	□	□	□	□	□
86. It's a problem that I have to eat according to a timetable	□	□	□	□	□	□

Fig. 1: Sample items "Questionnaire of daily problems with diabetes" (DPD).

insulin. Information was also collected on age, sex, work, method of treatment, indices of acute complications including HbA_1 scores and reported diagnoses of long term complications. In order to assesss quality of life, we administered a short scale [26] with which the subjects rated subjective importance and satisfaction in 8 aspects of life and 8 aspects of health.

The mean age of our subjects was 59 years. 56% of the subjects were women, 47% were retired. The groups' sociodemographic variables were very comparable (Tab. 1). Regarding illness-related variables, however, they differed in many respects (Tab. 1). Compared with the non-insulin dependent subjects the insulin-treated subjects had a longer disease duration and poorer metabolic control. More of the insulin-treated subjects had a history of a hypoglycemic episode or diabetic coma. They tested their urine and blood glucose more often than the non-insulin treated subjects. The percentages of patients with long-term complications, however, were about the same. The insulin-treated group had significantly higher overall levels of day-to-day stress than the NIDDM group (total score 1.27 ± 0.7 vs. 0.85 ± 0.7, $t = 4.32$, $p < .01$) and significantly higher levels on 7 of 10 scales (Fig. 2). The most stressful factors for the insulin-treated patients were "fear of long-term complications", "diet", "problems with treatment regimen" and "reduction in level of performance". For the NIDDM group too, the aspect producing the most stress was "fear of long term complications", then "diet", "performance" and "treatment regimen".

For the insulin treated patients the total stress score correlated with the duration of disease ($r = .27$, $n = 86$, $p < .01$), whereas for the non-insulin treated patients the total stress score was more strongly associated with HbA1 levels ($r = .21$,

Table 1: Description of the sample

Personal	Type II diabetes	
	insulin-treated N = 90	non-insulin-treated N = 117
Age (years)	59.8 (± 9.6)	59.0 (± 9.7)
Gender (% female)	56%	56%
Pensioner (%)	50%	44%
Medical		
Duration of disease (years)	12.8 (± 8.3)	8.7 (± 6.6)
BMI (kg/m2)	26.3 (± 4.5)	28.6 (± 6.3)
Weight reduction diet (% yes)	34%	50%
Blood-glucose % $\geq 1 \times$/day	48%	26%
Urine-testing % $\geq 1 \times$/day	55%	34%
a HbA_1 normal (% of subjects)	19%	33%
acceptable (%)	37%	38%
unacceptable (%)	44%	30%
b Hypoglycemic coma (% yes)	24%	5%
c Diabetic coma (% yes)	14%	3%
d Days hospitalized	33.0 (±34.6)	21.4 (±26.2)
Long-term complications (% of ss.)	50%	47%

a: normal $\leq$8.0%; acceptable = 8.0% – 10.0%; unacceptable >10.0%
b: reported frequency within the last two years
c: reported frequency within the last two years
d: reported frequency within the last five years

n = 110, $p < .05$). These different correlations suggested different problems sources in the two groups. Problems with illness were associated with poor metabolic control only in the NIDDM group, and because 70% of the NIDDM group had normal HbA_1 scores, these patients were not stressed by diabetes. Among the insulin-treated patients, problems with illness and self-control correlated with the duration of the disease. It might have been that coping with handling regimen demands became – much harder in the long term – i.e. coping with the risk of hypoglycemia and altered hypoglycemic symptoms [8].

In both groups, the connection between the total score of "day-to-day stress" with the quality of life varied depending on the aspect of life being considered (Tab. 2). Problems with diabetes were associated with "physical health" and "financial security", but they were not connected very strongly to other aspects of life such as "leisure", "family" or "living arrangements". Clearly patients with diabetes discriminate between diabetes related problems and aspects of life not affected by diabetes.

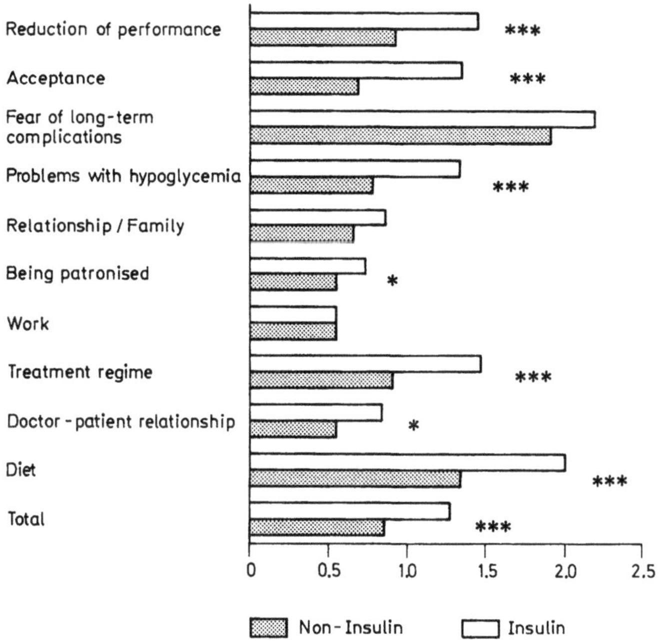

Fig. 2: Stress scales for 90 patients with insulin-treated and 117 patients with non-insulin-treated type II diabetes mellitus.

Table 2: Correlations of "Daily problems with diabetes" (DPD) and aspects of "Quality of life" (QOL)

N = 207 Quality of life (QOL)	DPD total
Friends/Social contacts	– .14
Leisure/Hobbies	– .07
Physical health	– .43
Income/Financial security	– .33
Work/Household	– .18
Living situation	– .09
Family/Children	– .06
Partner/Sex	– .21
Physical performance	– .48
Ability to relax	– .51
Energy/Joy	– .45
Mobility	– .23
Visual/Auditory performance	– .28
Freedom from anxiety	– .42
Freedom from complaints/Pain	– .35
Independence of care	– .23

Psychological treatment strategies

The "day-to-day stress" associated with diabetes mellitus can provide general topics for treatment intervention and also important ideas for specific treatment goals. In the development of treatment strategies, careful functional analyses can reveal the relevant psychobiological interdependences. Diet is one of the main problems for all patients with type II diabetes. Therefore, dietary problems serve here as an example of how to develop possible treatment strategies.

Using some items from our scales, patients scoring high in "diet" find it a very heavy burden:
- having to avoid tasty foods,
- not being able to eat according to their wishes,
- having to eat according to a timetable,
- having to eat without hunger or appetite,
- having to put the diet together oneself,
- not being able to keep to the diet.

In other words, patients with diabetes mellitus experience their dietary demands as a "restrained eating pattern". This is an eating pattern that is characterized by a voluntary, cognitively directed restriction of caloric intake in quantitative, qualitative and temporal aspects. It is often employed by young women to keep their body weight within socially accepted limits [42]. There is much evidence that this eating pattern triggers psychopathological symptoms of eating disorders, particularly binge attacks [42]. Restrained eating can alter insulin resistance, disturb normal weight regulation and interoceptive perception of hunger or satiety [21], and influence neurotransmitter systems (serotonergic system, central norepinephrine system), with a negative effect on mood and appetite [5, 48, 58].

Several studies have shown that eating disorders are twice as high in young diabetic women as in control groups [33, 45, 49]. These observations, together with the fact that most diabetic patients with a clinical eating disorder developed the eating disorder after diabetes manifestation [50], led to the hypothesis that some aspects of diabetes can trigger eating disorders. Dietary restriction may be one major risk factor.

Therefore, in a study of young diabetic women we tested the hypothesis that certain characteristics of "eating disorder psychopathology" become more pronounced as the extent of "restrained eating" increases [32]. The patients with diabetes had higher scores than the normal restrained and unrestrained eaters on scales that measure "drive for leanness", "concerns about body shape and weight", "preoccupation with food and dieting", and "bulimic tendencies". Furthermore, the diabetics reported more feelings of ineffectiveness, more depression and distorted introceptive awareness. These results supported the hypothesis of IDDM as a specific risk factor for the development of an eating disorder. In particular, the diabetes specific dietary behavior appears to enhance the probability of binge-eating attacks. This may also be true for patients with type II diabetes. Wing et al. [57] studied 98 obese type II diabetic patients who were participating in a behavioral weight-control program. The patients completed the Binge-Eating Scale [20] pre- and post-treatment and at 1-year follow-up. Twenty-one percent of the females and 9% of the males met the criteria for having a serious binge-eating problem. "Restrained eating" or other types of eating patterns were not assessed in this study. Correlations were found between binge-eating severity and depressive symptomatology. Scores on the Binge-Eating Scale decreased significantly during the weight control program and were associated with improvements in mood but not with weight loss or improvements in glycemic control.

If we have to consider the dietary regimen as a risk factor for binge-eating and other dietary disturbances, then it is not enough to tell patients what they should or should not eat. In addition to educating patients about diet, we have to teach them to cope with the dietary restrictions and to acquire strategies to prevent stressful situations. Behavioral training programs should be introduced in two stages. In the first stage short-term strategies aimed at restructuring eating pattern to both meet physical needs and fit reasonably well into the daily routine should be taught. Practice in structured eating behavior can be offered: for example, how to eat at least five meals a day, using variable food, not omitting meals to reduce caloric intake but eating less at each meal and trying to include food that tastes good.

In a second stage, long-term strategies for coping with stressful situations should be introduced. The reasons for binges and eating problems should be explored by means of self-monitoring. Patients can be trained in relaxation techniques, in the strategy of planning and in assertive behavior. Cognitive restructuring health beliefs and beliefs about self-efficacy can help to establish a stable level of motivation for self-management. Finally, patients should be given advice on how to communicate effectively with their doctors.

In spite of a long tradition of behavioral interventions in the form of weight control programs [19], up to now there have been only a few attempts to offer patients extensive training such as just described. From those reports on these attempts, however, we can postulate that long-term treatment effects will improve with the introduction of stress-reducing and cognitive-behavioral interventions [30, 31, 44, 55]. By considering psychological aspects as important in achieving the twofold treatment goal – improving the quality of the patients' life and controlling the metabolic disease – we will gain not only a better understanding of the patients but also an additional effective treatment strategy.

References

[1] Alonga, N.: Perception and severity of disease and health locus of control in compliant and noncompliant patients. Diabetes Care *3* (1980) 533 – 534.

[2] Anderson, L. A., R. F. DeVellis, B. Boyles et al.: Patients' perceptions of their clinical interactions: development of the multidimensional desire for control scales. Health Education Research *4* (1989) 383 – 397.

[3] Ary, D. V., D. Toobert, W. Wilson et al.: Patient perspective on factors contributing to nonadherence to diabetic regimen. Diabetes Care *9* (1986) 168 – 172.

[4] Beck, A. T., C. H. Ward, M. Mendelson et al.: An inventory for measuring depression. Archives of General Psychiatry *4* (1961) 53 – 63.

[5] Blundell, J.: Serotonin and appetite. Neuropharmacology *23* (1984) 1537 – 1551.

[6] Connell, C. M.: Psychosocial predictors of morale among older adults with diabetes. Psychology & Health *4* (1990) 91 – 98.

[7] Connell, C. M., J. J. O'Sullivan, E. B. Fisher et al.: Variables predicting adherence and metabolic control among retirement community residents with non-insulin-dependent Diabetes mellitus. Journal of Compliance in Health Care *3* (1988) 135 – 149.

[8] Cox, J. D., L. A. Gonder-Frederick, L. W. Clarke: Blood glucose discrimination training in insulin-dependent diabetes-mellitus patients. Biofeedback & Self-Regulation *13* (1988) 201 – 207.

[9] Davidson, J. K., H. K. Delcher, A. Englund: Spin-off cost/benefits of expanded nutritional care. Journal of American Dietary Association *75* (1979) 251 – 255.

[10] Davidson, J. K.: The Grady Memorial Hospital diabetes unit ambulatory care program. In: I. P. Assal, M. Berger, N. Gay (eds.): Diabetes education. Excerpta Medica, Amsterdam, Oxford, Princeton 1983.

[11] Davis, W. K., G. E. Hess, R. G. Hiss: Psychosocial Correlates of survival in diabetes. Diabetes Care *11* (1988) 538 – 545.

[12] Davis, W. K., G. E. Hess, R. Van Harrison et al.: Psychosocial Adjustment on and control of Diabetes Mellitus: Differences by Disease Type and Treatment. Health Psychology *6* (1987) 1 – 14.

[13] Demers, R. Y., A. V. Neale, N. J. Wenzloff et al.: Glycosylated hemoglobin levels and self-reported stress in adults with diabetes. Behavior Medicine *15* (1989) 167 – 172.

[14] Dichmann, R., R. Handreg, G. Libner et al.: Untersuchungen über die Bedeutung einer gezielten Patientenaufklärung auf die Güte der Stoffwechselführung in einer Meßstelle für Diabetes mellitus. Zeitschrift für die Gesamte Innere Medizin *36* (1981) 491 – 494.

[15] DiMatteo, M. R.: Physician-patient communication: Promoting a positive health care setting. In: J. C. Rosen, L. J. Soloman (eds.): Prevention in health psychology, pp. 328 – 365. University Press, New England 1985.

[16] Dunn, S. M., J. R. Turtle: The myth of the diabetic personality. Diabetes Care *4* (1981) 640 – 646.

[17] Glasgow, R. E., D. J. Toobert: Social environment and regimen adherence among type II diabetic patients. Diabetes Care *11* (1988) 377 – 386.

[18] Gonder-Frederick, L. A., D. J. Cox: Behavioral responses to perceived hypoglycemic symptoms. Diabetes Educator *12* (1986) 105 – 109.

[19] Goodman, J. I., E. D. Schwartz, L. Frankel: Group therapy of obese diabetic patients. Diabetes *4* (1953) 280 – 284.
[20] Gormally, J., S. Black, S. Daston et al.: The assessment of binge eating severity among obese persons. Addictive Behaviors *7* (1982) 47 – 55.
[21] Hales, C. N., P. J. Randle: Effects of low-carbohydrate diet and diabetes on plasma concentrations of glucose, nonesterified fatty acid and insulin during oral glucose tolerance test. Lancet *1* (1963) 790.
[22] Hampson, S. E., R. E. Glasgow, D. J. Toobert: Personal models of Diabetes and their relations to self-care activites. Health Psychology *9* (1990) 632 – 646.
[23] Haynes, R. B.: A critical review of the "determinants" of patients compliance with therapeutic regimes. In: D. L. Sackett, R. B. Haynes (eds.): Compliance with therapeutic regimes, pp. 26 – 39. John Hopkins, Baltimore (1976).
[24] Hopper, S. V., K. Schechtman: Factors affecting diabetes control in a low-income population. Patient Education Counsel *7* (1985) 275 – 288.
[25] House, W. C., L. Pendleton, L. Parker: Patients' versus physicians' attributions of reasons for diabetic patients' noncompliance with diet. Diabetes Care *9* (1986) 302.
[26] Huber, D., G. Henrich, P. Herschbach: Measuring the quality of life: A comparison between physically and mentally chronically ill patients and health persons. Pharmacopsychiatry *21* (1988) 453 – 455.
[27] Jacobson, A. M., A. G. Adler, J. I. Wolfsdorf, B. Aderson et al.: Psychological characteristics of adults with IDDM. Diabetes Care *13* (1990) 375 – 381.
[28] Jacobson, A. M., L. I. Rand, S. T. Hauser: Psychologic stress and glycemic control: A comparison of patients with and without proliferative diabetic retinopathy. Psychosomatic Medicine *47* (1985) 372 – 381.
[29] Jenny, J. L.: Differences in adaptation to diabetes between insulin-dependent and non-insulin-dependent patients: Implications for patients education. Patient Education and Counseling *8* (1986) 39 – 50.
[30] Kaplan, R. M., C. J. Atkins: The behavioral management of type II diabetes mellitus. In: R. M. Kaplan, M. H. Criqui (eds.): Behavioral Epidemiology and Disease Prevention, pp. 353 – 358. Plenum Press, New York 1985.
[31] Kulzer, B.: Verhaltensmedizinische Aspekte der Therapie des Typ II-Diabetes. Verhaltensmodifikation und Verhaltensmedizin *11* (1990) 317 – 339.
[32] Laessle, R. G., S. Waadt, G. Duran et al.: Psychologische Merkmale von Eßstörungen bei jungen Frauen mit Diabates mellitus: Erste Ergebnisse einer empirischen Untersuchung. Verhaltensmodifikation und Verhaltensmedizin *11* (1990) 229 – 242.
[33] Lautenbacher, St.: Anorexia und Bulimia nervosa bei Diabetes mellitus (Typ-I): Epidemiologie, Symptomatik und Pathogenese. Verhaltensmodifikation und Verhaltensmedizin *11* (1990) 258 – 280.
[34] Levine, S. P., J. H. Shah, L. Bell et al.: Psychological factors affecting adherence to diet in male diabetic patients. Psychological Reports *59* (1986) 439 – 445.
[35] Linn, M. W., B. S. Linn, J. S. Skyler et al.: The importance of self-assessed health in patients with diabetes. Diabetes Care *3* (1980) 599 – 606.
[36] Lustman, P. J., L. S. Griffith, R. E. Cluse et al.: Psychiatric illness in diabetes mellitus. The Journal of Nervous and Mental Disease *174* (1986) 736 – 742.
[37] Marble, A.: The natural history of diabetes. In: International Symposium on Lipid Metabolism, Obesity and Diabetes mellitus: Impact upon Atherosclerosis, Wiesbaden/

Oberursel 13. – 15. 4. 1972. 2. Hormone and Metabolic Research, Suppl. 4. Thieme, Stuttgart 1974.

[38] Marteau, T. M., M. Johnston, J. D. Baum et al.: Goals of treatment in diabetes: A comparison of doctors and parents of children with diabetes. Journal of Behavioral Medicine *10* (1987) 33 – 48.

[39] Mühlhauser, J., U. Jörgens, M. Berger et al.: Bicentric evaluation for a teaching and treatment programme for type I (insulin-dependent) diabetic patients improvement of metabolic control and other measures of diabetes care for up to 22 month. Diabetologie *25* (1983) 470 – 476.

[40] Pauli, P., F. Strian, S. Lautenbacher et al.: Emotionale Auswirkungen der autonomen Deafferentierung bei Diabetes Neuropathie. Zeitschrift für Klinische Psychologie *18* (1990) 268 – 277.

[41] Pirart, J.: Diabetes mellitus and its degenerative complications: a prospective study of 4400 patients observed between 1947 and 1973. Diabetes Care *1* (1978) 168 – 252.

[42] Polivy, J., C. P. Herman: Dieting and binging: A causal analysis. American Psychologist *40* (1985) 193 – 201.

[43] Popkin, M. K., A. L. Callies, R. D. Lentz et al.: Prevalence of major depression, simple phobia and other psychiatric disorders in patients with long-standing type-I-diabetes. Archives of General Psychiatry *45* (1988) 64 – 68.

[44] Rainwater, N., T. Ayllon, L. W. Frederiksen et al.: Teaching self-management skills to increase diet compliance in diabetes. In: R. B. Stuart (eds.): Adherence, compliance and generalisation in behavioral medicine, pp. 304 – 328. Bruner/Mazel, New York 1982.

[45] Rosmark, B., C. Bere, S. Holmgren et al.: Eating disorders in patients with insulin-dependent diabetes mellitus. Journal of Clinical Psychiatry *47* (1986) 547 – 550.

[46] Sackett, D. L., R. D. Haynes: Compliance with therapeutic regimes. John Hopkins University Press, Baltimore 1976.

[47] Sammler, A.: Katastrophale Zustände. Medical Tribune, deutsche Ausgabe, *23* (1986) 44 – 45.

[48] Schweiger, U.: Diabetes mellitus und Eßstörungen. In: F. Strian, R. Hölzl, M. Haslbeck (Hrsg.): Verhaltensmedizin und Diabetes mellitus, S. 203 – 214. Springer Verlag, Berlin, Heidelberg, New York, London, Paris, Tokyo 1988.

[49] Steel. J. M., R. J. Young, G. G. Lloyd et al.: Abnormal eating attitudes in young insulin-dependent diabetics. British Journal of Psychiatry *155* (1989) 515 – 521.

[50] Waadt, S., G. Duran, R. G. Laessle et al.: Eßstörungen bei Patienten mit Diabetes mellitus: Eine Übersicht über Falldarstellungen und Therapiemöglichkeiten. Verhaltensmodifikation und Verhaltensmedizin *11* (1988) 281 – 305.

[51] Waadt, S., P. Herschbach, G. Duran et al.: Entwicklung eines Fragebogens zu Behandlungsproblemen und Therapiezuweisung bei Patienten mit Diabetes mellitus. Praxis der Verhaltensmedizin und Rehabilitation in press.

[52] Watkins, J. D., D. E. Roberts, T. F. Williams et al.: Obervation of medication errors made by diabetic patients in the home. Diabetes *16* (1967) 882 – 885.

[53] Williams, G., J. Pickup, H. Keen: Psychological factors and metabolic control: Time for reappraisal. Diabetic Medicine *5* (1988) 211 – 215.

[54] Williams, T. F., D. A. Martin, M. D. Hogan et al.: The clinical picture of diabetic controll studied in four settings. American Journal of Public Health 57 (1967) 441–451.
[55] Wilson, W., D. V. Ary, A. Biglan et al.: Psychological predictors of self-care behaviors (compliance) and glycemic control in non-insulin-dependent diabetes mellitus. Diabetes Care *9* (1986) 614–622.
[56] Wing, R. R.: Behavioral strategies for weight reduction in obese type II diabetic patients. Diabetes Care *12* (1989) 139–144.
[57] Wing, R. R., M. D. Marcus, L. H. Epstein et al.: Binge Eating in obese patients with type II diabetes. International Journal of Eating Disorders *8* (1989) 671–679.
[58] Wing, R. R., M. D. Marcus, E. H. Blair et al.: Depressive symptomatology in obese adults with type II diabetes. Diabetes Care *13* (1990) 170–172.
[59] Wurtman, R. J., J. J. Wurtman (eds.). Nutrition and the Brain. Vol. 7. Raven Press, New York 1986.

Well-being in non-insulin-dependent diabetic patients (NIDDM) – a long-term follow-up

M. Toeller

The Duesseldorf-Paris-Naples Intervention Trial in NIDDM Patients

The aim of the "Duesseldorf-Paris-Naples (DPN) Intervention Trial in NIDDM Patients" is to evaluate the influence of different diabetes care programmes on the metabolic control and the quality of life of NIDDM patients [34]. Participating centres are the Diabetes Research Institute at Duesseldorf University, Germany (Dr. Monika Toeller et al.), the Department of Diabetes of Hotel Dieu Hospital in Paris, France (Prof. Gérard Slama et al.) and the Institute of Internal Medicine and Metabolic Diseases of Naples University, Italy (Dr. Gabriele Riccardi et al.).

Table 1 gives an overview of the study design of this multinational multi-centre trial. Patients were randomly assigned to different diabetes care programmes and followed up over 36 weeks. The main aims were to study the effects of intervention on hemoglobin A_{1c} and the quality of life of the patients. In addition, the centre in Duesseldorf is looking at the effects of intervention on insulin sensitivity as measured by the hyperinsulinemic euglycemic clamp technique. Several other parameters characterizing the metabolic syndrome ("Syndrome X") were docu-

Table 1: Study design of the Duesseldorf-Paris-Naples (DPN) Intervention Trial in NIDDM Patients

Study design Patients were randomly assigned to different diabetes care programmes

0	4	8	12	16	20	24	28	32	36	weeks
•	•	•	•	•	•	•	•	•	•	
△			△			△			△	
□						□				

Target parameters		
	•	HbA_{1c} (%)
	△	*Quality of life* (Sum score of tests)
	□	Insulin sensitivity (hyperinsulinemic euglycemic clamp, MCR mg/kg x min)

Further parameters to observe:
BW, BP, FIRI, FBG, 2 hr pp BG, TG, CH, HDL, LDL, BG AND IRI after 100 g oral glucose and 1 g i. v. tolbutamide, dietary intake (4 day records) etc.

mented in the study and also the nutritional intake of the patients was assessed by analysis of 4-day dietary records which were filled in by the patients before intervention and at specific intervals during the follow-up study [34].

Characteristics of patients who were followed up in the Duesseldorf centre

In this report some quality of life aspects of the Duesseldorf part of the study will be presented. Table 2 shows some of the initial characteristics of the manifest NIDDM patients who were included in the study in the Duesseldorf centre. There were a total number of 66 patients with a mean age of 58 years and a mean duration of diabetes of 8 years. At entry all of them were insufficiently controlled by diet and sulfonylurea drug treatment. They were overweight and showed elevated hemoglobin A_{1c} levels as well as high fasting and postprandial blood glucose values. In addition most of them had high blood pressure and elevated serum-cholesterol and triglyceride levels. Many of them were smokers.

Selection of instruments to measure quality of life

By selection of the instruments to measure quality of life in the study it was necessary to keep in mind that the study was going to be performed in adult or elderly patients and that quality of life could possibly mean something different to patients living in Duesseldorf, Paris or Naples. As we wanted to study whether the quality of life of the patients could be changed or improved by our intervention procedures, measuring instruments which are specifically sensitive to changes were needed [1, 5, 7, 9, 11, 15, 16, 18, 19, 20, 27, 35, 36, 41, 42, 48]. In this context it was also the goal to apply only test instruments which fulfilled the test theoretical conditions as far as possible.

Table 2: Characteristics of patients followed up in the Duesseldorf centre

Initial data of manifest NIDDM patients	
Total number (n)	66
Sex (m/f)	31/35
Age (years)	58 ± 7
BMI (kg/m^2)	29 ± 3
Duration of diabetes (years)	8 ± 5
OAD (tablets/day)	2 ± 1
HbA_{1c} (%)	9.1 ± 1

Table 3: Instruments to measure quality of life in the DPN Intervention Trial in NIDDM Patients

Measuring instruments – sensitive to changes – were selected to provide information on the following components of quality of life
Subjective mental condition Mental and physical stress Social integration/activity Subjective physical condition Subjective stress caused by antidiabetic therapy Conviction regarding the necessity to control diabetes by adequate therapy (individual life change events were controlled before and during the study)

All measuring instruments selected for the study are particularly sensitive to changes. They are able to provide information on the following components of quality of life: the subjective mental condition of the patients, the mental and physical stress, the social integration and activity, the subjective physical condition, the subjective stress caused by the diabetes therapy and the conviction regarding the necessity to control diabetes by adequate therapy [3, 12, 14, 22, 23, 39, 40, 44–47]. In addition, life-changing events had to be controlled for in the long-term study in order to ascertain whether such serious events would occur and whether they were equally or similarly distributed in the different intervention groups (Tab. 3) [26, 27, 29, 31, 43, 48]. All instruments which were applied in the study to measure quality of life will be described and some of the results at long-term follow-up will be presented.

State of mind scale

Firstly, the "State of mind scale" (Befindlichkeitsskala, Bf-S', Zerssen 1976) was used to record short-term changes in general emotional disturbances [25, 45, 46]. Zerssen State of Mind scale is a self-record inventory with 28 items (Tab. 4). The patients record e. g. whether they feel now more "outgoing" or more "inhibited" or "neither nor". From other items information can be obtained as to whether patients feel "in a good mood" or "gloomy" or whether they feel "lacking in drive" or "motivated".

Figure 1 shows the distribution of sum scores in the "State of mind scale" in our study sample of 66 NIDDM patients before intervention compared to the sum-scores of a sample of non-diabetic controls of comparable age. It may seem surprising that the mean of sum scores does not show statistically significant differences between the diabetic patients and the non diabetic controls. However it can be concluded from these results that – using the "State of mind scale" –

Table 4: Assessment of quality of life in the DPN study

State of mind scale

(Befindlichkeitsskala, Bf-S', Zerssen 1976)
to record short-term changes in general emotional disturbances
Self-report inventory with 28 items

I am feeling now:

more	more	neither nor
outgoing	inhibited	
in a good mood	gloomy	
lacking in drive	motivated	

etc.

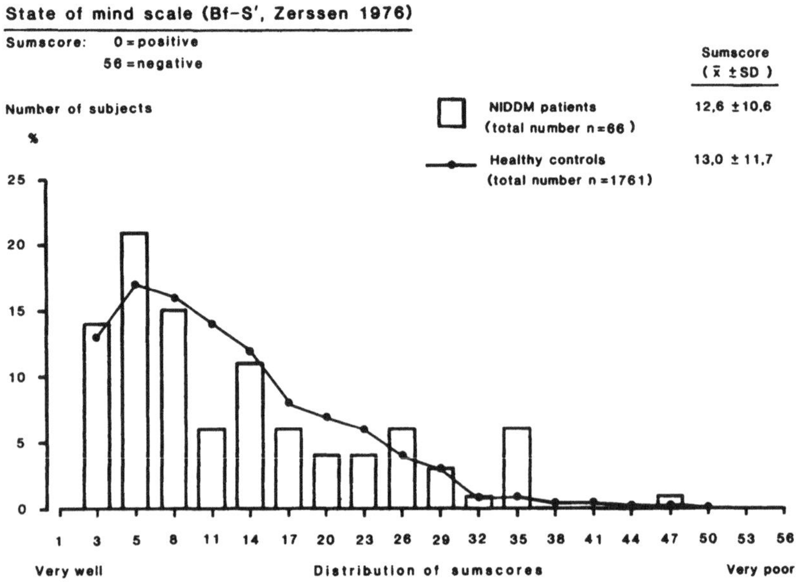

Fig. 1: Results by the "State of mind scale" of 66 NIDDM patients at entry compared to results obtained from 1761 non-diabetic controls of a comparable age.

NIDDM patients do not feel worse compared to the non-diabetic population of comparable age. In both groups there were persons who were close to the more active and optimistic pole of the scale and others who were closer to the passive and depressive state of mind pole. But it should also be noted that in general the well-being of both, NIDDM patients and non-diabetic controls, was rather close to the positive pole of the scale with a mean of sum scores of 12.6 in the diabetic

Table 5: Results by the "State of mind scale" at start of the study and after 12, 24 and 36 weeks of intervention in the Duesseldorf centre

State of mind scale (Bf-S', 28 items, Zerssen 1976)

Sum score: 0 = positive
56 = negative

I am feeling now:

Week	More positive (0) n%	More negative (2) n%	Neither/ Nor (1) n%	Patients total n	Sum score $\bar{x} \pm SD$
0	71	17	12	66	12.6 ± 10.6
12	74	12	14	66	10.7 ± 9.6
24	73	9	18	63	10.6 ± 10.0
36	72	10	18	61	11.0 ± 10.5

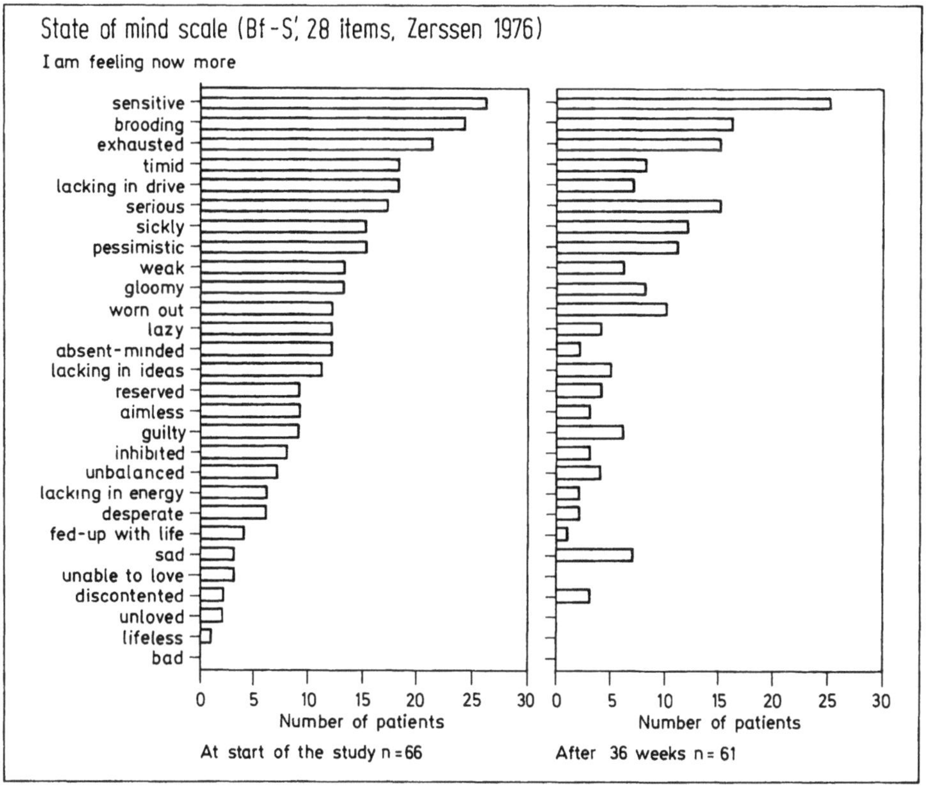

Fig. 2: Number of patients with negative feelings in the "State of mind scale" at entry compared to the results after 36 weeks of intervention.

patients and a mean of sum scores of 13.0 in the controls. The maximal negative score possible in the "State of mind scale" is 56.

The decrease of the sum scores during the follow-up demonstrates that there is a decrease of negative mental feelings in the patients over the time of the 36-week intervention period (Tab. 5). Figure 2 illustrates which severe negative feelings were markedly reduced during the study. At entry a higher number of patients had felt brooding, exhausted, timid, lacking in drive, weak, lazy etc. compared to the 36-week results. Such symptoms are specifically crucial in the treatment and control of NIDDM patients who present very often with a rather sedentary life-style. By means of the intervention measures the study patients have achieved a step forward into the direction of a healthier life-style [38].

At this point it should be mentioned that we could not obtain data from 3 patients at the 24-week examination (n = 63) and of further 2 patients at the 36-week examination (n = 61). A detailed analysis of the reasons, however, did not give any indication that these missing values could have changed the results.

List of complaints

The "List of complaints" (Beschwerdenliste, B-L', Zerssen 1976) was used to record the degree of subjective impairment by physical and general complaints [10, 44]. The "List of complaints" is a self-report inventory with 24 items, such as: "I am suffering from headaches, fatigue, balance disturbances" etc. The degree of severity of a symptom can be marked in a 4 step rating scale (Tab. 6). Table 7 demonstrates the results of sum scores obtained at the start of the study compared to those after 12, 24 and 36 weeks of intervention. The decrease of sum scores during the follow-up study shows a change in a positive direction, which means that an improvement of physical complaints or symptoms could be

Table 6: Assessment of quality of life in the DPN study

List of complaints
(Beschwerdenliste, B-L', Zerssen 1976)
to record the degree of subjective impairment by physical and general complaints

Self-report inventory with 24 items

I am suffering from the following:

	severely	moderately	scarcely	not at all
Headaches				
Fatigue				
Balance disturbances				
etc.				

Table 7: Results by the "List of complaints" at start of the study and after 12, 24 and 36 weeks of intervention in the Duesseldorf centre

List of complaints (B-L', Zerssen 1976)

Sum score: 0 = positive
72 = negative

Week	Sum score $\bar{x} \pm$ SD (Min.-Max.)	Patients total n
0	16 ± 10 (0–46)	66
12	13 ± 11 (0–42)	66
24	11 ± 9 (0–34)	63
36	11 ± 10 (0–42)	61

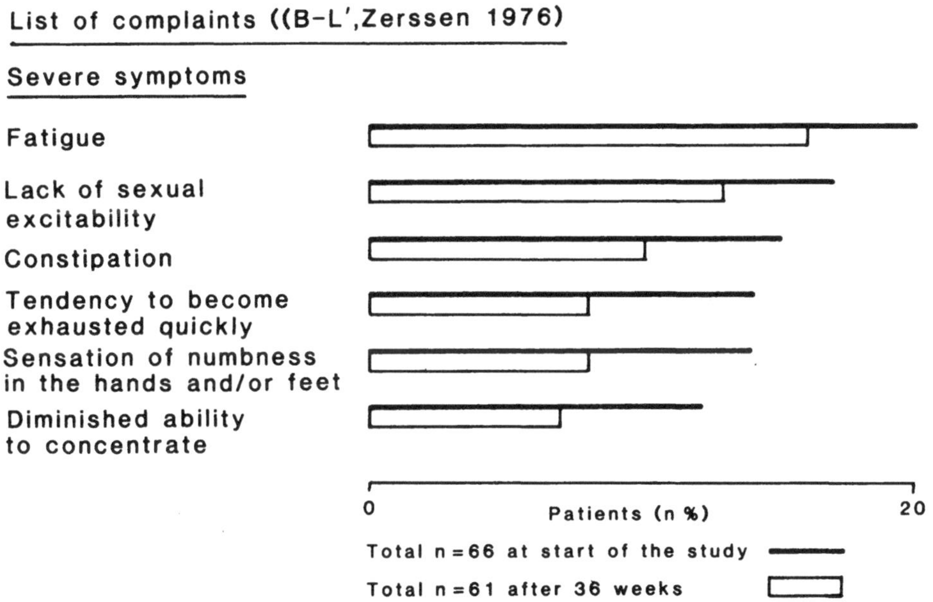

Fig. 3: Number of patients with severe symptoms in the "List of complaints" at entry compared to the results after 36 weeks of intervention.

achieved. Figure 3 gives an impression which of the initially severe symptoms of the patients were reduced. After 36 weeks fewer patients complained "to have a sensation of numbness in the hands and/or feet", "to become exhausted quickly" and "to have a diminished ability to concentrate". Also the number of patients with constipation, lack of sexual excitability and fatigue decreased.

Diabetes locus of control scale

The "Diabetes locus of control scale" was used to assess the degree of commitment and self-responsibility in the diabetes therapy [4, 6]. This "Diabetes locus of control scale" was developed on the basis of the "Health locus of control scale" published by Wallston and Wallston and Kaplan and Maides in 1976 [17, 21, 24, 28, 30, 32, 33, 39, 49]. The "Diabetes locus of control scale" was validated in a large sample of diabetic patients by Möhlmann et al. in 1988 [23]. The "Diabetes locus of control scale" is a self-report 6-point rating scale with 11 items. Patients record whether they agree or disagree to statements like: "If I take care of my diabetes, I can avoid complications" (Tab. 8).

Table 9 gives a summary of the results which were achieved during follow-up. The mean score of the patients at the start of the study was 29.1. During the intervention period a decrease of the scores in the direction of internal control was observed. The shift to increased internal control in the patients is particularly well illustrated in Figure 4.

Table 8: Assessment of quality of life in the DPN study

Diabetes locus of control scale
(on the basis of the Health locus of control scale, Wallston, Wallston, Kaplan and Maides 1976) to assess the degree of commitment and self-responsibility in antidiabetic therapy

Self-report rating scale with 11 items

If I take care of	Yes, I agree			No, I disagree		
my diabetes, I can	3	2	1	1	2	3
avoid complications	very much	average	a little	a little	average	very much

Table 9: Results by the "Diabetes locus of control scale" at start of the study and after 12, 24 and 36 weeks of intervention in the Duesseldorf centre

Diabetes locus of control scale
(Wallston, Wallston, Kaplan and Maides 1976)
internal = 11
external = 66

Week	Patients total n	Sum score $\bar{x} \pm$ SD (Min.-Max.)
0	66	29.1 ± 8.1 (13–54)
12	66	25.5 ± 9.3 (12–48)
24	63	25.9 ± 9.3 (11–45)
36	61	25.8 ± 10.2 (12–52)

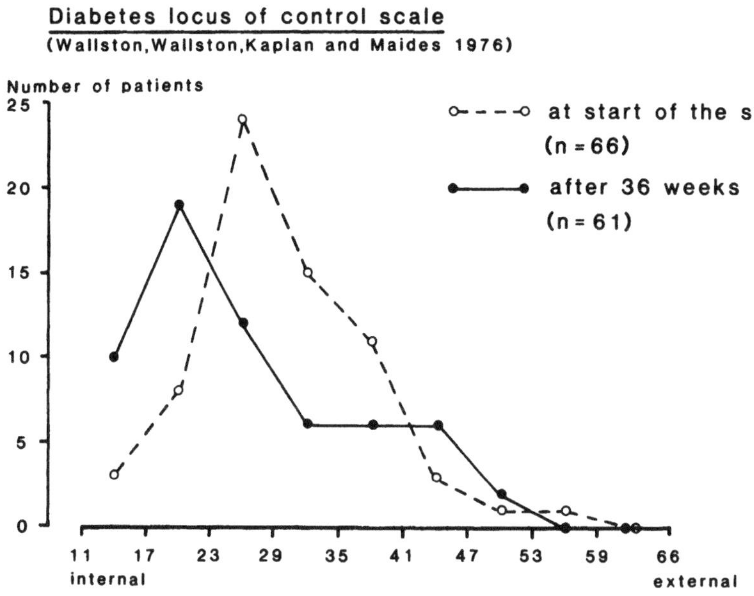

Fig. 4: Distribution of patients in the "Diabetes locus of control scale" at entry compared to the results after 36 weeks of intervention.

Questionnaire on the management of diabetes in daily life

A "Questionnaire on the management of diabetes in daily life "was used to assess especially crucial components of diabetes and its treatment and their impact on daily life. The questionnaire is a self-report rating scale with 11 items (Tab. 10). This questionnaire has been used in many studies with IDDM and NIDDM patients [35, 37]. Patients can give their ratings on a 7-point scale to questions such as "Are you troubled by your diabetes in everyday life?" etc.

Table 10: Assessment of quality of life in the DPN study

Questionnaire on management of diabetes in daily life
(Toeller et al. 1985, Diabetes Research Institute Düsseldorf)
to assess especially crucial components of diabetes and its treatment and their impact on daily life

Self-report rating scale with 11 items

Are you troubled by your diabetes in everyday life?	−3 very much	−2	−1	0	1	2	3 not at all
etc.							

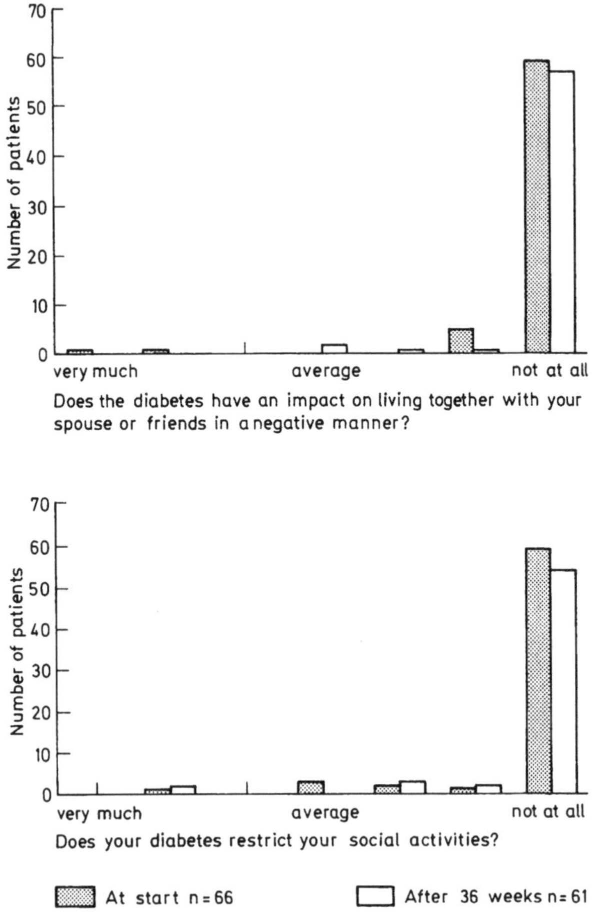

Fig. 5: Distribution of patients in the "Questionnaire on management of diabetes in daily life" at entry compared to the results after 36 weeks of intervention.

It is interesting to see that NIDDM does not seem to have much negative impact on living together with the family or friends and that NIDDM patients do not feel seriously restricted in their social activities by the disease (Fig. 5). This has also been shown in other studies. However, it could also be questioned whether NIDDM patients who very often have a rather sedentary lifestyle without many social activities will not miss these because they are not aware of the pleasure of having leisure activities with their friends [35].

Several of the patients said that the management of diabetes does not represent a burden to them. But there were also some patients who felt under strain because of the management of diabetes in daily life (Fig. 6). However, compared to the start of the study, after 36 weeks more patients felt that they could reach good

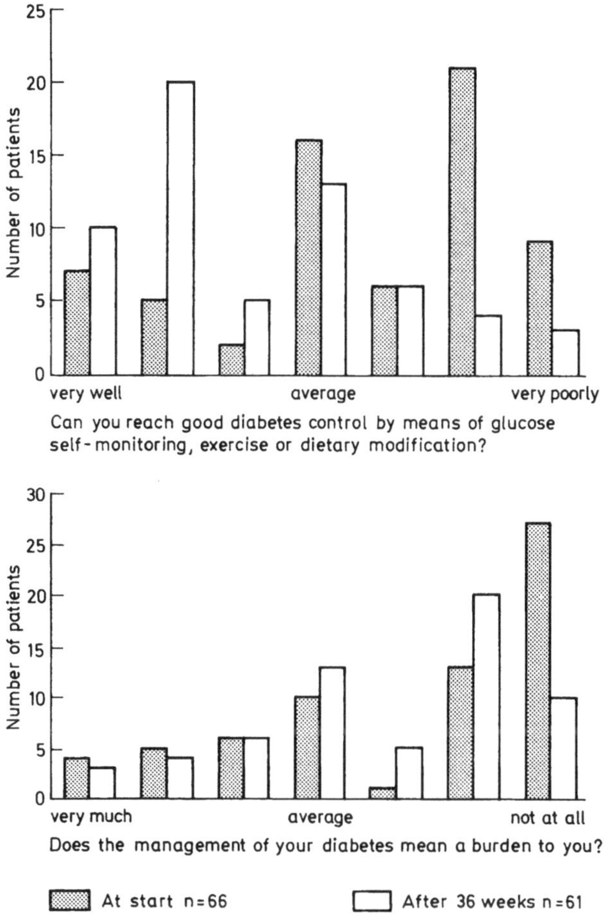

Fig. 6: Distribution of patients in the "Questionnaire on management of diabetes in daily life" at entry compared to the results after 36 weeks of intervention.

diabetes control by means of blood glucose self-monitoring, exercise or dietary modification. An increase in their own actions and commitment to the management of the disease was observed in many patients in the follow-up study [34].

Questionnaire on changes in experience and behaviour

Changes in experience and behaviour were assessed by retrospective questioning using the "Questionnaire on changes in experience and behaviour" by Zielke and Kopf-Mehnert (Tab. 11). This self-report questionnaire contains 42 items [47]. By bipolar rating on a 7 point scale patients express their feelings e. g.: "I feel less hard pressed" or "I no longer get excited about many things". Table 12 gives

Table 11: Assessment of quality of life in the DPN study

Questionnaire on changes in experience and behaviour
(Veränderungsfragebogen des Erlebens und Verhaltens, VEV, Zielke und Kopf-Mehnert 1978) to assess bipolar changes through retrospective questioning

Self-report questionnaire with 42 items

	Change		
	+3 +2 +1	0	−1 −2 −3
I feel less hard pressed. *I no longer get excited about many things* etc.	in the same direction	no	in the opposite direction

Table 12: Results by the "Questionnaire on changes in experience and behaviour" after 36 weeks of intervention in the Duesseldorf centre

Questionnaire on changes in experience and behaviour
(VEV, Zielke and Kopf-Mehnert 1978)

0 → 36 weeks	Number of patients
Changes in a positive direction	48
Changes in a negative direction	11
Unchanged	2

an overview of the number of patients with changes in experience and behaviour in a positive direction (n = 48) and with changes in a negative direction (n = 11). There was no change in two patients only.

Life change index scale

Individual stress produced by serious life changing events was assessed by the "Life change index scale" by Holmes and Rahe, modified by Siegrist and Dittmann in 1976 (Tab. 13) [13, 26, 27, 31, 32]. This checked whether a patient or somebody in his family became seriously ill during the study, whether a family member or a close friend had died or whether major familial or financial problems occurred during the intervention period etc.

More than half of the patients did not record any serious life changing events during the intervention study (Fig. 7). However 45% of the patients had such events. Most patients recorded one life change event, however, a few patients reported more than 5 life change events over 36 weeks. In general, the number of life change events reported was lower during the intervention study compared

Table 13: Assessment of quality of life in the DPN study

Life change index scale
(Holmes and Rahe 1967, modified by Siegrist and Dittmann 1976)
to assess the individual stress produced by life change events

Checklist with 38 items

	happened no/yes
Have you been seriously ill?	
Has a member of your family died?	
Have you had financial problems?	
etc.	

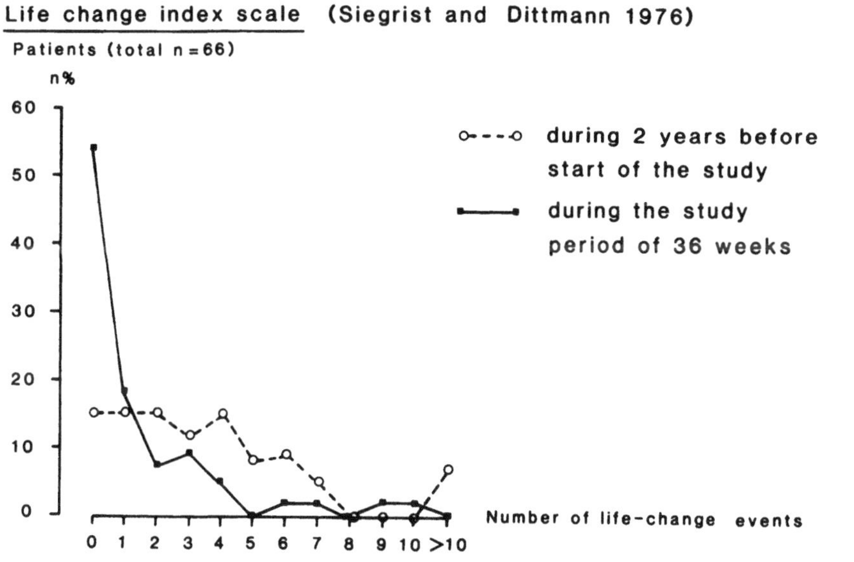

Fig. 7: Number of patients who recorded life change events during the study period compared to the results of a 2-year period before start of the study.

to the results of a two-year period before start of the study (Fig. 7). This could mean that fewer events occurred or that the patients with an improved general well-being did not feel stressed as much as before by such events [2, 8].

Summary

The results of the Duesseldorf Intervention Trial in non-insulin-dependent diabetic patients (NIDDM), where quality of life was assessed by different scales and questionnaires, can by summarized as follows:

During an intervention period of 36 weeks, changes in a positive direction were shown by all instruments measuring quality of life. Attention should be drawn to the most fascinating issue of the study. Some of the scales demonstrated that at the start of the study the NIDDM patients felt the same as non-diabetic

Table 14: Summary of the results by the instruments applied to measure quality of life in the Duesseldorf Intervention Trial in NIDDM Patients

0 → 36 weeks (n = 66) (n = 61)	Changes in a positive direction
• List of complaints	yes
• State of mind scale	yes
• Questionnaire on management of diabetes in daily life	yes
• Diabetes locus of control scale	yes
• Questionnaire on changes in experience and behaviour	yes

controls with regard to many aspects of their quality of life. However, during the intervention study a significant improvement in all aspects of quality of life was achieved in the NIDDM patients. In conclusion it would seem that non-insulin-dependent diabetic patients who get sufficient care and attention from their doctor will end up with a better quality of life than that which is generally present in the non-diabetic population of comparable age.

Acknowledgements

Antonie Klischan, Ph. D., Waltraud Schumacher, R. D., Karin Lange, Ph. D. and Julia Schilling, M. D. assisted in performing this study and analysing the "quality of life" data. We thank all diabetic patients who have participated in the Duesseldorf Intervention Trial in NIDDM Patients.

References

[1] Alogna, M.: Perception of severity of disease and health locus of control in compliant and non-compliant diabetic patients. Diabetes Care *3* (1980) 533–534.

[2] Bebbington, P., C. Tennant, E. Sturt et al.: The domain of life events: A comparision of two techniques of description. Psychological Medicine *14* (1984) 219–222.

[3] Bradley, C., C. R. Brewin, D. S. Gamsu et al.: Development of scales to measure perceived control of diabetes mellitus and diabetes-related health beliefs. Diabetic Medicine *1* (1984) 213–1218.

[4] Craig, A. R., J. A. Franklin, G. Andrews: A scale to measure locus of control of behaviour. Brit. J. of Med. Psychology *57* (1984) 173–180.

[5] Deyo, R. A.: Measuring functional outcomes in therapeutic trials for chronic disease. Controlled Clin. Trials *5* (1984) 223–240.

[6] Edelstein, J., M. W. Linn: Locus of control and the control of diabetes. Diabetes Education *13* (1987) 51–54.

[7] Epstein, L. H., P. A. Cluss: A behavioural medicine perspective on adherence to long-term medical regiments. J. Consult. Clin. Psychol. *50* (1982) 950–971.

[8] Evans, C. L., I. A. Hughes: The relationship between diabetic control and individual and family characteristics. Journal of Psychosomatic Research *31* (1987) 367–374.

[9] Felton, B. J., T. A. Revenson: Coping with chronic illness: A study of illness controllability and the influence of coping strategies on psychological adjustment. Journal of Consulting and Clinical Psychology *52* (1984) 343–353.

[10] Good, L. R., C. C. Parker: Physical anxiety questionnaire. Psychosomatics *12* (1971) 371–379.

[11] Guyatt, G. H., C. Bombardier, P. X. Tugwell: Measuring disease-specific quality of life in clinical trials. CMA J. *134* (1986) 889–895.

[12] Harris, R., M. W. Linn, L. Pollack: Relationship between health beliefs and psychological variables in diabetic patients. Brit. J. of Medical Psychology *57* (1984) 253–259.

[13] Holmes, T.: The Holmes and the Rahe social readjustment rating scale. Journal of Psychosomatic Research *11* (1967) 213–218.

[14] Johnson, J. H., I. G. Sarason: Life stress, depression and anxiety: Internal-external control as a moderator variable. Journal of Psychosomatic Research *22* (1978) 205–208.

[15] Jordan-Marsh, M., R. Neutra: Relationship of health locus of control to lifestyle change programs. Research in Nursing and Health *8* (1985) 3–11.

[16] Kaplan, R. M., J. W. Bush, C. C. Berry: Health status: types of validity and the index of well-being. Health Serv. Res. *11* (1976) 478–507.

[17] Kaplan, R. M., C. J. Atkins, R. M. Timms: Validity of a quality well-being scale as an outcome measure in chronic obstructive pulmonary disease. J. Chron. Dis. *37* (1984) 85–95.

[18] Kaplan, R. M., S. L. Hartwell, D. K. Wilson et al.: Effects of diet and exercise interventions on control and quality of life in non-insulin-dependent diabetes mellitus. J. Gener. Int. Med. *2* (1987) 220–228.

[19] Kaplan, S. H.: Patient reports of health status as predictors of physiologic health measures in chronic disease. J. Chron. Dis. *40* (Suppl. 1) 27S–35S.

[20] Kincey, J.: Compliance with a behavioural weight-loss programme: Target setting and locus of control. Behaviour Research and Therapy *21* (1983) 109–114.

[21] Levenson, H.: Activism and powerful others: Distinction within the concept of internal-external control. Journal of Personality Assessment *38* (1974) 377–383.

[22] Mechanic, D.: The experiences and reporting of common physical complaints. J. Health. Soc. Behav. *21* (1980) 146–155.

[23] Möhlmann, B.: Vergleich zweier Erhebungsmethoden von 'Health Locus of Control' bei Diabetikern und Gesunden. Diplom-Arbeit im Fach: Angewandte Psychologie. Heinrich-Heine-Universität Düsseldorf 1988.

[24] Nagy, V. T., G. R. Wolfe: Chronic illness and health locus of control beliefs. Journal of Social and Clinical Psychology *1* (1983) 58–65.

[25] Querski, K. N., H. M. Hodkinson: Evaluation of a ten question mental test in the institutionalized patient. Age Ageing *3* (1974) 152–157.

[26] Rahe, R. H., J. L. Mahan, R. J. Arthur: Prediction of near-future health change from subject's preceding life changes. Journal of Psychosomatic Research *14* (1970) 401–406.

[27] Rahe, R. H., J. D. Mc Kean, A. J. Arthur: A longitudinal study of life change and illness patterns. Journal of Psychosomatic Research *10* (1967) 355–366.

[28] Ruzicki, D. A.: Relationship of participation preference and health locus of control in diabetes education. Diabetes Care 7 (1984) 372–377.

[29] Sarason, I. G., J. H. Johnson, J. M. Siegel: Assessing the impact of life changes: Development of the life experiences survey. Journal of Consulting and Clinical Psychology *46* (1978) 932–946.

[30] Schlenk, E. A., L. K. Hart: Relationship between health locus of control, health value and social support and compliance of persons with diabetes mellitus. Diabetes Care *7* (1984) 566–574.

[31] Siegrist, J.: Die Bedeutung von Lebensveränderungen für den Ausbruch einer Krankheit. Med. Klin. *75* (1980) 770–777.

[32] Siegrist, J., K. Dittmann, K. Siegrist et al.: Soziale Belastungen und Herzinfarkt. Enke, Stuttgart 1980.

[33] Slenker, S. E.: Health locus of control of joggers and nonexercisers. Perceptual and Motor Skills *61* (1985) 323–328.

[34] Toeller, M., A. Klischan, W. Schumacher et al.: The Duesseldorf intervention trial in NIDDM patients. Diabetes *40* (1991) (Suppl. 1) 479A.

[35] Toeller, M.: Diätbehandlung, Schulung und Compliance des nicht-insulinbehandelten Typ II-Diabetikers. Diabetespraxis 2 (1986) 2–6.

[36] Toeller, M.: Diabetikerschulung: Ziele, Durchführung und Effizienz. Med. Klin. *81* (1986) 181–186.

[37] Toeller, M.: Mögliche Eigenleistung des Diabetikers in der Behandlung. Eine prospektive Untersuchung bei Typ I-Diabetikern. In: F. Strian, R. Hölzl, M. Haslbeck (Hrsg.): Verhaltensmedizin und Diabetes mellitus, S. 444–455. Springer, Berlin, Heidelberg, New York, London, Paris, Tokyo 1988.

[38] Toeller, M.: Diabetesschulung. Internist *31* (1990) 208–217.

[39] Wallston, K. A., S. A. Maides, B. S. Wallston: Health related information seeking as a function of health-related locus of control and health value. Journal of Research in Personality *10* (1976) 215–222.

[40] Wallston, K. A., B. S. Wallston, G. D. Kaplan et al.: Development and validation of the health locus of control scale (HCL). Journal of Consulting and Clinical Psychology *44* (1976) 580–585.

[41] Williams, G., J. Pickup, H. Keen: Psychological factors and metabolic control: Time for reappraisal. Diabetic Medicine *5* (1988) 211–217.

[42] Wilson, W., D. V. Ary, A. Biglan et al.: Psychosocial predictors of self-care behaviours (compliance) and glycaemic control in non-insulin-dependent diabetes mellitus. Diabetes Care *9* (1986) 614–622.

[43] Wyler, A. R., M. Masuda, T. H. Holmes: Magnitude of life events and seriousness of illness. Psychosomatic Medicine *33* (1971) 115–122.

[44] Zerssen, D. v.: Die Beschwerdenliste als Test. Therapiewoche *21* (1971) 190–1914.

[45] Zerssen, D. v.: Selbstbeurteilungs-Skalen zur Abschätzung des "subjektiven Befundes" in psychopathologischen Querschnitt- und Längsschnitt-Untersuchungen. Arch. Psychiart. Nervenkr. *217* (1973) 299–314.

[46] Zerssen, D. v., D. M. Koeller, E. R. Rey: Die Befindlichkeits-Skala (B-S) – ein einfaches Instrument zur Objektivierung von Befindlichkeitsstörungen, insbesondere im Rahmen von Längsschnitt-Untersuchungen. Arzneimittel-Forsch. *20* (1970) 915–918.

[47] Zielke, M.: Diagnostik in der Psychotherapie, Kohlhammer, Stuttgart 1981.

[48] Zimmermann, M., B. Pfohl, D. Stange: Life events assessment of depressed patients: A comparison of self-report and interview formart. Journal of Human Stress *12* (1986) 13–19.

III Studies with acarbose

Acarbose monotherapy in non-insulin-dependent diabetes mellitus – the German experience

M. Hanefeld

Introduction

Non-insulin-dependent diabetes mellitus (NIDDM) is a common disease in middle-aged sedentary people and the elderly with a steadily increasing prevalence rate in Germany [20] as well as in western European countries.

As shown by the Diabetes Intervention Study (DIS) (Tab. 1) [11, 13] and other epidemiologic investigations [24, 35], NIDDM is associated with a cluster of risk factors and diseases that strongly contribute to the excessive cardiovascular morbidity of these patients [11]. There now exists a bulk of evidence that NIDDM and coronary heart disease are fostered by a common set of risk factors [37]. These risk factors are intricately interrelated and act as a vicious cycle. This led us in 1973 to the concept of the metabolic syndrome (Fig. 1) [10, 14]. From the view point of diabetology, insulin resistance as basal defect became the hallmark

Table 1: Prevalence of coronary risk factors (%) among DIS patients and the general population (Dresden study, n = 1216) [13]

	Type II diabetics	Population	Limits
Hyperlipoproteinemia	17.6	7.6	TG > 2.8 mmol/l and/or Chol. > 7.76 mmol/l
Hypertriglyceridemia	11.3	3.4	
Hypercholesterolemia	3.5	3.7	
Mixed HLP	2.8	0.5	
Hypertension	53.0	17.3	BP > 160/95 mmHg and/or Antihypertensive drugs
Smoking	34.0	30.3	Tobacco > 1 g/day
Obesity	49.0	8.2	IBWI M > 1.2 F > 1.3

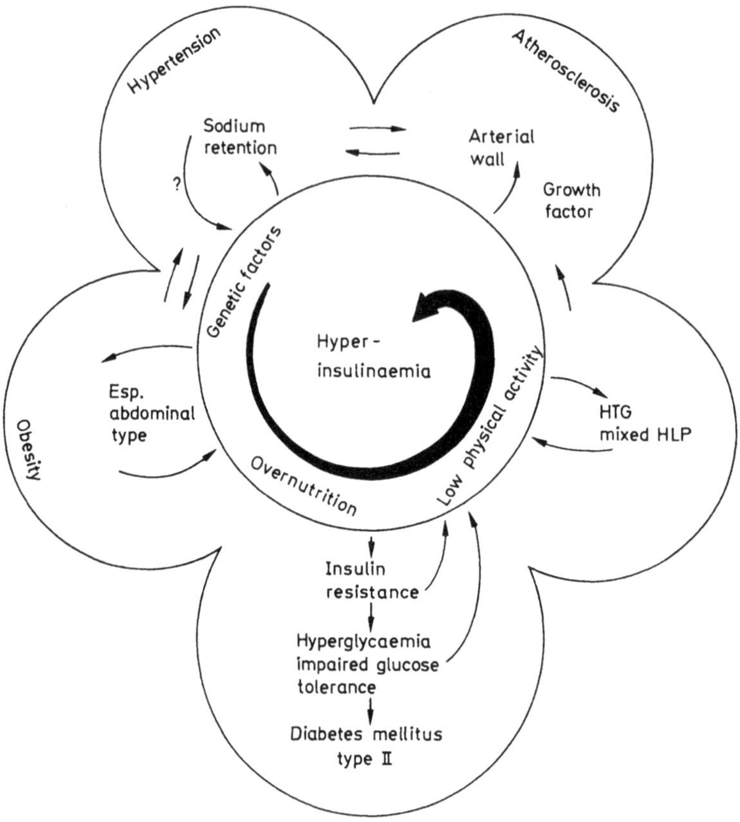

Fig. 1: The metabolic syndrome [14].

of this syndrome [26, 25] which, as Syndrome X, is discussed in detail by Dr. H. Lebovitz in this proceedings volume. On the other hand, recent results of obesity research [3] favor the hypothesis that abdominal obesity with (or due to) disturbances in steroid metabolism is of crucial importance for insulin resistance and development of NIDDM, hypertriglyceridemia and hypertension. Dyslipoproteinemia, in particular anomalies in synthesis, conversion and removal of triglyceride-rich lipoproteins, acts as a risk factor for both NIDDM and cardiovascular diseases [32, 15]. Therefore, the treatment of NIDDM requires an integrated approach with the correction of overweight, dietary advice and regular adequate physical activity of the endurance type as prime measures. Optimal therapy of dyslipoproteinemia and choice of antihypertensive drugs with positive impact on metabolic control are important aids in achieving the goals for acceptable or good metabolic control. Some leading diabetologists argue that with intensified dietary advice by structured education programs and inclusion of modern behaviour modification techniques, better compliance to recommendations for a

Table 2: Distribution of insulin, oral antidiabetic drugs, and diet treatment according to group: The Diabetes Intervention Study, 5-yr follow-up [11]

	Controls (%)	IHE plus placebo (%)	IHE plus clofibric acid (%)
n	329	316	238
Insulin	21 (6.4)	15 (4.7)	9 (3.8)
Oral antidiabetic drugs	156 (47.4)	89 (28.2)*	81 (34.0)*
Diet	152 (46.2)	212 (67.1)*	148 (62.2)*

IHE, intensified health education
* $P < 0.01$ vs. control subjects

healthier lifestyle will dramatically reduce the necessity for oral antidiabetics. The reality in Germany, however, is that still more than 50% of the NIDDM are treated with oral antidiabetics [20]. Currently in the USA nearly 40% of the NIDDM are given sulfonylureas [19].

In a controlled study with newly diagnosed NIDDM [11] that were classified as diet-controlled after a 6-week screening phase with diabetes diet at the 6th year, more than one third of the participants of the intervention trial had to be treated with oral antidiabetics or insulin despite best efforts with intensified health education, in particular comprehensive dietary advice (Tab. 2). Nevertheless, Table 2 demonstrates that intensified health education is a potent tool in reducing drug consumption.

The data of the 8 years follow up (Tab. 3) in the Diabetes Intervention Study confirm both the increasing percentage of treatment with oral antidiabetics with increasing duration of NIDDM and the potentials of health education.

Table 3: Distribution of insulin, oral antidiabetic drugs, and diet treatment according to group: The Diabetes Intervention Study. 8-yr follow-up (preliminary results)

	Controls (%)	Intervention (%)
n	208	461
Insulin	51 (24.5)	68 (14.7)
Oral antidiabetic drugs	111 (53.4)	216 (46.9)
Diet	46 (22.1)	177 (38.4)

Principles of treatment in NIDDM

The goals of treatment in NIDDM are primarily directed at relieving symptoms, improving the quality of life, and avoiding acute complications such as hyperosmolar coma, infectious diseases etc. With increasing life expectancy particularly in patients with an onset of the disease before the age of 65 years, the risk for long term complications such as premature atherosclerosis, nephropathy and retinopathy adds more and more weight to the definition of therapeutic goals. Besides good glucose control and reduction of overweight, correction of dyslipoproteinemia and near to normal adjustment of blood pressure should be given attention to prevent or delay late complications. The European NIDDM Policy Group [1] as well as the American Diabetes Association [27] recommend target levels of metabolic parameters and body mass index for evaluating the adequacy of diabetes control. As recently reviewed by Gerich [8], in the USA, about one third of unselected patients with NIDDM do not achieve satisfactory glycemic control with sulfonylureas.

If we apply these criteria to the patients of the Diabetes Intervention Study treated with (sulfonylureas) glibenclamide (Tab. 4), it becomes obvious that most patients fail to attain good control.

Table 4: Distribution (%) of quality of glucose control by the categories of the NIDDM Policy Group in patients treated with insulin, sulfonylureas, and diet: The Diabetes Intervention Study, 5-yr follow-up [15]

FBG mmol/l	good 4.4 – 6.7	acceptable <7.8	poor >7.8	p
Controls (n = 328)				
Insulin	9.5	4.5	75.7	<0.01
Sulfon.	7.7	14.7	77.6	
Diet	30.5	14.6	55.0	
Intervention (n = 638)				
Insulin	25.9	7.4	66.7	<0.01
Sulfon.	12.2	9.1	78.7	
Diet	34.3	17.6	48.1	

It is of particular interest to look at the quality of metabolic control and level of coronary risk factors of the treatment regimen among NIDDM. As shown with the data of the Diabetes Intervention Study, (Tab. 5) neither good glycaemic control nor correction of risk factors were achieved with sulfonylurea prescription.

Table 5: Distribution (%) of body mass index and triglycerides by the categories of the NIDDM Policy Group in patients treated with insulin, sulfonylureas, and diet: The Diabetes Intervention Study, 5-yr follow-up [15]

	good	acceptable	poor	p
BMI kg/m^2 M/F	<25/<24	<27/<26	>27/>26	
Controls (n = 328)				
Insulin	28.6	14.3	57.1	n. s.
Sulfon.	15.5	23.3	61.3	
Diet	19.2	18.5	62.3	
Intervention (n = 638)				
Insulin	40.7	11.1	48.1	<0.01
Sulfon.	11.7	13.7	74.6	
Diet	17.9	20.3	61.8	
TG mmol/l	<1.7	<2.3	>2.3	
Controls (n = 328)				
Insulin	25.0	35.0	40.0	n. s.
Sulfon.	46.3	18.1	35.6	
Diet	39.5	23.1	37.4	
Intervention (n = 638)				
Insulin	50.0	30.8	19.2	n. s.
Sulfon.	43.0	20.4	36.6	
Diet	45.8	25.4	28.8	

Oral sulfonylureas have held the stage as the leading oral antidiabetics for more than three decades in Germany. Monodrug therapy with biguanides is forbidden in our country due to their association with lactic acidosis. Sulfonylureas primarily enhance insulin secretion and probably, to some degree, insulin sensitivity. However, as demonstrated in the Diabetes Intervention Study data, it is general clinical experience that good glucose control cannot be achieved with these drugs in many patients. Furthermore, the rate of secondary sulfonylurea failure is high. Their prescription frequently causes weight gain and increased plasma triglyceride levels. Hypertriglyceridemia has been shown to be an important independent coronary risk factor in NIDDM [7, 31]!

The most common complication of sulfonylurea treatment is hypoglycemia. In Sweden, the incidence of severe episodes was 0.22/1000 [2]. This is particularly dangerous in the elderly.

Therefore, other approaches to the treatment of NIDDM and the prevention of macroangiopathy are needed.

Acarbose as a first line drug in NIDDM insufficiently treated with diet

Besides peripheral insulin resistance and overproduction of glucose by the liver in the fasting state, NIDDM is characterized by the inability to adequately respond to ingested carbohydrates and glucose load resp., despite long lasting postprandial hyperinsulinemia in most NIDDM. This can be prevented by lowering the absorption of glucose in the small intestine. The terminal digestion of carbohydrates is achieved by alpha-glucosidases at the surface of the brush border of the small bowel. By delaying glucose release from disaccharides, oligosaccharides and complex carbohydrates, intestinal glucosidase inhibitors [23] can adapt glucose increment in the blood to delayed insulin secretion in patients with NIDDM who are being insufficiently treated with diet or sulfonylureas. The primary assumption of intensive research in this field for more than 15 years was that this could be achieved by inhibition of alpha glucosidases [4]. This finally was successful and the BAYER pharmaceutical company was the first to produce a commercially available disaccharidase inhibitor i.e. acarbose (Glucobay®) which has been on the market in Germany since October 1st, 1990.

Acarbose, a pseudotetrasaccharide of microbial origin reversibly inhibits alpha-glucosidases. Its chemical structure is similar to natural carbohydrates and it binds competitively to the saccharidases at the surface of the brush border. Thus, the release of glucose from complex carbohydrates is reduced up to 80% in the upper part of the small bowel [5]. In striking analogy to the mode of action of cholestyramine [9], this should cause a cascade of events:

reduction of postprandial blood glucose increment, diminished stimulation of insulin release, reduction of postprandial hyperinsulinemia, improved insulin sensitivity by correction of hyperglycemia and hyperinsulinemia, and – last, but not least – diminished postprandial triglyceride synthesis in the liver.

Clinical investigations on acarbose as monodrug therapy

Data of clinical trials available so far suggest a 10% reduction of fasting blood glucose and 20% reduction of postprandial blood glucose for monodrug therapy [34]. These pooled data are mainly derived from clinical observation studies without placebo control. Because of its effectiveness in glycemic control and presumed positive impact on insulin resistance and hypertriglyceridemia, acarbose may prove to be a first line drug for patients with mild to moderate type II diabetes.

We therefore evaluated in a randomized placebo controlled double-blind clinical trial the efficacy and safety of acarbose as a first line drug for patients with

NIDDM insufficiently treated with diet alone. Details of this study have been published elsewhere [12].

The patients were 100 consecutive NIDDM from five Dresden outpatient clinics who were considered as candidates for treatment with oral hypoglycaemic agents by their responsible metabolic physician. Great efforts were undertaken to improve dietary compliance. Therefore, in every case a reinforcement of dietary advice was performed before entry in the study by an experienced dietitian. It has to be emphasized that all patients were on diabetes diet, for at least three months before drug treatment was considered. The average diet pretreatment time in an established diabetes clinic for the acarbose treatment group was 70 months. Four subjects had to be excluded because the inclusion criteria concerning blood glucose levels had been broken. One patient did not tolerate acarbose and a second had to be excluded because he was only able to take 100 mg acarbose per day due to gastrointestinal complaints.

Effect on glucose control

Acarbose significantly improved glucose control in the fasting as well as in the postprandial state (Tab. 6). It is remarkable that postprandial hyperglycemia and

Table 6: Blood glucose fasting, 1 h pp, and HbA_1 after 24 week treatment with acarbose (n = 47) or placebo (n = 47). Adjusted mean values (Study BAYg 5421/0620)

	Acarbose	Placebo	p
Blood glucose (mmol/l)			
fasting	8.5	9.6	<0.01
1 h pp	10.5	13.5	<0.01
HbA_1 (%)	8.68	9.29	<0.01

hyperinsulinemia can be reduced for at least five hours after a test meal (Fig. 2). A smoothing effect on circadian glucose levels has been described by Willms [36]. The persistent improvement of glycaemic control is confirmed by significant reduction of HbA_1. As shown in Figure 3, acarbose was most effective in patients with poor HbA_1 values. Out of 13 patients in the acarbose group with HbA_1 > 10% at the beginning, only three did not reach acceptable HbA_1 values at the 24th week. In contrast, in the placebo group at the 24th week, only one of 13 had achieved acceptable values.

Effect on C-peptide and insulin

Fasting insulin concentrations remained unchanged during the observation period. Postprandial insulin, however, was significantly lower at the 24th week of acarbose treatment. Fasting and postprandial C-peptide levels exhibited no significant changes [12].

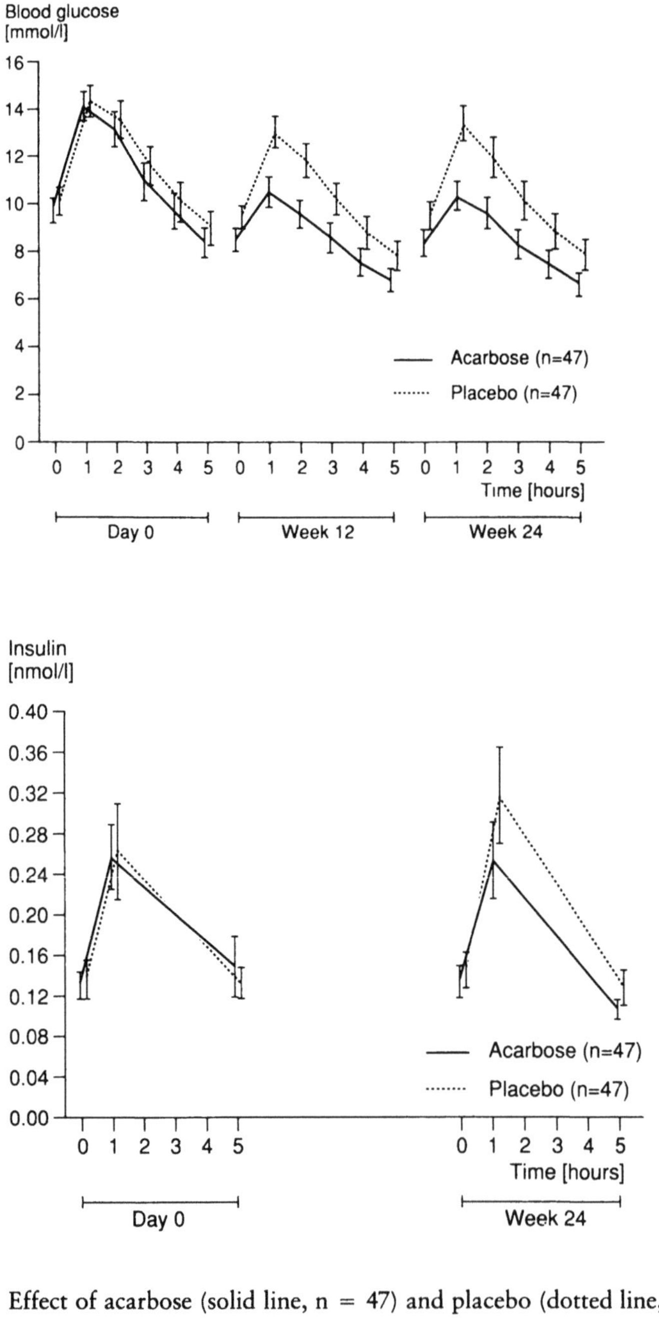

Fig. 2: Effect of acarbose (solid line, n = 47) and placebo (dotted line, n = 47) on: blood glucose and insulin concentrations; fasting postprandial levels after a test meal (means with 95 % confidence limits) [12].

With respect to postprandial insulin increment, a significantly lower increase was seen after a test meal in the acarbose treated group (Δ IRI 0.095 nM) versus the placebo group (Δ IRI 0.135 nM $p < 0.05$). Fasting level was 0.11 nM in each group. This finding is in accordance with previously published data in the literature [28, 29].

The lower increment in postprandial insulin should be the consequence of lower postprandial glucose enhancement. This, however, does not explain the reduction in fasting blood glucose at the same level of C-peptide and serum insulin.

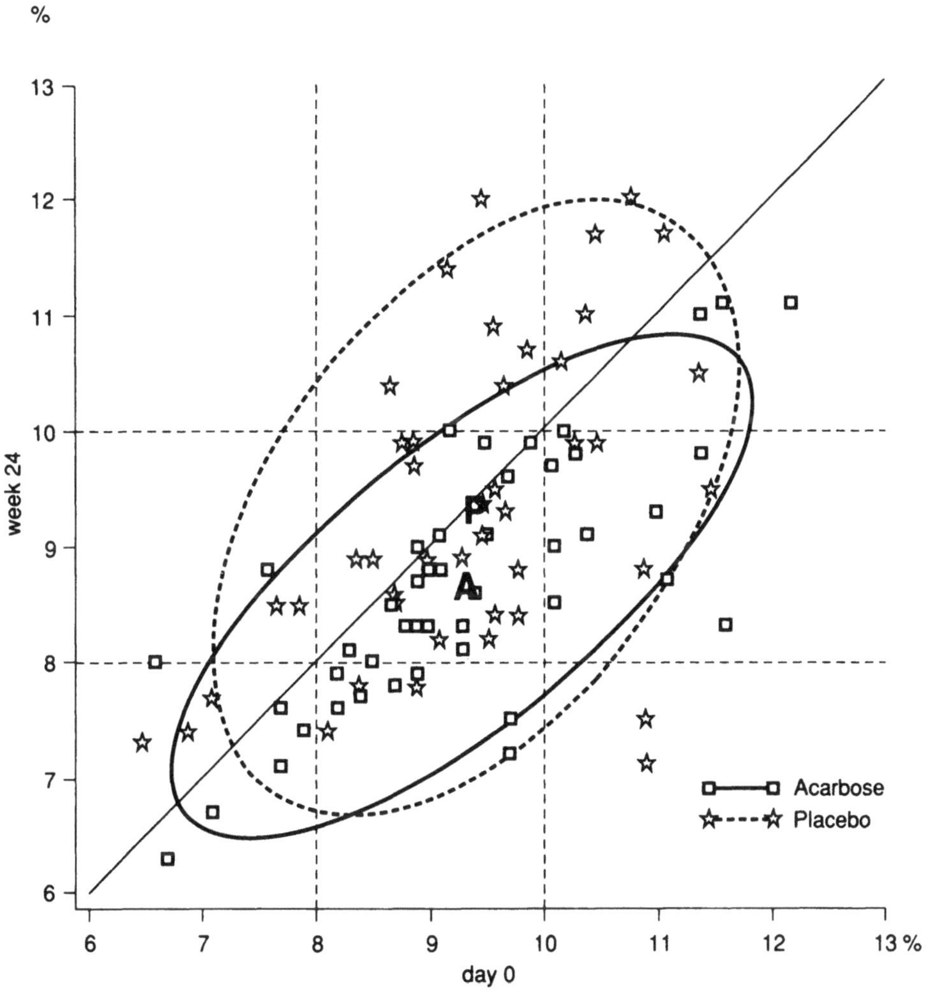

Fig. 3: Effect of acarbose on hemoglobin A_1 concentration versus placebo, correlation plot with concentration ellipsoid on day 0 versus concentration after 24 weeks treatment (Study BAY g 5421/0620).

By extrapolation this can be interpreted as indicative of improved peripheral insulin action. Hyperglycemia is of prime importance for the action of insulin. According to the concept of "glucotoxicity", impaired β-cells responses recover when fasting blood concentration is reduced in NIDDM [6]. Even more important, peripheral insulin sensitivity is improved if circadian glucose levels are reduced to near normal by substantial reduction of weight [17, 16] or intensified insulin treatment [33]. Our data suggest that peripheral insulin resistance, a hallmark of NIDDM, is down regulated by acarbose via reduced circadian levels of glucose and postprandial hyperinsulinemia resp.

Effect on blood lipids

Acarbose has no effect on major cholesterol fractions e.g. LDL-cholesterol and HDL-cholesterol. However, in the present study, the one hour postprandial hypertriglyceridemia was significantly reduced (Tab. 7). Since FFA levels remained unaffected by acarbose intake, this is probably due to diminished hepatic triglyceride synthesis by lower levels of insulin.

Steiner and Vranic [32] have shown that insulin level significantly contributes to hepatic VLDL-triglyceride production. This assumption is supported by investigations by Nestel [21] on the impact of acarbose on triglyceride kinetics. In healthy normolipidemic men, acarbose significantly reduced VLDL-triglyceride production in the liver.

Triglycerides have been proven to be an independent risk factor for coronary heart disease in NIDDM [31, 7, 15]. There is accumulating evidence that the increase in postprandial triglyceride-rich-lipoproteins, in particular the so called remnants of chylomicron and VLDL-catabolism, is highly atherogenic.

Effect on energy balance and dietary behaviour

In accordance with long-term clinical experience, body weight was not reduced by acarbose intake [5]. Calorie consumption and food composition remained unaffected. Even more, the patients learned that eating sucrose and other disaccharides enhances gastrointestinal side effects. Thus, acarbose to some degree may help to improve diet compliance.

Side-effects

The most frequently reported adverse effects were flatulence, meteorism and diarrhea. However, as previously mentioned, only one patient dropped out

Table 7: Effect of acarbose on triglycerides, total cholesterol, and fibrinogen [12]

	Acarbose (n = 47)		Placebo (n = 46)		
	week 0	week 24	week 0	week 24	p*
Triglycerides (mmol/l)+ fasting	2.2 (1.2 – 4.1)	1.8 (1.0 – 3.3)	2.1 (1.3 – 3.3)	1.9 (1.1 – 3.2)	0.11
1 hr postprandial	2.4 (1.4 – 4.2)	1.9 (1.1 – 3.3)	2.2 (1.5 – 3.3)	2.2 (1.5 – 3.2)	<0.01
5 hr postprandial	2.3 (1.3 – 4.0)	2.0 (1.3 – 3.3)	2.2 (1.5 – 3.3)	2.2 (1.5 – 3.2)	0.20
Total cholesterol (mmol/l)	5.7 (4.6 – 6.9)	5.8 (4.9 – 6.7)	5.8 (4.9 – 6.8)	6.0 (4.7 – 7.3)	0.39
Fibrinogen (g/l)	3.2 (2.2 – 4.3)	2.9 (2.2 – 3.6)	3.1 (2.4 – 3.9)	2.8 (2.4 – 3.3)	0.67

* Test results for group comparison concerning changes from wk 0 to wk 24

+ Values in geometric means

because of gastrointestinal complaints. In general the percentage of patients who cannot tolerate the drug is below 3% [5]. In our study [12], 78% of the patients in the acarbose group as well as 28% in the placebo group suffered from flatulence during the first four weeks of treatment with 100 mg acarbose thrice daily. After that time the frequency of side-effects steadily decreased.

Thus, in the 24th week, only 31% had minor complaints. Enzymatic adaptation in the small bowel might lead to a reduction of side-effects. Adaptation of the colonic bacterial flora to increased inflow of carbohydrates may further contribute to the relief of complaints.

Diarrhea was reported in 14% of cases with no clear time related tendendy to disappear. A more detailed dietary history revealed that the major reasons for diarrhea are preexisting enteritis, excessive intake of disaccharides and consumption of dietary foods containing sugar alcohols as sweeteners. No symptoms of hypoglycemia were observed. Considering the mode of action, reduction of hyperinsulinemia inclusive, this should not be expected with acarbose monodrug therapy. Liver enzymes such as GPT, GOT and gamma-glytamyltransferase were not affected by acarbose.

Comparative investigations with sulfonylureas and biguanides

In Germany glibenclamide is the dominating oral hypoglycemic drug. Two studies [18, 30] have been published comparing acarbose and glibenclamide as monodrug therapy in patients with NIDDM insufficiently treated with diet alone. Both do not include a placebo group, both were multicenter open clinical trials. In the study published by Hoffmann [18], 95 patients in five private practices insufficiently treated with diet alone were randomly allocated to 3 × 100 mg acarbose daily or 3.5 mg glibenclamide once, twice or trice daily. In the study by Spengler [30], 72 NIDDM were treated according to that design for 24 weeks with either acarbose or glibenclamide. The results were very consistent: acarbose and glibenclamide had comparable blood glucose lowering efficacy. In the study by Hoffmann [18], HbA_1 decreased from 10.7 to 7.5% and from 10.8 to 7.6% following treatment with acarbose and glibenclamide resp. The corresponding values in the study by Spengler [30] were 10.8% to 8.5% and 11.0% to 8.7% after treatment with acarbose and glibenclamide resp. In acarbose-treated patients, gastrointestinal complaints (14 out of 48) was the major adverse effect; and in the glibenclamide group, symptoms of hypoglycemia (9 out of 47) were the major adverse effects [18]. No comparative investigations with biguanides were performed in Germany since monotherapy with this group of oral hypoglycemic agents is not allowed by the national authorities. In the international literature only scarce information exists about comparative studies [22]. By extrapolation these preliminary data suggest that acarbose is at least as effective as biguanides.

Summary and conclusions

Acarbose proved to be an effective and safe non-systemic drug for the treatment of NIDDM insufficiently treated with diet alone. In comparison with sulfonylureas it has the advantage of reducing postprandial hyperinsulinemia and postprandial hypertriglyceridemia, two hormonal-metabolic abnormalities which are considered to contribute to excessive and accelerated atherogenesis in type II diabetes. Lower levels of fasting and postprandial blood glucose together with reduced postprandial insulin levels suggest a down regulation of peripheral insulin resistance. No serious side-effects have been reported so far. In contrast to sulphonylureas, acarbose monotherapy cannot provoke hypoglycemic attacks. Therefore, it should be considered as a first line drug in NIDDM patients who cannot longer be controlled with diet alone (Fig. 4).

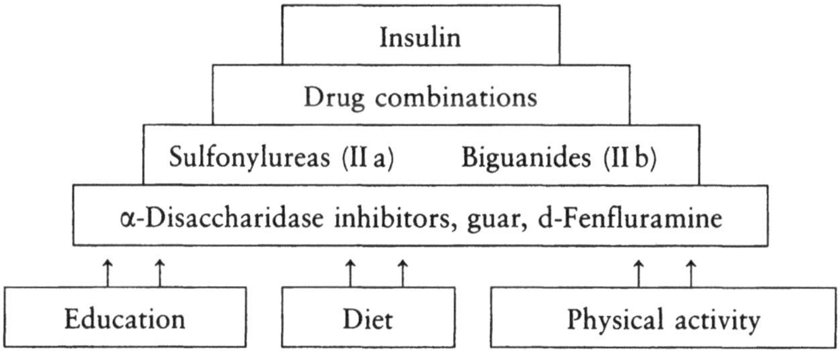

Fig. 4: Stepwise treatment of NIDDM.

References

[1] Alberti, K., F. Gries: Management of non-insulin-dependent diabetes mellitus in Europe: a consensus view. Diabetic Med. *5* (1988) 275–281.

[2] Berger, W.: Incidence of severe side-effects during therapy with sulfonylureas and biguanides. Horm. Metab. Res. *17* Suppl. 15 (1985) 111–115.

[3] Björntorp, P.: Obesity and diabetes. In: K. G. M. M. Alberti, L. P. Krall (eds.): The diabetes annual 5, pp. 373–395. Elsevier, New York 1990.

[4] Caspary, W. F., S. Graf: Inhibition of human intestinal alpha-glucosidehydrolases by new complex oligosaccharide. Res. Exp. Med. *175* (1979) 1–6.

[5] Clissold, S. P., C. Edwards: Acarbose, a preliminary review of its pharmacodynamic and pharmacokinetic properties, and therapeutic potential. Drugs *35* (1988) 214–243.

[6] Ferner, R., M. D. Rawlins, K. G. M. Alberti: Impaired β-cell responses improve when fasting blood glucose concentration is reduced in non-insulin-dependent diabetes. Q. J. Med. *66* (1988) 137–146.

[7] Fontbonne, A., E. Eschwege, F. Cambien et al.: Hypertriglyceridaemia as a risk factor of coronary heart disease mortality in subjects with impaired glucose tolerance or diabetes. Results from the 11-year follow-up of the Paris Prospective Study. Diabetologia *32* (1989) 300–304.

[8] Gerich, J. E.: Oral hypoglycemic agents. New England J. Med. *321* (1989) 1231–1245.

[9] Goldstein, J. L., Brown, M. S.: Receptor regulation: New approach to the therapy of hypercholesterolemia. In: L. A. Carlson, A. G. Olsson (eds.): Treatment of hyperlipoproteinemia, pp. 103–108. Raven Press, New York 1984.

[10] Hanefeld, M.: Thesis. Untersuchungen über Wechselbeziehungen zwischen Lipidstoffwechsel und Leberkrankheiten, pp. 191–192. Medical Academy "C. G. Carus", Dresden 1973.

[11] Hanefeld, M., S. Fischer, J. Schmechel et al.: Diabetes Intervention Study. Multiintervention trial in newly diagnosed NIDDM. Diabetes Care *14* (1991) 308–317.

[12] Hanefeld, M., S. Fischer, J. Schulze et al.: Therapeutical potentials of acarbose as first line drug in non-insulin-dependent diabetes insufficiently treated with diet alone. Diabetes Care *14* (1991) 732–737.

[13] Hanefeld, M., H. Haller, J. Schulze et al.: Die Diabetesinterventionsstudie (DIS) – eine multizentrische Multiinterventionsstudie bei Typ II-Diabetikern. I. Mitteilung. Dtsch. Gesundheitswes. *39* (1984) 1889–1894.

[14] Hanefeld, M., W. Leonhardt: Das metabolische Syndrom. Dtsch. Gesundheitswes. *36* (1981) 545–551.

[15] Hanefeld, M., H. Schmechel, U. Julius et al.: Five year incidence of coronary heart disease in relation to major risk factors and quality of metabolic control in newly diagnosed non-insulin dependent diabetes: The Diabetes Intervention Study. NMCD – Nutr. Metab. Cardiovasc. Dis. *1* (1991) 135–140.

[16] Hanefeld, M., M. Weck: Very low calorie diet therapy in obese non-insulin dependent diabetes patients. Int. J. Obesity *13* (Suppl. 2) (1989) 33–37.

[17] Henry, R. R., G. Brechtel, K. Griver: Secretion and hepatic extraction of insulin after weight loss in obese non-insulin-dependent diabetes mellitus. J. Clin. Endocrinol. Metab. *66* (1988) 979–986.

[18] Hoffmann, J.: Acarbose und Glibenclamid bei Typ-II-Diabetes. Eine Vergleichstudie zu Wirksamkeit und Nebenwirkungen. Münchner Med. Wschr. *132* (1990) 49–51.

[19] Kennedy, D. L., J. M. Piper, C. Baum: Trends in the use of hypoglycemic agents, 1964–1986. Diabetes Care *11* (1988) 558–562.

[20] Michaelis, D., E. Jutzi: Epidemiologie des Diabetes mellitus in der DDR-Bevölkerung. Alters- und geschlechtsspezifische Inzidenz- und Prävalenztrends im Zeitraum 1960–1987. Z. Klin. Med. *46* (1991) 59–64.

[21] Nestel, P. J.: Lower triglyceride production with carbohydrate-rich diet during treatment with acarbose. In: W. Creutzfeldt (ed.): Acarbose for the treatment of diabetes

mellitus. 2nd International Symposium on Acarbose, Berlin/Germany, November 12. – 14., 1987, p. 68. Springer-Verlag, Berlin 1988.
[22] Pagano, G., P. Cavallo-Perin: Glucosidase-inhibitors and biguanides in the treatment of non-insulin dependent diabetic patients. Diab. Nutr. Metab. *3* (Suppl. 1) (1990) 69 – 76.
[23] Puls, W., H. Bischoff, H. Schutt: Pharmacology of amylase- and glucosidase-inhibitors. In: W. Creutzfeldt, U. R. Fölsch (eds.): Delaying absorption as a therapeutical principle in metabolic diseases, pp. 70 – 78. Stuttgart – New York 1983.
[24] Pyöräla, K., M. Laakso, M. Uusitupa: Diabetes and atherosclerosis: an independent epidemiologic view. Diabetes Metab. Rev. *3* (1987) 463 – 524.
[25] Reaven, G. M.: Role of insulin resistance in human disease. Diabetes *37* (1988) 1595 – 1607.
[26] Reaven, G. M., M. S. Greenfeld: Diabetes hypertriglyceridemia. Evidence for three clinical syndromes. Diabetes *30* (Suppl. 2) (1981) 66 – 75.
[27] Rifkin, H. (ed.): Physician's guide to non-insulin-dependent (type II) diabetes: diagnosis and treatment. 2nd ed. Alexandria, Va.: American Diabetes Association 1988.
[28] Sachse, G., B. Willms: Effect of the alpha-glucosidase inhibitor Bay g 5421 on blood glucose control of sulphonylurea-teated diabetrics. Diabetologia *17* (1979) 287 – 290.
[29] Scott, R. S., R. L. Knowles, D. W. Reaven: Treatment of poorly controlled non-insulin dependent diabetic patients with acarbose. Aust. N. J. Med. *14* (1984) 649 – 654.
[30] Spengler, M., G. Hänsel, K. Boehme: Acarbose und Glibenclamid bei Typ-II-Diabetes. Z. für Allgemeinmedizin *66* (1990) 606 – 610.
[31] Standl, E. L., H. Stiegler, H. U. Janka et al.: Risk profiles of macrovascular disease in diabetes mellitus. Diab. Metab. *14* (1988) 505 – 511.
[32] Steiner, G., M. Vranic: Hyperinsulinemia and hypertriglyceridemia, a vicious cycle with atherogenic potential. Intern. J. Obesity 6 (Suppl. 1) (1982) 117 – 124.
[33] Taskinen, M. R., T. Kuusi, E. Helve et al.: Insulin therapy induces antiatherogenic changes of serum lipoproteins in non-insulin-dependent diabetes. Atherosclerosis *8* (1988) 168 – 177.
[34] Tuomilehto, J.: Acarbose monotherapy in the treatment of non-insulin-dependent diabetes mellitus – a review. In: W. Creutzfeldt (ed.): Acarbose for the treatment of diabetes mellitus. 2nd International Symposium on Acarbose, Berlin/Germany, November 12 – 14, 1987, pp. 104 – 116. Springer-Verlag, Berlin 1988.
[35] Uusitupa, M. J., L. K. Niskanen, O. Siitonen et al.: 5-year incidence of atherosclerotic vascular disease in relation to general risk factors, insulin level, and abnormalities in lipoprotein composition in non-insulin-dependent diabetic and nondiabetic subjects. Circulation *82* (1990) 27 – 36.
[36] Willms, B.: Acarbose in non-insulin-dependent diabetes mellitus: Short-term studies in combination with oral agents. In: W. Creutzfeldt (ed.): Acarbose for the treatment of diabetes mellitus. 2nd International Symposium on Acarbose, Berlin/Germany, November 12 – 14, 1987, pp. 79 – 91. Springer-Verlag, Berlin 1988.
[37] Wilson, P. W. F., W. B. Kannel, K. M. Anderson: Lipids, glucose intolerance and vascular disease: the Framingham study. In: R. W. James, D. Pometta (eds.): Dyslipoproteinaemias and Diabetes, pp. 1 – 11. Karger, Basel 1985.

Acarbose in non-insulin-dependent diabetes mellitus: combination with sulfonylureas and interaction with diet

B. Willms

Combination with sulfonylureas

Acarbose was first evaluated in combination with sulfonylureas [5]. The aim of this type of treatment was to improve the control of diabetes in patients with imminent secondary failure of sulfonylureas, especially in those who are reluctant to change to insulin.

Indication

In most sulfonylurea treated type II diabetic patients the combination with acarbose is – besides diet, exercise, and weight control – the only choice they have due to the long list of contraindications to biguanides. The majority of type II diabetic patients are rather old where an age-dependent decrease in glomerular filtration rate or a "liability to cardiac failure" is common. Both conditions are contraindications to biguanides listed in the drug record of metformin in Germany. Even old age itself (more than 65 years) is listed as contraindication.

Acarbose has a lot of side-effects due to the delay of the absorption of carbohydrates. Some carbohydrates reach the colon and are fermented by colonic bacteria to CO_2 and H_2 resulting in meteorism and flatulence. But life threatening side-effects of acarbose are not known and therefore acarbose is licensed for diabetes in general without major contraindications.

Short-term study

More than 10 years ago [10] we showed the effectiveness of acarbose in the treatment of type II diabetes. We studied acarbose in 12 sulfonylurea-treated type II diabetic patients. Acarbose (6 × 50 mg), given in a double-blind crossover experiment for a period of 7 days, lowered the mean and the maximal blood glucose concentration, the integrated blood glucose response, and the amplitude of glycemic excursions (Fig. 1).

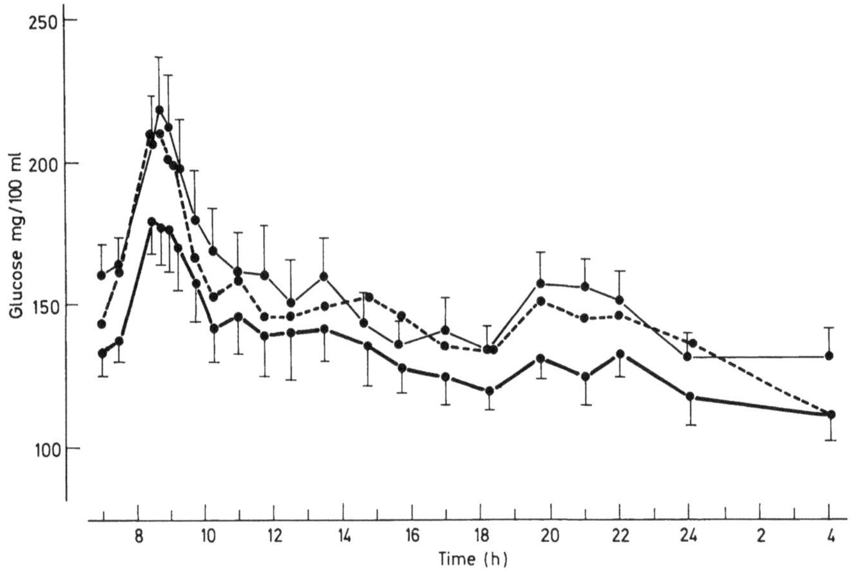

Fig. 1: Mean diurnal blood glucose values of 12 sulfonylurea-treated diabetics before treatment (thin solid line) and after 7 days of therapy with acarbose (thick solid line) or placebo (dotted line). The bars represent 1 SD.

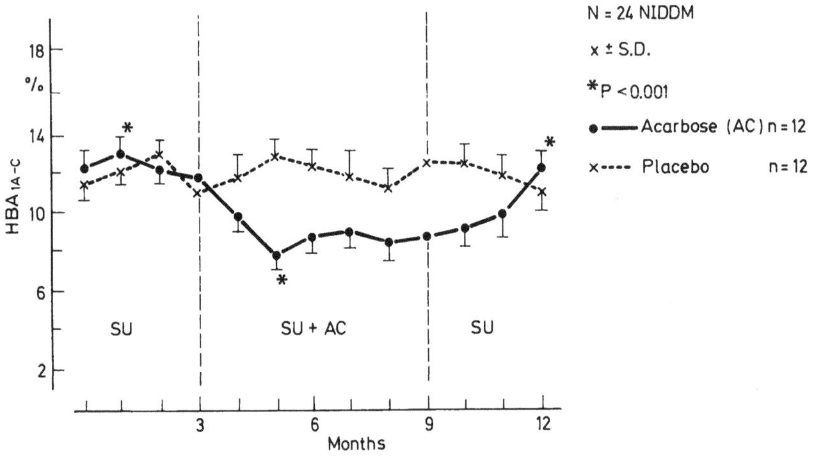

Fig. 2: Effect of acarbose on HbA_{1A-C} levels in NIDDM treated with sulfonylurea.

Long-term study

Sachse et al. [11] later (1982) studied the long-term efficacy of acarbose in combination with sulfonylureas. After a 3-month pretreatment period, 24 sulfonylurea-treated patients received acarbose in addition (3 × 100 mg daily) or placebo for 6 months. Only patients with postprandial blood glucose values of more than 200 mg/100 ml were included in the study.

Acarbose significantly lowered the postprandial blood glucose values, the mean daily blood-glucose values and the HbA_1 values (Fig. 2). Fasting blood glucose, serum insulin, blood lipids and body weight did not change during the study period. In the placebo group there was no significant change in the entire 12 months. The side-effects, flatulence and meteorism, subsided after 4 weeks and did not recur again during the rest of the experimental period.

Vierhapper et al. [15] described a waning of the acarbose effect in type II diabetes during prolonged treatment.

Long-term crossover study

We extended and varied the original study by Sachse et al. [11] from 1982. We treated 14 sulfonylurea-treated type II diabetic patients with acarbose who had been admitted to our hospital due to poor control of their diabetes. The drug was administered individually according to efficacy and tolerability between 300 and 600 mg daily (mean 414 ± 146 mg). Acarbose was given in addition to glibenclamide for 3 months, followed by a placebo period of 3 months, and then was given again for 3 months. All patients checked their blood glucose with a memory glucometer before and after breakfast and supper. HbA_{1c} was measured at the end of the 3 periods and could nearly be normalized by the additional treatment with acarbose (Fig. 3). Home blood glucose monitoring showed an improvement of the mean blood glucose concentration and the postprandial blood glucose differences. The preprandial blood glucose values before breakfast and supper were not influenced by acarbose. Glycosuria was also decreased.

The effect of acarbose on diabetes control was reproducible in both test periods. No loss of efficacy during the test periods was observed.

The effect of acarbose on the HbA_{1c} value can be estimated by comparison of the placebo period with both acarbose periods: acarbose decreased HbA_{1c} by 0,5 resp. 0,7%. The decrease from the intial value (8,5%) to the value at the end of the first acarbose period (6,5%) therefore, is mainly due to our teaching and dieting program. Thus, teaching and intensive dieting is more effective than acarbose alone.

In this study acarbose was well tolerated. The hematological and biochemical safety parameters as well as pulse and blood pressure showed no adverse reac-

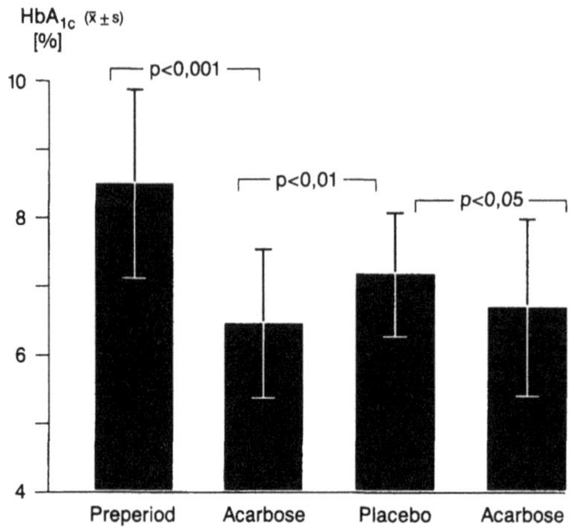

Fig. 3: HbA_{1c} values in NIDDM treated with sulfonylureas at the time of the admission to hospital (preperiod), after 3 months treatment with sulfonylureas and acarbose, after 3 months with sulfonylureas and placebo and again after 3 months treatment with sulfonylureas and acarbose.

tions. No improvement in lipid metabolism (cholesterol and triglyceride concentrations) could be observed. Body weight did not decrease. Meteorism and flatulence were frequently observed, but decreased during the study in frequency and intensity without loss of the antidiabetic efficacy of acarbose.

Thus, acarbose is an effective, well tolerated drug in type II diabetic patients who are not adequately controlled with diet and sulfonylureas alone.

Interaction with diet

The dietary therapy of diabetic patients has mainly two goals: to beneficially influence the control of diabetes and to prevent atherosclerosis which threatens diabetics more than non-diabetics.

Carbohydrate content

For this reason different diabetes associations [1, 2, 3, 4, 6, 7] have recommended a low fat content of the diet and – as the protein content should also be kept low – a corresponding high carbohydrate content (Tab. 1). According to these recommendations the carbohydrate content of the diet should be 50–60% of total calories.

Table 1: Dietary recommendations for diabetic patients

Diabetes association	Year	Carbohydrates %	Fat %	Protein %
American Diabetes Association	1979	50 – 60	max. 30	12 – 20
British Diabetes Association	1980	50	35	
Canadian Diabetes Association	1984	50	30	
American Diabetes Association	1986	55 – 60	max. 30	0,8 g/kg
Diabetes and Nutrition Study Group of the EASD	1987	50 – 60	25 – 30	
Deutsche Diabetes-Gesellschaft	1990	50	35	15

Acarbose has been studied with different amounts of carbohydrates in the diet of non-diabetics and in type II diabetic patients. Seiberling et al. [12] demonstrated in non-diabetics a decrease of the postprandial blood glucose increase after breakfast and supper (not after lunch) with diets containing 60% carbohydrates as well as 43% carbohydrates. The dose of acarbose used was 3 × 200 mg per day.

Oerter et al. [9] studied the efficacy of 3 × 100 mg of acarbose in type II diabetic patients. The postprandial blood glucose increase after breakfast was significantly decreased in patients eating a diet of 55% carbohydrates as well as with those eating a diet of 40% carbohydrates. When the carbohydrate content of the diet was lowered to 25%, the postprandial blood glucose increase was so small that no additional acarbose effect could be demonstrated.

Thus, acarbose is effective for patients eating diets with a recommended high (50 – 60%) carbohydrate content as well as for patients eating a diet with a moderate carbohydrate content of just 40%.

Dietary fibre

One argument against acarbose that is often raised is that a modern diabetic diet which is rich in dietary fibre and slowly absorbable carbohydrates with a low glycemic index is as effective as enzymatic inhibition of carbohydrate absorption. Therefore we studied the effects of a muesli and α-glucosidase inhibition. This has been studied both with miglitol (BAY m 1099) [13] and with acarbose [14].

The postprandial blood glucose increase was significantly lower after the dietary fibre rich muesli than after a standard breakfast consisting of bread and marmalade. However, addition of the α-glucosidase inhibitor further decreased the postprandial blood glucose rise significantly. Addition of the α-glucosidase inhibitor to the muesli did not further decrease the postprandial blood glucose values compared to those with bread and α-glucosidase inhibitor.

Thus pharmacological delay of carbohydrate absorption by α-glucosidase inhibition is even more effective in decreasing postprandial blood glucose concentration than a diet with fewer refined carbohydrates, low glycemic index, and rich in dietary fibre.

Of course, we would not recommend that all our type II diabetic patients take an α-glucosidase inhibitor instead of following a diabetic diet. But some, especially older patients, may have problems with a modern diabetic diet, partly due to intestinal side effects and partly due to chewing problems caused by their "third teeth". For these patients acarbose may be an alternative.

Milk and milk products in the diabetic diet

Acarbose does not inhibit the β-glucosidase lactase and therefore should not inhibit the absorption of lactose. It has been argued that acarbose is an ineffective drug for diabetics consuming high amounts of milk and milk products. On the other hand, milk is very useful for us as it supplies calcium and helps preventing osteoporosis.

To study the interaction of acarbose with milk and milk products in the diet, we tested the blood glucose increase after a breakfast consisting of milk and yoghurt and compared this to a standard breakfast of bread and marmalade. Both breakfasts were given in random order with and without 200 mg of acarbose. The composition of the breakfast meals is shown in Table 2.

12 type II diabetic patients participated in this study. Their mean age was 57 years, mean duration of diabetes 8 years, mean height 170,8 cm, and mean weight 87,4 kg. Thus all were overweight. Two were treated with diet alone, 10 with diet and glibenclamide. Their diet contained in average 1278 Kcal with 141 g of carbohydrates.

Table 2: Composition of the breakfast meals

1. Standard breakfast
   - 50 g graham bread (wheat)
   - 10 g margarine
   - 60 g white cheese
   - 25 g marmalade with fructose
   - 269,8 Kcal (1128,4 KJ)
   - 33,3 g carbohydrates
     - 18,0 g starch
     - 11,4 g fructose
     - 1,9 g lactose
     - 1,5 g saccharose
     - 0,5 g glucose
   - 12,3 g protein
   - 8,7 g fat
   - 3,2 g dietary fibre

2. Yoghurt milk breakfast
   - 150 g Ehrmann diet yoghurt
   - 400 g milk, 3,5 g fat/100 ml
   - 373,5 Kcal (1562,9 KJ)
   - 29,5 g carbohydrates
     - 1,5 g fructose
     - 23,0 g lactose
     - 2,5 g saccharose
     - 2,5 g glucose
     - no starch
   - 18,7 g protein
   - 18,4 g fat
   - 0,0 g dietary fibre

The results are shown in Table 3 and Figure 4. 200 mg of acarbose significantly decreased the postprandial blood glucose increase after the standard breakfast with bread and marmalade. The blood glucose increase after the milk yoghurt breakfast was, as expected, not influenced by acarbose. But the blood glucose increase after the milk yoghurt breakfast was, on the other end, significantly lower than the postprandial blood glucose increase after bread and marmalade. The glycemic index of milk is only 50% compared to that of bread and marmalade. The postprandial blood glucose after milk and yoghurt is the same as after bread and marmalade with acarbose.

Acarbose is ineffective after consumption of milk and milk products, but this is meaningless, as the glycemic index of milk is much lower than that of bread and marmalade.

Table 3: Maximal blood glucose concentrations (max), time of the maximum (T max), postprandial difference (Δ pp) and area under the curve (AUC) after a standard breakfast, a milk yoghurt breakfast, a standard breakfast with 200 mg acarbose and a milk yoghurt breakfast with 200 mg acarbose.
n = 12, given are mean and SEM.

	Standard breakfast	Milk yoghurt, breakfast	Standard breakfast + 200 mg acarbose	Milk yoghurt breakfast + 200 mg acarbose
max	245.7	205.7***	191.6***	204.2***
(mg/dl × min)	± 12.1	± 12.2	± 13.5	± 13.2
T max	68.8	63.8	68.8	67.5
(min pp)	± 2.9	± 7.2	± 5.4	± 10.8
Δ pp	96.1	50.2***	35.4***	52.5***
(mg/dl)	± 8.3	± 5.8	± 3.8	± 7.4
AUC	7792.5	3433.1**	2114.4***	3295.6**
(mg/dl × min)	± 1083.4	± 707.7	± 646.8	± 1196.2

** $p < 0.01$ compared to standard breakfast
*** $p < 0.001$ compared to standard breakfast

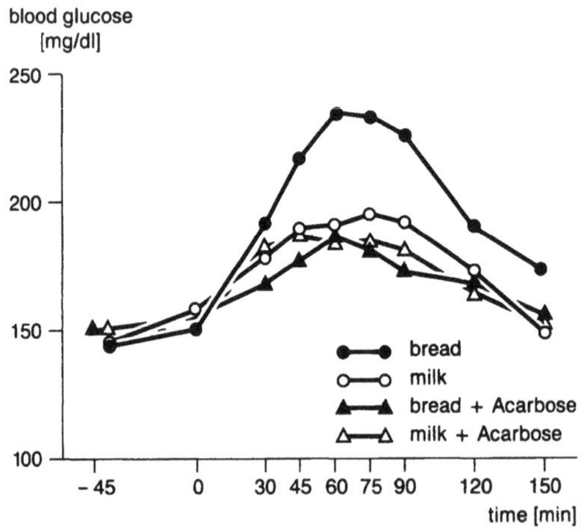

Fig. 4: Postprandial blood glucose increase in NIDDM after a standard breakfast (bread and marmalade), a milk yoghurt breakfast and both breakfasts with 200 mg acarbose. n = 12.

Saccharose

Table 4 shows recommendations of different associations concerning the consumption of saccharose for diabetic patients [1, 2, 6, 7]. It can be seen that the strict rejection of the consumption of saccharose has been weakened during the years (with exception of the Deutsche Diabetes-Gesellschaft). To evaluate the effect of saccharose and fructose and the interaction of acarbose with these sugars, we studied the effect of a breakfast marmalade with 30 g saccharose in comparison to a breakfast marmalade with 30 g fructose and the effect of 3 × 100 mg acarbose on these diets.

Table 4: Dietary recommendations for diabetic patients concerning saccharose

Association	Year	Recommendation
American Diabetes Association	1979	Glucose and glucose-containing disaccharides (sucrose, lactose) are restricted
American Diabetes Association	1986	In some individuals, modest amounts of sucrose and other refined sugars may be acceptable, contingent to metabolic control and body weight
Diabetes and Nutrition Study Group, EASD	1988	... suggest that total intake of added sucrose is limited to 30 g/l
Deutsche Diabetes-Gesellschaft	1990	Diabetic patients are principally advised to avoid saccharose and the consumption of low molecular carbohydrates

8 type II diabetic patients with a mean age of 67 years and a mean duration of diabetes of 6,3 years participated in this study. All were treated with diet and glibenclamide. Their mean height was 162,5 cm, their mean weight 74,6 kg. They had a diet of 1270 kcal with 141 g carbohydrates. In random order they consumed for breakfast a strawberry marmalade which contained, besides the carbohydrates of the fruit an additional 30 g saccharose and 30 g fructose respectively. Both breakfasts were evaluated with a treatment of 3 × 100 mg acarbose. A blood glucose profile was taken on the fourth day of treatment.

The results are given in Table 5 and Figure 5.

The results show that the blood glucose increase after the breakfast with marmalade containing saccharose was significantly higher than after the breakfast with marmalade containing fructose. 100 mg acarbose given at the breakfast meals, could decrease the blood glucose increase after saccharose significantly. Also, the blood glucose increase after the breakfast with marmalade containing

Table 5: Maximal blood glucose concentrations (max) and postprandial difference (Δ pp) after a breakfast with saccharose containing marmalade, a breakfast with fructose containing marmalade, a breakfast with saccharose containing marmalade and 100 mg acarbose and a breakfast with fructose containing marmalade and 100 mg acarbose. The marmalade contained per portion 30 g added saccharose resp. 30 g added fructose (n = 8, given are mean and SEM).

	Saccharose marmalade	Fructose marmalade	Saccharose marmalade + 100 mg acarbose	Fructose marmalade + 100 mg acarbose
Max (mg/dl)	292 ± 19.6	256* ± 19.6	217*** ± 14.8	223** ± 16.0
Δ pp (mg/dl)	131 ± 13.0	100 ± 11.6	63*** ± 12.0	62** ± 13.1

*** $p < 0.001$ in comparision to the saccharose containing marmalade
* $p < 0.05$ in comparison to the saccharose containing marmalade
** $p < 0.05$ in comparison to the fructose containing marmalade

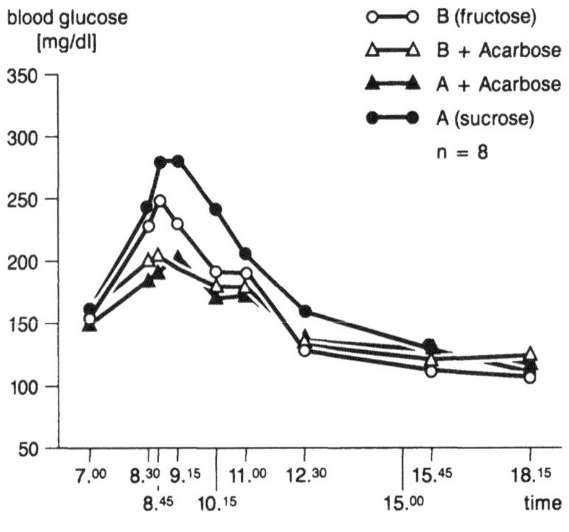

Fig. 5: Blood glucose profile in NIDDM who had a breakfast with the following additions: A = a marmalade with 30 g saccharose added; B = a marmalade with 30 g fructose added; and boths diets with 3 × 100 mg acarbose per day. n = 8.

fructose could be decreased significantly. As the resorption of fructose is not influenced by acarbose, the explaination may be that the acarbose inhibited the postprandial blood glucose increase after the absorption of starch resulting from the bread in the breakfast. With acarbose, the blood glucose profiles after saccharose and after fructose are nearly identical.

In summary, the addition of saccharose to the diabetic diet with marmalade has unfavourable effects on the blood glucose profile compared to the addition of fructose. This harmful effect of saccharose can be compensated by acarbose.

Beer, with and without alcohol

Alcoholic beverages are not mentioned in any recommendation of diets for diabetic patients. However, in non-diabetic men 12,4% of the total calories are derived from alcohol [8]. Also diabetic patients, especially men, consume considerable amounts of alcohol. Alcoholic beverages contain carbohydrates, in beer mainly maltose.

It has been argued that a lacking effect of acarbose in some patients may be due to their beer drinking habits, as maltase is present in the human intestine in much higher amounts than saccharase and therefore cannot be blocked as completely by acarbose as saccharase.

We therefore studied the effect of two types of beer on the carbohydrate metabolism and the influence of acarbose thereupon.

Römer Pils, normal beer with alcohol

9 type II diabetic patients, treated with sulfonylureas, participated in a study in which 500 ml of pils beer was given in addition to a supper consisting of 30 g rye bread, 10 g butter and 15 g protein as cheese. The beer had 3,9% w/vol alcohol and 1,4 g of maltotriose and higher maltose compounds pro 100 ml, in the total volume of 500 ml 7,075 g of maltose compounds. In random order, this evening meal was given with and without beer and with and without 200 mg of acarbose. Blood glucose was measured before supper and up to 150 min after the meal. The results are shown in Figure 6. This Figure shows that the blood glucose increase is much lower after supper than after breakfast. A significant effect of acarbose on this small blood glucose increase could only be demonstrated at 90, 120 and 150 min after the meal. This shows that acarbose is mainly indicated at breakfast and should be started with a single dose in the morning [13].

As the carbohydrate content of 500 ml of pils beer is only 7 g, no significant difference between the blood glucose increase after bread and beer can be shown. A significant effect of 200 mg of acarbose on this blood glucose increase can only be demonstrated at 30 and 45 min after the supper when the starting value is set to zero.

In summary: The blood glucose increase after supper is so small that acarbose is not necessary. The blood glucose increase after this supper together with 500 ml

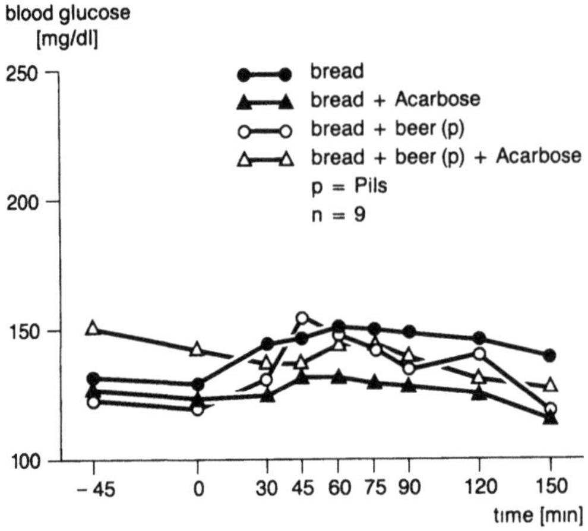

Fig. 6: Postprandial blood glucose increase in NIDDM after supper with 30 g carbohydrates as rye bread, the same supper with 500 ml of normal pils beer and both suppers with 200 mg of acarbose. n = 9.

beer is not different from that of bread alone. Acarbose is also not necessary in this case. Acarbose's lack of effect cannot be explained by the consumption of pils beer.

Clausthaler beer, beer without alcohol

6 type II diabetic patients didn't want to drink alcohol. Thus they tested a popular alcohol-free beer named Clausthaler. This beer has more carbohydrates than the normal alcohol containing beer: total 3,6 g/100 ml, 2,6 g of that are maltose. A total of 18 g carbohydrates (13 g maltose) were consumed with one bottle of 500 ml of Clausthaler beer.

The type of the study was the same as the previous study with pils beer. The results are given in Figure 7. It can be seen that the postprandial blood glucose after supper with the alcohol-free beer is much higher than after the normal beer. This may be explained by the high carbohydrate, especially the maltose, content. 200 mg of acarbose significantly decreased this postprandial blood glucose concentration, but not to the same level without this type of beer.

In summary: Even with such a diet, which is very unusual for diabetics, a significant acarbose effect can be demonstrated.

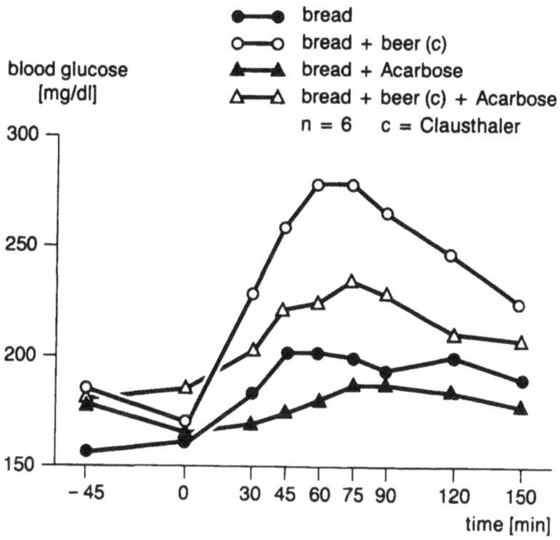

Fig. 7: Postprandial blood glucose increase in NIDDM after supper with 30 g carbohydrates as rye bread, the same supper with 500 ml Clausthaler beer (alcohol-free, maltose rich) and both suppers with 200 mg of acarbose. n = 6.

Summary

Acarbose is an effective drug in *combination with sulfonylureas* for patients with non-insulin-dependent diabetes mellitus. This has been shown in short-term studies (1 week), long-term studies (6 months) and long-term cross-over studies (2 × 3 months with a 3 month placebo period in between). Acarbose lowers the postprandial blood glucose concentration, the mean blood glucose concentration, the area under the blood glucose curve and the HbA_1 resp. HbA_{1c} values.

The acarbose effect is dependent on the *diet* given: The higher the carbohydrate content the more effective acarbose is. Acarbose is more effective than a fibre rich diet with low glycemic index (muesli). Acarbose does not affect the postprandial blood glucose after milk and milk products, but, due to the low glycemic index of milk, the latter is the same as after a standard breakfast with acarbose. The deleterious effect of saccharose (in comparison to fructose) can be compensated for with acarbose. Normal beer has a very low glycemic index and does not need acarbose. Alcohol free maltose rich beer produces a much higher blood glucose increase which can significantly be reduced by acarbose.

References

[1] American Diabetes Association: Nutritional recommendations and principles for individuals with diabetes mellitus: 1986. Diabetes Care *10* (1987) 126 – 132.

[2] American Diabetes Association: Principles of nutrition and dietary recommendation for individuals with diabetes mellitus: 1979. Diabetes *28* (1979) 1027 – 1030.

[3] British Diabetic Association, Nutrition Sub-Committee: Dietary recommendations for diabetics for the 1980's. Hum. Nutr. Appl. Nutr. *36A* (1982) 378 – 394.

[4] Canadian Diabetes Association, Special Report Committee: 1980. Guidelines for the nutritional management of diabetes mellitus. J. Canad. Assoc. *42* (1981) 110 – 118.

[5] Creutzfeldt, W. (ed.): First international symposium on acarbose. Excerpta Medica, Amsterdam 1982.

[6] Deutsche Diabetes-Gesellschaft: Grundlagen der Ernährung und Diätempfehlungen für Diabetiker. Akt. Ernährung *15* (1990) 27 – 38.

[7] Diabetes and Nutrition Study Group of the European Association of the Study of Diabetes: Nutritional recommendations for individuals with diabetes mellitus. Diab. Nutr. Metab. *1* (1988) 145 – 149.

[8] Ernährungsbericht 1984, herausgegeben von der Deutschen Gesellschaft für Ernährung e. V., Frankfurt.

[9] Oerter, E., H. Pfeffer, U. Keller et al.: Zum Stoffwechseleffekt von Diabetesdiäten mit unterschiedlichem Gehalt an Kohlenhydraten und Ballaststoffen. Der Einfluß von Acarbose. Akt. Endokr. Stoffw. *10* (1989) 117.

[10] Sachse, G., B. Willms: Effect of the α-glucosidase-inhibitor BAY g 5421 on blood glucose control of sulfonylurea treated diabetics and insulin treated diabetics. Diabetologia *17* (1979) 287 – 290.

[11] Sachse, G., E. Mäser, H. Laube et al.: Effect of long-term acarbose therapy on the metabolic situation of sulfonylurea-treated diabetics. In: W. Creutzfeldt (ed.): First international symposium on acarbose. Excerpta Medica, Amsterdam 1982.

[12] Seiberling, M., M. Toeller, A. R. Baunack et al.: Beeinflußt der Kohlenhydrat-Anteil der Mahlzeit die Insulin- und Blutglukose-Antwort unter Acarbosegabe? 30. Tagung der Dt. Ges. für Pharm. u. Tox. 1989, Naunyn-Schmiedebergs Archiv Pharmacol. *339* (1989), Abstract 301 (Springer-Verlag).

[13] Willms, B.: Acarbose in Non-insulin-dependent Diabetes Mellitus: Short-term Studies in Combination with Oral Agents. In: W. Creutzfeldt (ed.): Acarbose for the Treatment of Diabetes Mellitus, pp. 79 – 91. Springer-Verlag, Berlin Heidelberg New York 1988.

[14] Willms, B.: Stellenwert der Acarbose im Rahmen der aktuellen Diätempfehlungen für Diabetiker. Akt. Endokr. Stoffw. *12* (1991) 1 – 10.

[15] Vierhapper, H., P. Bratusch-Marrain, W. Waldhäusl: Effect of long-term treatment with acarbose (BAY g 5421) on postprandial blood glucose concentrations in type-II-diabetics. In: W. Creutzfeldt (ed.): First international symposium on acarbose. Excerpta Medica, Amsterdam 1982.

Clinical efficacy of BAY g 5421 (acarbose) in non-insulin-dependent diabetes mellitus (NIDDM) – a placebo-controlled double-blind comparative study

Yuichiro Goto, Yoshio Goto, S. Nakagawa, H. Orimo, Y. Ikeda, N. Sakamoto, I. Fukui, S. Tarui, S. Baba, T. Kaneko, G. Mimura

Introduction

The α-glucosidase inhibitor acarbose (BAY g 5421) inhibits salivary and pancreatic α-amylase as well as disaccharidases; sucrase and maltase in the intestinal microvilli [2, 7, 12]. When this drug is taken orally with a meal, it inhibits carbohydrate digestion and suppresses or delays absorption of the final breakdown products, glucose and fructose. As a result, postprandial hyperglycemia is reduced. Therefore, clinical usefulness of acarbose is anticipated mainly in the patients with NIDDM when adequate blood glucose control cannot be achieved with diet and exercise therapy. Several clinical trials have already been conducted in Western Europe [1, 8, 10] and revealed the effectiveness of the drug.

This is a multicentric, placebo-controlled double-blind group comparison trial to elucidate the clinical efficacy and safety of acarbose more objectively in NIDDM. This study was carried out from January 1987 through March 1988.

Methods

Subjects

Subjects eligible for this trial were patients with NIDDM of both sexes, 35–75 years, ambulatory or hospitalized, kept only on a constant diet therapy for a 4-week observation period and whose 1-hour and/or 2-hour postprandial baseline blood glucose level was 200 mg/dl or more.

Excluded were: 1. patients who have been treated with insulin or oral hypoglycemic agents, 2. pregnant women or women with childbearing potential, and 3. patients who were judged to be unsuitable by the doctor in charge. The concomitant use of dietary fiber (guar gum, pectin, etc.) and digestive enzyme preparations (diastase, pancreatin, etc.) was prohibited. The addition of hypolipidemic drugs were also prohibited during the study.

Prior to the trial, the nature and the purpose of the trial were explained to the patients and consent was obtained.

Test drug and administration schedule

Patients were assigned randomly to receive either 100 mg of acarbose tablet (BAY), 3 times daily with meals for 8 weeks or placebo tablet (PLA). The daily energy intake was kept constant throughout the study.

Clinical laboratory testing

Patients were evaluated with fasting blood glucose (FBG), 1-hour postprandial blood glucose (PBG1hr), 2-hour postprandial blood glucose (PBG2hr), HbA_1, HbA_{1c}, total cholesterol, triglycerides and HDL-cholesterol at 4 weeks and 8 weeks versus baseline data at the end of observation.

To determine the safety of the test drug, hematological (RBC, Hb, Ht, WBC, Pt), blood biochemistry tests (GOT, GPT, γ-GTP, Al-P, LDH, total bilirubin, BUN, serum creatinine, uric acid, Na, K, Cl, serum total protein, serum albumin) and urinanalysis (glucose, ketone body, protein, urobilinogen, sediment) were performed at the end of the observation and treatment periods.

Evaluation criteria

a) Improvement rating and global improvement rating

The degree of improvement of each item was rated in the following 5-step scale: 1. marked improvement, 2. moderate improvement, 3. slight improvement, 4. no change, 5. aggravation, (6. normal → normal).

The global improvement rating for assessment of the efficacy of acarbose on the glycemic control was evaluated according to the formulated criteria (Fig. 1). The degree of improvement in postprandial blood glucose was weighted taking into account the pharmacological action of acarbose.

In calculating the improvement rating in HbA_{1c}, we used either HbA_{1c} values measured by HPLC or "converted HbA_{1c} values" from the HbA_1 values using the conversion formulas by Sanoyama et al. [11] when only HbA_1 values were measured. "Converted HbA_{1c} values" were obtained in 23 of the BAY group and 18 of the PLA group, respectively.

	Absolute reduction Score A		+	*Post-treatment value* Score B	
PBG (mg/dl)	50 ≦	: 1	+	< 150	: 1
	30 ~ 49	: 2		150 ~ 199	: 2
	10 ~ 29	: 3		200 ~ 249	: 3
	± 9	: 4		250 ~ 299	: 4
	≦ − 10	: 5		300 ≦	: 5
FBG (mg/dl)	20 ≦	: 1	+	< 120	: 1
	10 ~ 19	: 2		120 ~ 139	: 2
	5 ~ 9	: 3		140 ~ 159	: 3
	± 4	: 4		160 ~ 179	: 4
	≦ − 5	: 5		180 ≦	: 5
HbA_{1c} (%)	1.2 ≦	: 1	+	< 5.5	: 1
	0.7 ~ 1.1	: 2		5.5 ~ 6.6	: 2
	0.4 ~ 0.6	: 3		6.7 ~ 7.8	: 3
	± 0.3	: 4		7.9 ~ 9.0	: 4
	≦ − 0.4	: 5		9.0 <	: 5

→ *Improvement rating*

Score A + B	Evaluation
2	Marked improvement
3 or 4	Moderate improvement
5 or 6	Slight improvement
7 or 8	No change
9 or 10	Aggravation

Fig. 1: Formulated criteria for global improvement rating in blood glucose: Calculation of "improvement rating" in each of PBG, FBG and HbA_{1c}.

b) Overall safety rating

The overall safety was rated by the attending physicians in 4 scales taking into account side effects and the results of clinical laboratory findings as follows: 1. no side effects at all, 2. side effects were present, but administration of the test drug was continued, 3. administration of the test drug was discontinued because of the side effects, 4. administration of the test drug was discontinued because the side effects required treatment.

c) Global utility rating

Global utility was rated, taking into account both improvement and overall safety, in 5-grades as follows: 1. very useful, 2. useful, 3. slightly useful, 4. useless, 5. use prohibited.

Blindness assessment

In this placebo-controlled double-blind study, the attending physicians were requested to guess whether their patients were taking acarbose or placebo, in order to assess, if the study was kept blind, because of characteristic abdominal symptoms caused by acarbose such as flatulence and meteorism.

Data compilation and analysis

The Mann-Whitney U-test, χ^2-test, Fisher's exact probability test, Student's t-test and single-sample χ^2-test were employed for statistical analysis. P values less than 5% were considered as significant and p values less than 10% were also provided as the reference for tendency. Correlation was evaluated by using Spearman's rank correlation coefficient.

Results

Patient characteristics at entry

246 patients were enrolled. Of these patients, 7 were ruled truly ineligible, 78 patients (BAY: 43, PLA: 35) were excluded from the efficacy analysis before breaking the key code in accordance with the exclusion criteria. Of the remaining 161 patients, 75 received acarbose and 86 received placebo.

In 239 patients analyzed, the degree and incidence of diabetic neuropathy and retinopathy were significantly higher ($p < 0.01$, $p < 0.05$, respectively) in the BAY group. However, there were no significant differences between the two groups regarding the other factors. Therefore, we considered the two groups homogeneous for the purpose of this study.

Effects on blood glucose levels

PBG1hr, PBG2hr and FBG *values* within each group versus baseline were reduced significantly only in the BAY group after treatment, but no significant reduction was observed in the PLA group. When the *degree of reduction* from baseline were compared between the two groups, there were significant changes in PBG1hr and 2hr in the BAY group (Fig. 2).

With regard to changes at 4- and 8-week treatment period, significant reductions in PBG1hr and 2hr were observed in the BAY group after 4- and 8-week treatment, FBG decreased significantly after 4-week treatment and also tended to decrease after 8-week treatment in the BAY group. There were no significant changes in any parameters in the PLA group (Fig. 3).

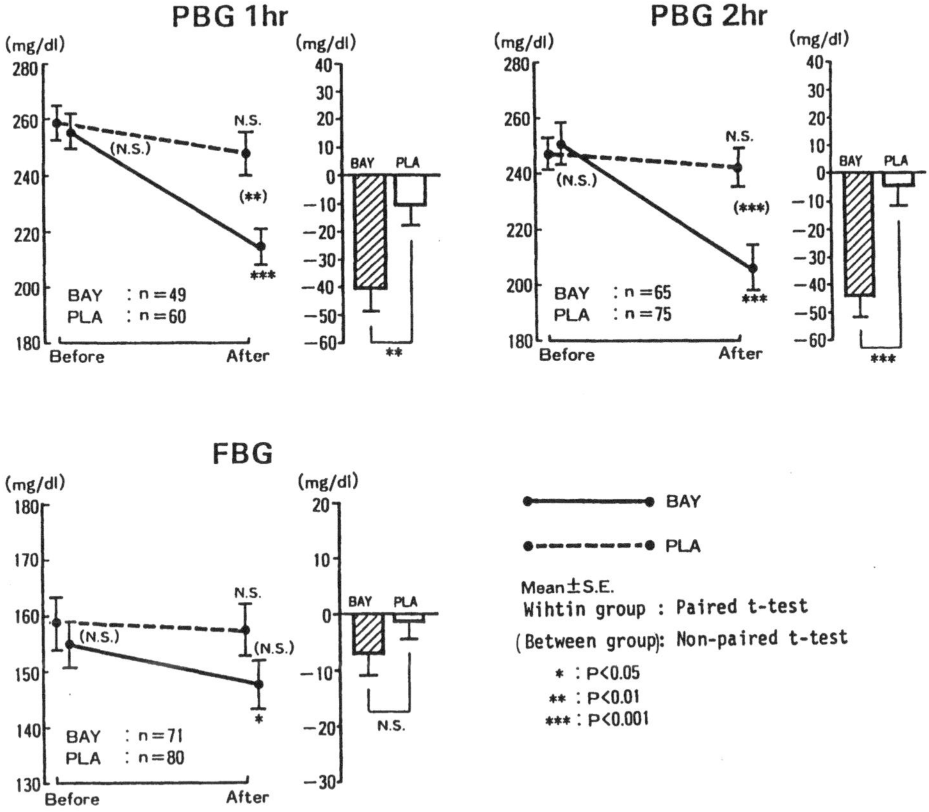

Fig. 2: Changes in blood glucose levels after treatment.

There was a significant difference ($p < 0.01$) between the baseline- and post-treatment-area under the blood glucose-time curve, in the patients whose FBG and PBG1hr and 2hr were measured at the same time, in the BAY group (Fig. 4).

HbA_1 and HbA_{1c}

Both HbA_1 and HbA_{1c} were significantly reduced after treatment compared with the baseline only in the BAY group (Fig. 5). Even after 4 weeks, the BAY group showed significant reductions in HbA_1 and HbA_{1c} compared with the baselines, and its degree of reduction was significantly larger than that of the PLA group (Fig. 6).

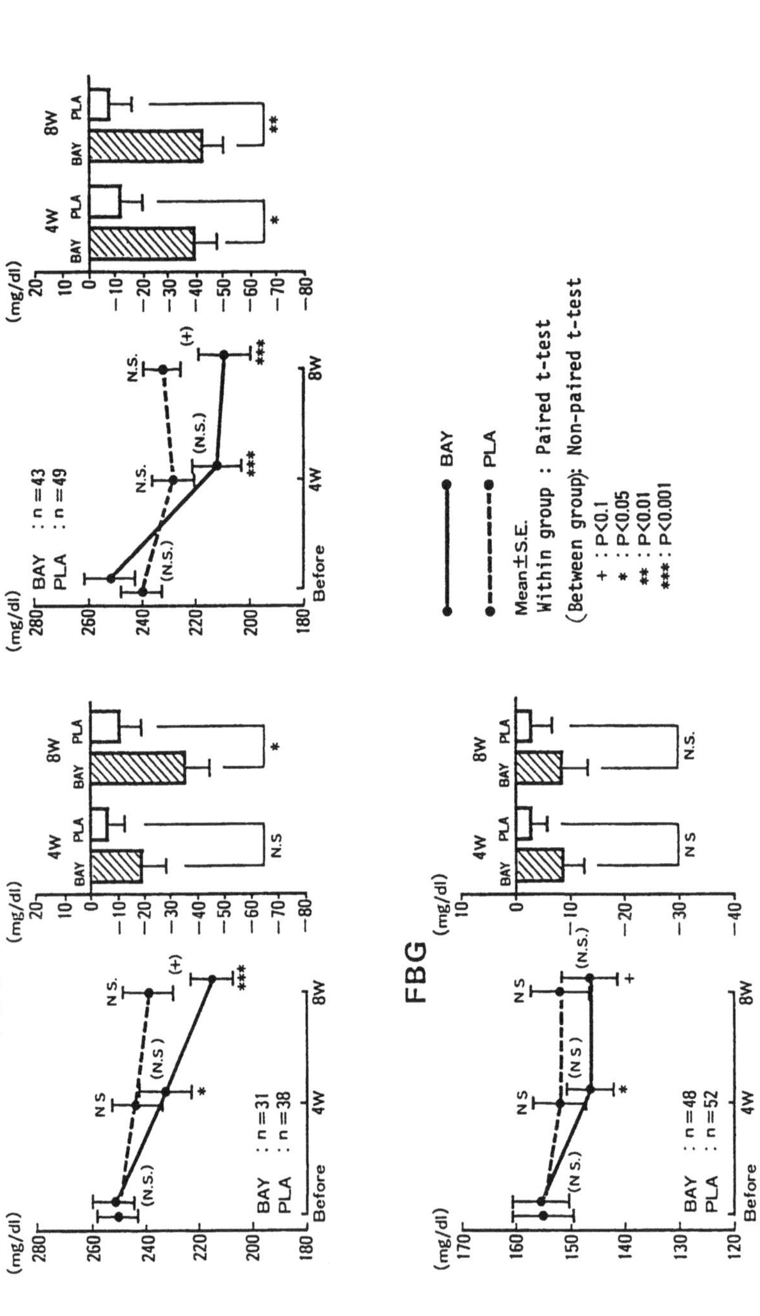

Fig. 3: Changes in blood glucose levels during the 8 week treatment period.

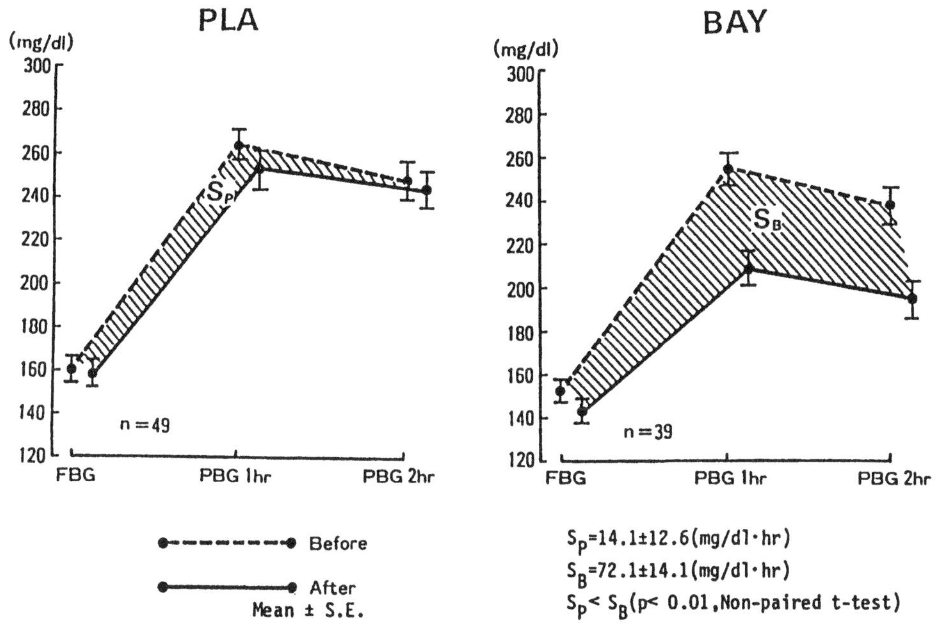

Fig. 4: Changes in fasting and postprandial blood glucose profiles after treatment.

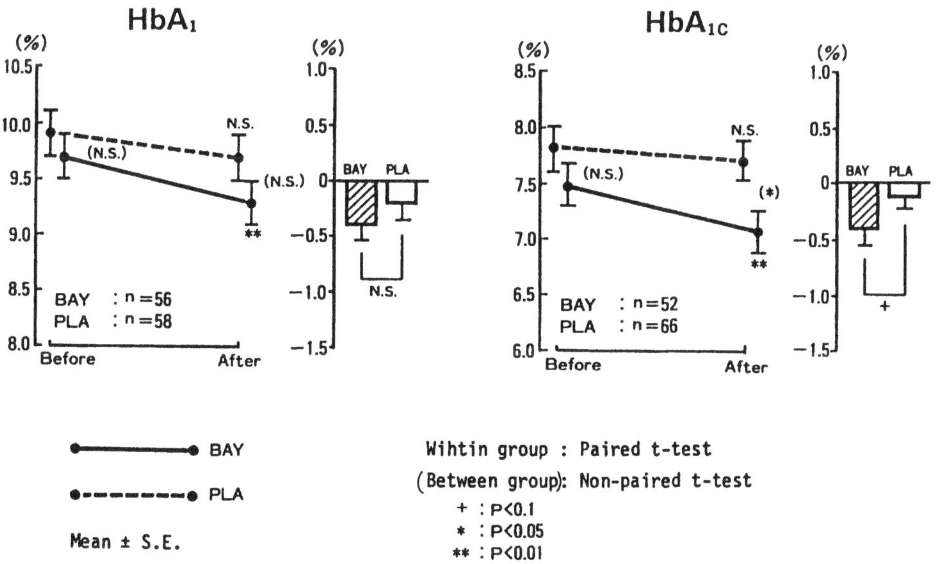

Fig. 5: Changes in HbA_1 and HbA_{1c} after treatment.

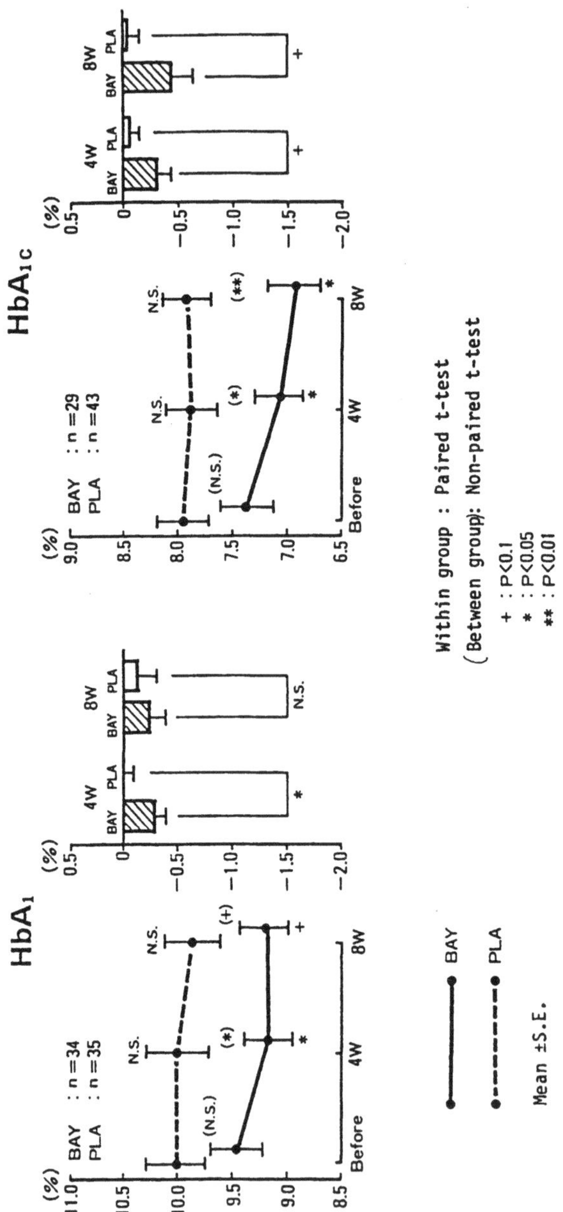

Fig. 6: Changes in HbA$_1$ and HbA$_{1c}$ during the 8 week treatment period.

Improvement rating evaluated by formulated criteria

PBG2hr values were used, as a rule, for calculating the PBG improvement rating. However, PBG1hr values were used only when PBG2hr values were missing or when PBG1hr values only fulfilled the criteria ($\geq$ 200 mg/dl).

The BAY group was significantly superior ($p < 0.01$) to the PLA group with respect to PBG improvement rating ($\geq$ "slight improvement"; BAY: 70.3%, PLA: 51.2%, $\geq$ "moderate improvement"; BAY: 51.2%, PLA: 19.0%). While no significant differences were found between the two groups in the improvement rating both for FBG and HbA_{1c}, the BAY group tended to be superior to the PLA group in HbA_{1c} ($p < 0.1$).

The rating for final global improvement of the BAY group was significantly higher ($p < 0.01$) than that of the PLA group ($\geq$ "slight improvement"; BAY: 66.2%, PLA: 52.4%, $\geq$ "moderate improvement"; BAY: 48.6%, PLA: 20.2%).

Changes in body weight and serum lipids

There was no significant difference in the extent of the body weight reduction between the two groups. However, body weight was reduced significantly ($p < 0.01$, $p < 0.05$) after treatment compared to the baseline in the BAY group (subgroup of $\geq$ 120% of ideal body weight: -1.1 kg; total: -0.47 kg).

No significant changes in total cholesterol, triglycerides and HDL-cholesterol were observed in either group.

Blindness assessment

In the BAY group, accuracy of the estimation of the categories "acarbose" or "probably acarbose" were 14.7% (11/75 cases) and 48.0% (36/75) respectively. This indicates that 62.7% (47/75) of the acarbose-treated patients were considered as receiving real drug. On the other hand, the estimation of the categories "placebo" or "probably placebo" in the PLA group were 8.1% (7/86) and 46.5% (40/86) respectively and the resultant accuracy rate was 54.7% (47/86). Based on the statistical analysis, the attending physicians' guess was significantly accurate for both groups ($p < 0.001$ or $p < 0.01$). However, the 95% confidence interval of accurate estimation was 50.8~66.0% as a whole.

Safety

Table 1 summarizes the symptoms and incidence of side-effects complained or observed throughout the treatment period.

Table 1: Side-effects

Symptoms	PLA		BAY		Test* (χ^2), (F)
	Cases	%	Cases	%	
Flatulence	14	11.6	47	39.8	$p < 0.001$
Meteorism	16	13.2	38	32.2	$p < 0.001$
Feeling hungry increased	1	0.8	5	4.2	N.S.
Soft stool	1	0.8	4	3.4	N.S.
Diarrhea	3	2.5	2	1.7	N.S.
Borborygmus	1	0.8	2	1.7	N.S.
Constipation	1	0.8	2	1.7	N.S.
Wooziness	1	0.8	1	0.8	N.S.
Stomach discomfort	1	0.8			N.S.
Nausea			1	0.8	N.S.
Vomiting			1	0.8	N.S.
Total number of patients	24/121 (19.8%)		58/118 (49.2%)		$p < 0.001$
Number of patients discontinued	3 (2.5)%		10 (8.5%)		$p < 0.05$

* (χ^2) = χ^2-test, (F) = Fisher exact probability test
N.S.: Not significant

A significantly higher incidence of side-effects (49.2%: 58/118) was observed in the BAY group compared to the PLA group (19.8%: 24/121). The most frequent side-effects for both groups were abdominal symptoms such as flatulence or meteorism (BAY > PLA; $p < 0.001$). The severity of those side-effects in both groups were mild-or-moderate in almost all patients. Administration was discontinued because of side-effects in 10 patients (8.5%) in the BAY group and 3 patients (2.5%) in the PLA group.

Abnormal clinical laboratory findings whose possibility of relation to the drugs was not excluded were observed 5.1% of the BAY group (7/99) and 6.6% of the PLA group (7/106), respectively.

Frequent abnormalities were increase of GPT (BAY: 2.0%, PLA: 2.8%), γ-GTP (BAY: 2.0%, PLA: 1.8%), GOT (BAY: 1.0%, PLA: 1.8%) and Al-P (BAY: 2.0%). There were no significant differences in the incidence or degree of abnormalities in laboratory data between the two groups. There were no severe cases and no withdrawals just because of abnormal findings. No intervention was necessary.

The overall safety rating evaluated by the attending physicians was 50.0% (59/118) in the BAY group and 20.7% (25/121) in the PLA group, and the rate of discontinuation because of side-effects was 8.5% (10/118) in the BAY group and 2.5% (3/121) in the PLA group, revealing a significantly higher rate in the BAY group than in the PLA group ($p < 0.001$, $p < 0.05$ respectively).

Global utility rating

The BAY group revealed significant superiority ($p < 0.001$) compared to the PLA group (≥ "slightly useful": BAY: 64.7%, PLA: 39.1%; ≥ "useful": BAY: 38.8%, PLA: 13.8%).

Discussion

In this placebo-controlled double-blind comparative study, no significant reductions were observed in FBG, PBG1hr, PBG2hr, HbA_1 and HbA_{1c} after treatment compared with their baseline levels in the PLA group. This demonstrated that the enrolled patients were already kept stable at the time of entry and also showed that patient selection was conducted properly.

Under the same conditions, significant reductions in those parameters observed in the BAY group showed that the trial revealed the objective clinical efficacy of acarbose.

When we compared the *degree of reduction* from baseline values between the two groups, significant differences in PBG1hr and PBG2hr were observed, while there were no significant differences in FBG, HbA_1 or HbA_{1c}. These results may well be explained by the inhibitory effects of acarbose on the postprandial hyperglycemia. Since significant reductions in FBG, HbA_1 and HbA_{1c} values compared to baseline were observed in the BAY group, it seemed that acarbose might improve glucose intolerance by its favorable effects on postprandial hyperglycemia. Thus, clinical efficacy of acarbose on glycemic control in NIDDM patients was objectively demonstrated.

No significant differences were observed between the two groups, however, in body weight, serum lipids and subjective symptoms. There was a significant decrease in body weight at the end of the treatment period in the BAY group, but mean reduction in body weight was merely 0.47 kg and was considered negligible in clinical practice. Sachse et al. [9] reported that there was no significant change in body weight in 12 NIDDM patients treated with 300 mg daily doses of acarbose for 6 months compared to placebo in controlled comparative study. Cook et al. [3] and Jörgens et al. [4] also indicated that significant body weight loss was not induced in obese patients by 300 mg or 600 mg daily doses of acarbose in a placebo-controlled double-blind study. Based on their reports and on our own findings in the present study, it appears that single doses of 100 mg suppress postprandial hyperglycemia, mainly by delaying absorption of carbohydrate. This means that the addition of acarbose to the patient's diet therapy can improve postprandial hyperglycemia without causing calorie loss. That is the reason acarbose is expected to be useful for diabetic treatment.

The incidence of side-effects was significantly higher in the BAY group than in the PLA group. However, when we looked into the details, we found that abdominal symptoms such as flatulence and meteorism were the most frequent symptoms in both groups and most of them were mild-to-moderate in severity. In the BAY group, these side-effects were considered a secondary effect of the pharmacologic action of acarbose: when small amounts of undigested carbohydrates reach the lower portion of the gastrointestinal tract, the intestinal flora breaks them down and results in the production of an excess amount of CO_2, CH_4, H_2, and organic acids such as acetic and butyric acids that may cause abdominal symptoms [5].

Body weight loss and diarrhea are two cardinal symptoms observed in carbohydrate malabsorption syndromes as manifested in disaccharidase enzyme deficiencies [6, 13]. Since negligible reduction in the body weight in the both groups was noted in our study, with extremely low incidence of diarrhea in both groups (1.7% in the BAY group and 2.5% in the PLA group), carbohydrate indigestion caused by acarbose at the 100 mg dose is considered negligible from the nutritional point of view. In addition, flatulence and meteorism occurred in 11.6% and 13.2% respectively even in the PLA group. These abdominal symptoms frequently observed in the BAY group were not considered as serious problems by the patients.

Abnormal clinical laboratory findings occurred in 5.1% (5/99) of the BAY group and 6.6% (7/106) of the PLA group, but none of them were considered serious in either group.

Attending physicians rated the PLA group significantly superior in terms of overall safety. Since the side-effects and abnormal laboratory findings in the BAY group were not particularly serious, acarbose may be considered a relatively safe drug. This affirmation can be made from the fact that the number of cases evaluated as "useless" or as "use prohibited" on the global utility was quite few.

Acarbose suppresses the process of carbohydrate hydrolysis in the intestine, and consequently delays glucose absorption and reduces postprandial hyperglycemia. This leads to good control in diabetic patients. In this way, the mechanism of the hypoglycemic action of acarbose is completely different from all of the currently available oral hypoglycemic agents or insulin. But the hypoglycemic effect of acarbose is not more prominent than that of those drugs. Therefore, acarbose is considered a drug which should be used in carefully selected patients whose adequate blood glucose control cannot be achieved with diet therapy and exercise therapy, but who are not yet severe enough to warrant oral hypoglycemics or insulin. Furthermore, acarbose may be the drug of choice when postprandial blood glucose control is inadequate despite drug therapy.

Conclusion

The α-glucosidase inhibitor, BAY g 5421 (acarbose) is considered a useful drug in the treatment of NIDDM and is expected to be applied clinically in the future.

References

[1] Aubell, R. et al.: Blood glucose concentrations and glycosuria during and after one year of acarbose therapy. Arzneim.-Forsch./Drug Res. *33* (II) (1983) 1314 – 1318.

[2] Caspary, W. F., S. Graf: Inhibition of human intestinal α-glucoside-hydrolases by a new complex oligosaccharide. Res. Exp. Med. (Berl.) *175* (1979) 1 – 6.

[3] Cook, R. F. et al.: A double-blind trial of an alpha-glucoside-hydrolase inhibitor in obese patients on a maintenance diet. La Clinica Dietologica *7* (1980) 431 – 432.

[4] Jörgens, V. et al.: The glycosidehydrolase inhibitor acarbose (BAY g 5421) in the treatment of obesity. La Clinica Dietologica *7* (1980) 438 – 439.

[5] Muto, Y.: Digestion and absorption, pp. 178 – 180. Daiichi press K. K., Tokyo 1988.

[6] Muto, Y.: Digestion and absorption, pp. 252 – 256. Daiichi press K. K., Tokyo 1988.

[7] Puls, W. et al.: Glucosidase inhibition: A new approach to the treatment of diabetes, obesity, and hyperlipoproteinaemia. Naturwissenschaften *64* (1977) 536.

[8] Rosenkranz, R. et al.: Improvement of carbohydrate metabolism by acarbose in maturity-onset diabetics not sufficiently treated with diet only. In: W. Creuzfeldt (ed.): Proceedings of first international symposium on acarbose, pp. 305 – 308. Excerpta Medica, Amsterdam 1981.

[9] Sachse, G. et al.: Diabetische Stoffwechsellage unter längerfristiger Acarbosetherapie. Therapiewoche *32* (1982) 3587 – 3590.

[10] Sailer, D., G. Röder: Treatment of non-insulin dependent diabetic adults with a new glycoside hydrolase inhibitor (BAY g 5421). Arzneim.-Forsch./Drug Res. *30* (II) (1980) 2182 – 2185.

[11] Sanoyama, K. et al.: Differences of HbA_1 values due to variant measurements and an attempt to calculate some conversion formulas into HbA_{1c} values. The clinical report *22* (1988) 1075 – 1078.

[12] Schmidt, D. D. et al.: α-glucosidase inhibitors. New complex oligosaccharides of microbial origin. Naturwissenschaften *64* (1977) 535.

[13] Tsuchiya, M., T. Morishita: Small intestine, pp. 147 – 162. Nagai press K. K., Osaka 1981.

Effects of long-term administration of acarbose in patients with NIDDM – a double-blind study with placebo

N. Sakamoto, N. Hotta, N. Koh, F. Sakakibara, T. Haga, M. Kobayashi, H. Kakuta, T. Sano, H. Yamada, H. Matsumae, S. Kitazawa

Introduction

Acarbose, a potent α-glucosidase inhibitor [4, 12] is known to reduce the postprandial rise of blood glucose [3, 7, 8]. It has been studied widely as a new means for glycemic control in insulin-dependent (IDDM) and non-insulin-dependent diabetes mellitus (NIDDM) [1, 5, 11, 13, 14]. In Japan, it was confirmed that glycemic control in NIDDM was improved by administering acarbose at an optimum dose of 100 mg 3 times a day [6]. The aim of this study was to evaluate the long-term effects of acarbose on glycemic control in mild NIDDM treated with diet therapy only.

Patients and methods

Patients

NIDDM out-patients, aged 35 to 75 without serious complications, insufficiently controlled (postprandial blood glucose ≧ 200 mg/dl) on diet therapy were included. All patients had given their informed consent.

Protocol

This was a double-blind study. After a 4-week run-in-period, patients received acarbose (100 mg, 3 times a day) or a matching placebo together with each meal for 24 weeks. The diet therapy was not changed throughout the study. To avoid the fluctuation of blood glucose level caused by variation in the volume of carbohydrate in the meal, patients were asked to bring the same volume rice ball when postprandial blood glucose levels were measured.

Fasting blood glucose, postprandial blood glucose and glycosylated hemoglobin (HbA_1) were determined at 0, 8, 16 and 24 weeks. Seventy-five-gram oral glucose tolerance tests (75 g OGTT) were performed before and at the end of the study. Blood glucose and serum insulin were determined before and 30, 60, 120 and 180 minutes after administration of acarbose or placebo. Body weight was measured at 0, 8, 16 and 24 weeks. Cholesterol, triglycerides and HDL-cholesterol were determined at 0, 8 and 24 weeks. Subjective symptoms and compliance with therapy were assessed by interviews with patients at each visit. Usual clinical laboratory tests and urinalysis were performed before, at 8 weeks and at the end of the study.

Data analysis

Values were given as mean ± SE. Statistical analyses were made using the Student's t-test, Chi square test and Fisher's exact test.

Results

Fourty cases, 20 acarbose (A) and 20 placebo (P) were included in the study. However, 3 cases were excluded from the analyses because of low compliance with therapy (1 case in group A, no side-effects occurred) and refusal to visit the hospital (2 cases in group P). The results of the six cases used only to evaluate safety were: group A, drop out because of side-effects (1 case), short run-in period (1 case) and PBG < 200 mg/dl at week 0 (1 case); in group P, PBG was not determined at week 0 (1 case), drop out because of leukemia (1 case), and low compliance (1 case, side-effects occurred).

Both groups had similar sex, age, body mass index and diabetes duration (Tab. 1). At the start of the study, no significant difference was observed between the two groups for all the test items (Tab. 2).

Blood glucose and HbA_1

Figure 1 and Table 2 show the changes in blood glucose and HbA_1. A significant decrease in PBG and HbA_1 was observed only in group A. The change of PBG at the end of the study was -48.5 ± 14.5 mg/dl in group A, and -3.8 ± 13.6 mg/dl in group P. The change of HbA_1 was $-1.4 \pm 0.4\%$ in group A, and $-0.4 \pm 0.4\%$ in group P. The changes in group A were larger than those in group P. However, with HbA_1, no significant difference was observed between the two groups.

75 g OGTT

Figure 2 shows the blood glucose and plasma IRI after 75 g OGTT. At the end of the study, a tendency for the blood glucose to decrease was observed in group A 60 minutes after administration. The AUC calculated by the trapezoid method

Table 1: Subjects

Items		Acarbose	Placebo	Test
Total cases		19	18	–
Sex	Male	14	14	NS (Fisher)
	Female	5	4	
Age (Years)	~ 39	2	4	–
	40 ~ 49	6	7	
	50 ~ 59	10	4	
	60 ~	1	3	
	Mean ± SE	49.8 ± 1.9	47.9 ± 2.5	NS (t-test)
In- or Out-patients	In	0	0	NS (Fisher)
	Out	18	17	
	In ↔ Out	1	1	
BMI	~ 19.9	1	3	–
	20 ~ 22.9	8	5	
	23 ~ 24.9	4	7	
	25 ~ 26.9	4	3	
	27 ~	2	0	
	Mean ± SE	23.5 ± 0.6	22.9 ± 0.6	NS (t-test)
Duration of diabetes (years)	< 1	4	1	–
	1 ~ 4	8	8	
	5 ~ 9	4	6	
	≧ 10	2	2	
	Mean ± SE	4.6 ± 1.0	4.8 ± 0.7	NS (t-test)
	Unknown	1	1	–
Complications	Absent	8	11	NS (χ^2-test)
	Exist	11	7	
Pretreatment	None	3	1	NS (Fisher)
	Diet	16	16	
	Diet + SU	0	1	

decreased from 792.1 ± 45.4 mg · hr/dl to 698.0 ± 58.3 mg · hr/dl in group A, whereas no change was observed in group P (from 764.5 ± 37.1 mg · hr/dl to 752.8 ± 34.5 mg · hr/dl). However, no significant difference was observed.

Table 2: Changes in blood glucose, HbA_1, body weight and serum lipids

	Items	Acarbose (n = 16)		Placebo (n = 15)
PBG (mg/dl)	Week 0	250.1 ± 11.7 (16)		257.3 ± 14.9 (15)
	Week 8	198.1 ± 18.0 (12)**		241.9 ± 18.2 (15)
	Week 16	207.4 ± 14.4 (16)**	*	255.4 ± 14.0 (14)
	Week 24	201.6 ± 15.6 (16)**	+	253.5 ± 20.8 (15)
FBG (mg/dl)	Week 0	158.9 ± 9.7 (16)		156.5 ± 11.0 (15)
	Week 8	142.2 ± 7.3 (13)$^{+}$		153.5 ± 11.7 (14)
	Week 16	146.6 ± 10.8 (16)		158.6 ± 12.9 (14)
	Week 24	146.1 ± 8.8 (16)		155.9 ± 10.0 (15)
HbA_1 (%)	Week 0	11.1 ± 0.5 (16)		10.3 ± 0.4 (13)
	Week 8	10.0 ± 0.5 (13)**		10.2 ± 0.5 (12)
	Week 16	10.0 ± 0.6 (15)*		10.4 ± 0.7 (11)
	Week 24	9.7 ± 0.6 (16)**		9.9 ± 0.5 (13)
Body weight (kg)	Week 0	60.7 ± 1.6 (16)		60.8 ± 2.3 (15)
	Week 8	59.5 ± 1.5 (12)		60.4 ± 2.1 (15)
	Week 16	59.6 ± 1.6 (16)		60.4 ± 2.4 (14)*
	Week 24	59.9 ± 1.6 (16)		60.0 ± 2.1 (15)*
Total cholesterol (mg/dl)	Week 0	210.9 ± 10.7 (16)		196.4 ± 8.2 (13)
	Week 8	214.4 ± 11.9 (12)		198.7 ± 10.4 (10)
	Week 24	212.3 ± 11.4 (16)		201.2 ± 9.7 (13)
Triglycerides (mg/dl)	Week 0	137.5 ± 22.2 (16)		154.6 ± 22.7 (13)
	Week 8	97.9 ± 8.4 (11)	*	159.7 ± 28.6 (10)
	Week 24	121.8 ± 16.1 (16)	+	168.1 ± 21.4 (13)
HDL-cholesterol (mg/dl)	Week 0	46.5 ± 2.6 (16)		45.2 ± 2.5 (12)
	Week 8	46.4 ± 2.0 (11)		43.8 ± 2.9 (9)
	Week 24	48.8 ± 2.2 (16)		50.9 ± 2.8 (12)*

t-test, $^{+}$: $p < 0.1$, *: $p < 0.05$, **: $p < 0.01$

Body weight

Table 2 shows the change in body weight. A significant reduction was observed only in group P. The change in body weight was -0.8 ± 0.8 kg in group A and -0.8 ± 0.3 kg in group P. No significant difference was observed between the two groups.

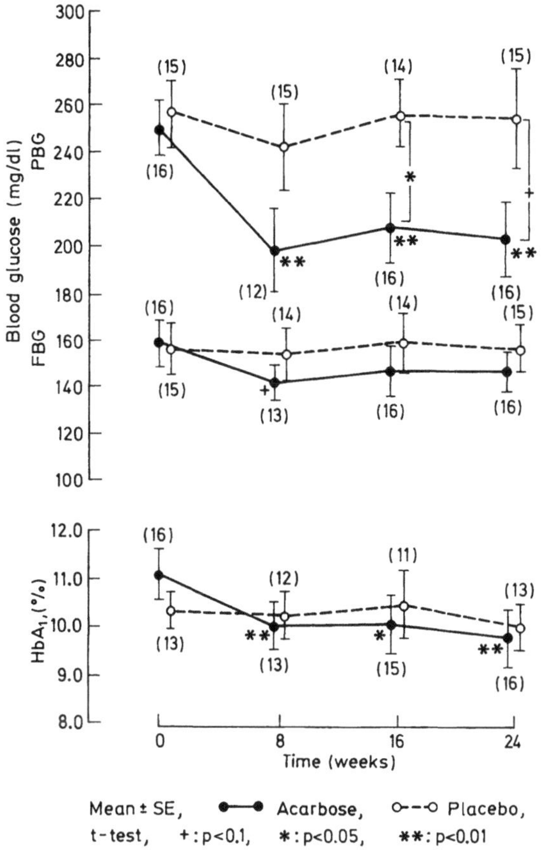

Fig. 1: Changes in blood glucose and HbA_1.

Serum lipids

Table 2 shows the changes in serum lipids. The values of the majority of the patients in both groups were within the normal limits. No significant difference was observed in total cholesterol. The triglycerides in group A showed a tendency to decrease in comparison to group P. A significant increase of HDL-cholesterol was observed only in group P.

Side-effects and abnormal changes in clinical laboratory findings

Table 3 shows the side-effects observed in the study. Almost all side-effects consisted of flatulence and abdominal distension. No significant difference was observed between the two groups. The symptoms were slight or moderate, and diminished gradually during administration without any specific treatment

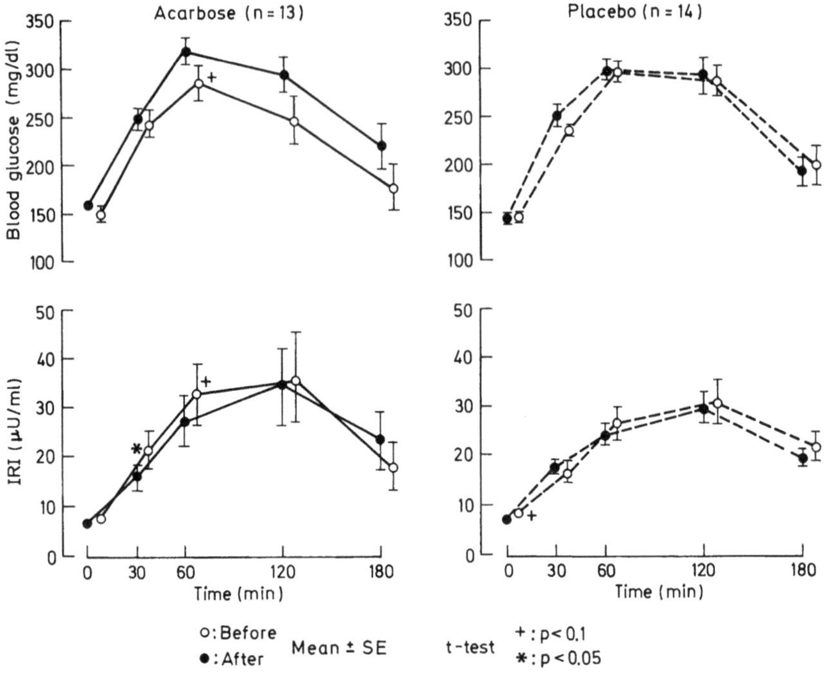

Fig. 2: Blood glucose and IRI after 75 g OGTT.

(Fig. 3). Treatment was discontinued in only one case due to complaints of vertigo. The symptom disappeared after the treatment was discontinued.

The abnormal changes in clinical laboratory findings were a slight rise in GPT and slight increase of WBC in urine sediment each of which occurred in one subject only in group A. No significant difference in the incidence of abnormal findings was observed between the two groups.

Discussion

The present study was conducted to confirm whether inhibitory effects of acarbose were reduced in a long-term administration and whether patient compliance was decreased by the frequent abdominal side-effects that have been reported with acarbose treatment.

A significant reduction in PBG and HbA_1 was observed in the acarbose group and the change was almost constant throughout the study, whereas almost all parameters in the placebo group remained similar to the pre-treatment values. Our data demonstrated that acarbose was able to maintain its effects for a long

Table 3: Side-effects

Symptoms	Acarbose (n = 19)	Placebo (n = 18)
Flatulence	10 (52.6%)	7 (38.9%)
Abdominal distension	7 (36.8%)	4 (22.2%)
Appetite increased	1 (5.3%)	1 (5.6%)
Vertigo	1 (5.3%)	
Soft stool	1 (5.3%)	
Borborygmus	1 (5.3%)	
Diaphoresis	1 (5.3%)	
Diarrhea		1 (5.6%)
Cases with side-effects	15 (78.9%)	11 (61.1%)
Cases of discontinuation	1 (5.3%)	

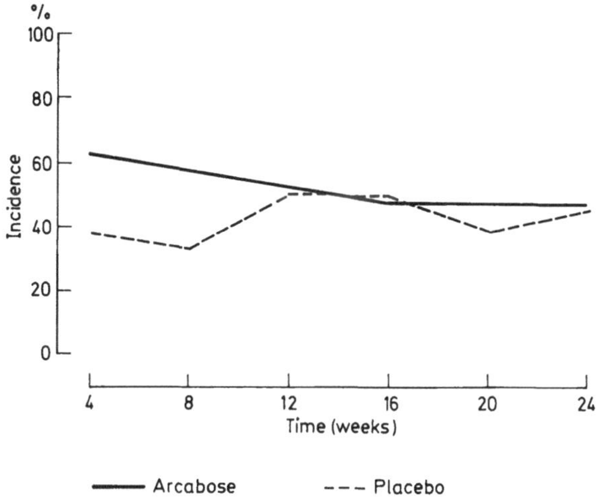

Fig. 3: Transition in the incidence of side-effects.

time. These results may be partially attributable to the selection of the patients and the constant volume of carbohydrates given at the determination of PBG. In spite of an apparent reduction of PBG, body weight was unchanged. This suggests that the effect of acarbose is not the inhibition of the absorption of saccharide, but a delay of it.

The change in HbA_1 was about 1.4% which is not greater than the change with insulin and oral hypoglycemic agents. Buchanan et al. [2] reported that acarbose was not an effective substitute for sulphonylureas. However, Klein et al. [10]

reported that HbA_1 is a strong and independent predictor of the incidence of development or progression of retinopathy. The threshold for a reduction in HbA_1 levels that slower the progression of retinopathy is not apparent and even a modest improvement of glycemic control may reduce the risk. For example, the risk of proliferative retinopathy was estimated to be roughly double when the difference of HbA_1 was 2%. Therefore, acarbose may be useful in mild diabetics for whom insulin or oral hypoglycemic agents are still unnecessary and for those whose glycemic control is insufficient even with those medications.

Side-effects were observed in 78.9% of the acarbose group and in 61.6% of the placebo group. Almost all of the side-effects in both groups consisted of flatulence and abdominal distension. These symptoms are caused by bacterial gas production from non-absorbed carbohydrates in the colon [9]. Such a high incidence may be related to the fact that questions about abdominal discomfort were systematically introduced in the interviews during the study. This explanation is supported by the high incidence of side-effects in the placebo group throughout the study, and the fact that no changes occurred with time. On the other hand, the incidence of side-effects in the acarbose group diminished gradually during the administration period. The hypothesis that the only symptoms that diminished during the administration of acarbose were the actual side-effects may be correct. This is because the incidence of side-effects in the acarbose group diminished to the same level as the placebo group at the end of the study. Tolerance was good and administration was discontinued only in one case in the acarbose group. No reduction in compliance was caused by the side-effects experienced in the acarbose group.

In conclusion, acarbose is effective in improving glycemic control in insulin-independent diabetics, and its effect is maintained for at least 24 weeks. Although abdominal side-effects occurred frequently, safety was equivalent to the placebo. Consequently, acarbose might be an useful adjunct to diabetic therapy.

References

[1] Aubell, R. et al.: α-Glucosidase inhibition on blood glucose control and insulin requirements in patients with insulin-dependent diabetes mellitus. Horm. Metabol. Res. *18* (1983) 253–255.

[2] Buchanan, D. R. et al.: Effectiveness of acarbose, and alpha-glucosidase inhibitor, in uncontrolled non-obese non-insulin dependent diabetes. Eur. Clin. Pharmcol. *34* (1988) 51–53.

[3] Caspary, W. F. et al.: Sucrose malabsorption in man after ingestion of α-glucoside-hydrolase inhibitor. Lancet *I* (1978) 1231–1233.

[4] Caspary, W. F. et al.: Inhibition of human intestinal α-glucosidehydrolases by a new complex oligosaccharide. Res. Exp. Med. (Berl.) *175* (1979) 1–6.

[5] Dimitriadis, G. D. et al.: Effects of prolonged (6 months) α-glucosidase inhibition on blood glucose control and insulin requirements in patients with insulin-dependent diabetes mellitus. Horm. Metabol. Res. *18* (1986) 253 – 255.

[6] Goto, Y. et al.: Utility of BAY g 5421 (acarbose) on NIDDM – Multicentric open study. The Clinical Report *23* (1989) 3949 – 3969.

[7] Hillebrand, I. et al.: The effect of the α-glucosidase inhibitor BAY g 5421 (acarbose) on meal-stimulated elevations of circulating glucose, insulin and triglyceride levels in man. Res. Exp. Med. (Berl.) *175* (1979) 81 – 86.

[8] Hillebrand, I. et al.: The effects of the α-glucosidase inhibitor BAY g 5421 (acarbose) on postprandial blood glucose, serum insulin and triglyceride levels: Dose-time-response relationships in man. Res. Exp. Med. (Berl.) *175* (1979) 87 – 94.

[9] Jenkins, D. J. A. et al.: Scope and specificity of acarbose in slowing carbohydrate absorption in man. Diabetes *30* (1981) 951 – 954.

[10] Klein, R. et al.: Glycosylated hemoglobin predicts the incidence and progression of diabetic retinopathy. JAMA *260* (1988) 2864 – 2871.

[11] Sachse, G. et al.: Effect of the α-glucosidase inhibitor BAY g 5421 on blood glucose control of sulphonylurea-treated diabetics and insulin-treated diabetics. Diabetologia *17* (1979) 287 – 290.

[12] Schmidt, D. D. et al.: α-glucosidase inhibitors. Naturwissenschaften *64* (1977) 535 – 536.

[13] Uttenthal, L. O. et al.: Long-term effects of intestinal alpha-glucosidase inhibition on postprandial glucose, pancreatic and gut hormon responses and fasting serum lipids in diabetics on sulphonylureas. Diabetic Medicine *3* (1986) 155 – 160.

[14] Walton, R. J. et al.: Improved metabolic profiles in insulin-treated diabetic patients given an alpha-glucosidehydrolase inhibitor. Br. Med. J. *1* (1979) 220 – 221.

Effects of acarbose on blood glucose control in insulin-dependent diabetes mellitus

Y. Ikeda, A. Tsuruoka, K. Izumi, M. Yoshida, Y. Nakata, Y. Omori, M. Sanaka, T. Kitagawa, Y. Miyamoto, H. Fujita, M. Kondo, T. Sato, A. Takeda, A. Tanae, K. Matsuoka, K. Murakami, S. Yamamoto

Introduction

Postprandial hyperglycemia in insulin-dependent diabetes mellitus (IDDM) is rarely corrected even with "intensive insulin therapy" [3, 5]. Acarbose, on the other hand, competitively inhibits α-glucosidases localized in the mucosa of the small intestine, distal to the duodenal bulb, and leads to delayed carbohydrate absorption [1]. Oral ingestion of acarbose with a meal is expected to reduce postprandial hyperglycemia [7]. The utility of acarbose in this respect has extensively been studied in patients with non-insulin-dependent diabetes mellitus (NIDDM). A number of investigators noted its favorable effect on blood glucose control [6, 10, 12, 13]. Patients with IDDM have also been studied for their responsiveness to acarbose used to normalize postprandial blood glucose levels [3, 9, 11]. The results available are also favorable.

In this study, IDDM patients were investigated whose daily insulin consumption remained relatively constant.

Patients and methods

Patients

The study included IDDM patients who had been treated with split/mixed injections of insulin and were adequately trained for blood glucose self-monitoring (SMBG) techniques. Before the study, informed consent was obtained orally from the patients. If the patient was under the age of 18, consent was also obtained from his/her parent or guardian.

Administration schedule

The study was designed as a multicentric, open study. Before administering of acarbose, the state of blood glucose control in each patient was observed for 4 weeks (observation period). In patients whose insulin consumption was found to be constant, 100 mg acarbose was administered with meals 3 times daily for 8 weeks (treatment period). In some cases, medication was continued for an additional 4 weeks.

Improvement rating in blood glucose control

The improvement rating in blood glucose control was assessed on the basis of blood glucose and glycohemoglobin (HbA_1 or HbA_{1c}) levels and SMBG data. These were measured at the outpatient clinic at 4-week intervals. Patients were instructed to perform SMBG at least 2 days of 6 times monitoring (before and after each of 3 meals) per month. All SMBG data values were measured at the same time of the day and were averaged.

Insulin consumption

Insulin consumption before acarbose administration was defined as the mean of insulin amounts (units/day) consumed in the observation period. Insulin consumption after acarbose administration was defined as the mean of insulin amounts consumed during the last 4 weeks of the treatment period.

Overall safety rating

The overall safety rating was assessed synthetically on the basis of adverse reactions, clinical laboratory findings and hypoglycemic symptoms.

Global utility rating

The global improvement rating was assessed mainly on the basis of the improvement rating in blood glucose control and the change in insulin consumption. Considering this global improvement rating and overall safety rating we assessed the global utility rating.

Statistical analysis

From measured values, the mean ± S. E. was calculated. The data were statistically analyzed by the Students' Paired t-Test and Wilcoxon's Signed Rank Test. The difference detected at $p < 0.05$ was considered to be significant.

Results

Patients included in analysis

Acarbose was administered to a total of 46 patients. One patient did not adhere to the indicated administration schedule throughout the study. The remaining 45 patients were included in the analyses. Their background factors are shown in Table 1. Five patients who received acarbose for only less than 2 weeks because of adverse reactions were excluded from the analysis of efficacy, which then included only 40 patients.

Improvement rating in blood glucose control

Measurements of HbA_1 in 38 patients and HbA_{1c} in 36 patients were taken both before and after administration of acarbose. The HbA_1 level decreased significantly from value of $10.84 \pm 0.34\%$ before administration, to a value of $10.42 \pm 0.31\%$ after administration. The HbA_{1c} level decreased from $8.85 \pm 0.26\%$ to $8.34 \pm 0.22\%$ ($p < 0.001$) (Fig. 1).

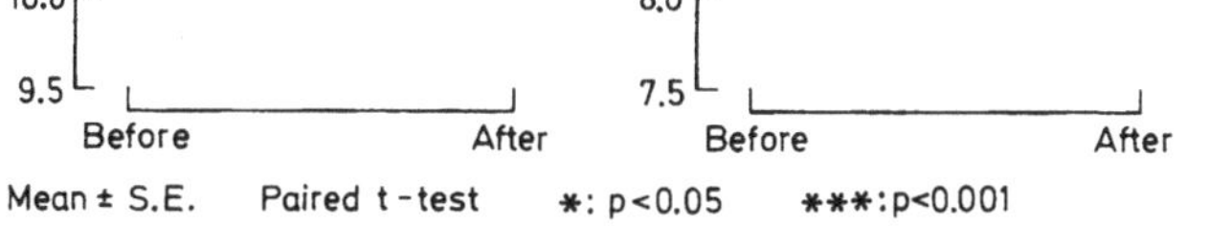

Fig. 1: Change of HbA_1 (left) and HbA_{1c} (right).

Diurnal variation in SMBG value was investigated by analyzing the data collected according to the time of the day (Tab. 2). After breakfast and after lunch, the blood glucose level was significantly ($p < 0.001$) lowered by acarbose. For 15 patients, SMBG data were obtained before and after acarbose, 7 times a day (before and after each 3 meals and before going to bed). Acarbose treatment significantly ($p < 0.01$) lowered blood glucose levels after breakfast and after

Table 1: Background factors of the patients

Number of patients handled: 45		
Sex:	male	13 patients
	female	32
Age:	16 – 19	7
(yr)	20 – 29	9
	30 – 39	9
	40 – 49	10
	50 – 68	10
	Mean	36.8
	± S. E.	± 3.5 (yr)
Duration of Diabetes (yr):		
	1 – 4	5
	5 – 9	14
	10 – 14	14
	15 – 19	9
	20 – 36	3
	Mean	11.6
	± S. E.	± 1.0 (yr)
BMI:	18.3 – 19	11
	20 – 24	31
	25 – 28.5	3
	Mean	21.6
	± S. E.	0.3
Daily insulin dose (U):		
	13 – 19	4
	20 – 29	10
	30 – 39	12
	40 – 49	7
	50 – 99	12
	Mean	40.6
	± S. E.	± 3.1 (U)
Diabetic complication:		
None		22
with 1 complication		11
with 2 complications		6
with 3 complications		6
retinopathy		23
nephropathy		6
neuropathy		12

Table 1: Background factors of the patients (continued)

HbA_1 (%):	7.4 – 7.9	3 patients
	8.0 – 9.9	15
	10.0 – 11.9	12
	12.0 – 16.8	14
	no measurement	1
	Mean	10.76
	± S.E.	± 0.31 (%)
HbA_{1c} (%):	6.5 – 6.9	2
	7.0 – 8.9	22
	9.0 – 10.9	12
	11.0 – 14.1	3
	no measurement	6
	Mean	8.82
	± S.E.	± 0.25 (%)
Duration of SMBG (yr):		
	less than 1	2
	$1 \leq yr < 2$	4
	$2 \leq yr < 3$	5
	$3 \leq yr < 4$	12
	$4 \leq yr < 5$	8
	$5 \leq yr < 9$	14
	Mean	4.1
	± S.E.	± 0.3 (yr)

lunch (Fig. 2). The M-value for these 15 patients tended to be reduced from a level of 22.03 ± 5.22 before administration to a level of 18.85 ± 5.8 after administration. This had no statistical significance.

In the doctor's assessment, 16 (40.0%) of the patients had a blood glucose level that was considered "improved". Twenty-nine (72.5%) of the patients had a blood glucose level which considered as at least "slightly improved".

Insulin consumption

Acarbose treatment significantly ($p < 0.01$) decreased insulin consumption from 42.3 ± 3.4 to 41.0 ± 3.5 units/day.

According to the doctor's assessment, insulin consumption was reduced during the treatment period for 16 patients (40.0%), and had to be increased for 3 patients (7.5%).

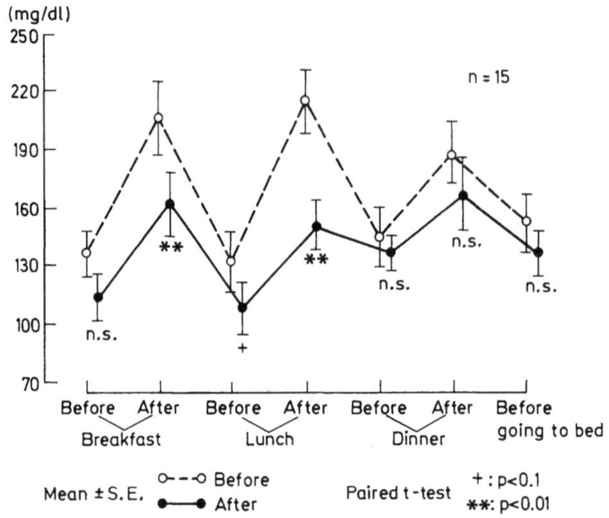

Fig. 2: Change of diurnal variation in SMBG value.

Table 2: Change of diurnal variation in SMBG value

Time	Before	After	Paired t-test
Before breakfast	134.3 ± 6.8	122.4 ± 7.0	p < 0.1
After breakfast	203.4 ± 12.8	161.5 ± 11.4	p < 0.001
Before lunch	121.1 ± 10.5	104.4 ± 9.9	p < 0.1
After lunch	210.6 ± 12.8	161.5 ± 11.4	p < 0.001
Before dinner	143.5 ± 9.1	137.7 ± 6.5	n. s.
After dinner	191.3 ± 14.6	175.4 ± 13.5	n. s.
Before going to bed	157.7 ± 10.1	137.9 ± 10.0	n. s.

Mean ± S.E. (mg/dl)

Other parameters

Body weight showed no significant change during acarbose treatment. Levels of serum lipids (total cholesterol, HDL-cholesterol, and triglyceride) were within the normal range before treatment, and showed no significant change during treatment.

Global improvement rating

Global assessment of efficacy revealed 16 "improved" or more favorable cases (40.0%) and 32 "slightly improved" or more favorable cases (80.0%) (Tab. 3).

Table 3: Doctor's assessment

1. Global improvement rating

Markedly improved	Improved	Slightly improved	Unchanged	Aggravated	Total
2	14	16	7	1	40
40.0%					
80.0%					

2. Overall safety rating

No ADR	Mild ADR, but able to continue	Discontinued due to ADR	Discontinued due to ADR, and needed care	Total
18	22	5	0	45
		11.1%		
	60.0%			

3. Global utility rating

Very useful	Useful	Sightly useful	Useless	Un-desirable	Total
3	11	19	10	2	45
31.1%					
73.3%					

Hypoglycemic episodes

Changes in the incidence of hypoglycemic episodes are shown in Figure 3. The incidence tended to increase until the 4th week of acarbose treatment ($p < 0.1$). No significant change was observed after that. The hypoglycemic symptoms were not serious in any of the cases, and were reduced promptly after oral ingestion of sucrose or another kind of sugar. None of the patients needed to be hospitalized.

Treatment period 0-4 W

Observation period	⧻	‡	+	–
⧻	1	0	1	0
‡	3	0	2	0
+	0	2	6	0
–	0	2	5	12

Increased: 12/34 (35.3%)
Unchanged: 19/34 (55.9%)
Decreased: 3/34 (8.8%)

Signed rank test: Observation period > Treatment period 0-4 W (p<0.1)

Treatment period 4-8 W

Observation period	⧻	‡	+	–
⧻	0	0	1	0
‡	2	1	2	0
+	1	2	5	2
–	0	1	5	14

Increased: 11/36 (30.6%)
Unchanged: 20/36 (55.6%)
Decreased: 5/36 (13.9%)

n.s.

Treatment period 8-12 W

Observation period	⧻	‡	+	–
⧻	0	0	2	0
‡	1	0	2	0
+	0	1	5	2
–	0	1	5	8

Increased: 8/27 (29.6%)
Unchanged: 13/27 (48.1%)
Decreased: 6/27 (22.2%)

n.s.

⧻: very many ‡: many +: few –: none

Fig. 3: Changes in the incidence of hypoglycemic episodes.

Adverse reactions

Adverse reactions appeared in 27 (60.0%) of 45 treated patients (Tab. 4). Most of them were gastrointestinal symptoms such as abdominal distention, flatulence, etc. Most reactions were not so serious and the study was continued with 22 of the 27 patients. In 17 of the 22 cases, the symptoms were spontaneously eliminated or reduced during the study. The study was discontinued for 5 patients (11.1%) because of adverse reactions (gastrointestinal symptoms, 4 patients and systemic pruritus, 1 patient). All these symptoms disappeared rapidly and never reappeared after acarbose was discontinued.

Global utility rating

Clinical utility of acarbose was assessed by the doctors in charge as "useful" or more favorable for 14 of 45 patients (31.1%), and as "slightly useful" or more favorable for 34 patients (75.6%) (Tab. 3).

Table 4: Adverse reactions

Symptoms	No. of cases	incidence (%)	Severity		
			severe	moderate	mild
Abdominal distention	23	51.1	3	12	8
Flatulence	16	35.6	2	5	9
Meteorism	12	26.7	1	2	9
Soft stool	4	8.9	1	1	2
Abdominal pain	3	6.7	2		1
Hypoglycemia	2	4.4	1	1	
Diarrhea	1	2.2	1		
Constipation	1	2.2	1		
Nausea	1	2.2	1		
Systemic pruritus	1	2.2	1		
Anorexia	1	2.2			1

Total number of patients handled:	45 patients
Total number of ADRs:	65 cases
Number of patients ADRs appeared:	27 patients (60.0%)
Treatment discontinued due to ADRs:	5 patients (11.1%)

Discussion

Improvement in blood glucose control

Postprandial blood glucose control in IDDM is known to be difficult. With an intention of correcting postprandial hyperglycemia and of reducing the amplitude of diurnal variation in the blood glucose level, we treated IDDM patients orally with acarbose, which is known to inhibit carbohydrate hydrolases.

Acarbose treatment significantly decreased HbA_1 (or HbA_{1c}). Reduction in postprandial blood glucose levels and decreased M-values were also noted from SMBG data. Thus, acarbose improved blood glucose control in these IDDM patients. Analysis of SMBG data disclosed significant reduction in postprandial blood glucose after breakfast and lunch and decrease in the amplitude of diurnal blood glucose variation. However, acarbose treatment failed to significantly inhibit blood glucose rises after dinner. A large individual difference in the composition of dinner may be responsible for this failing. Relatively high content of protein and fat may also be a cause. Strict regulation of the meal was impossible in the present study because only outpatients were included. It may have masked the post-dinner hyperglycemia reduction which otherwise would have been observed. According to other authors [2, 5, 14] as well, inhibitory effects of acarbose on postprandial hyperglycemia are not always evident at each meal. For patients given standardized meals, however, acarbose inhibits postprandial hyperglycemia at each meal [4].

Reduction in insulin consumption

Acarbose treatment significantly reduced the insulin consumption of IDDM patients. Studies using an artificial pancreas (Biostator®) also demonstrated that a single or one-day treatment with acarbose reduced the amount of automatically infused insulin [8, 9]. A 2- to 6-month treatment with acarbose also reduces insulin consumption [4, 5]. However, in short-term studies (5-day to 2-week treatment), acarbose has reportedly not changed insulin consumption [2, 14]. The duration chosen for these studies was certainly too short to finally adjust insulin dosage to an optimal level.

Hypoglycemia

The incidence of hypoglycemic episodes tended to increase up until the 4th week of treatment. This change was statistically insignificant. These symptoms were promptly eliminated after oral ingestion of saccharides, and never became serious. However, increases in the incidence of hypoglycemia have been noted in acarbose-treated IDDM patients [2, 5, 11]. Therefore, in some cases, when acarbose and insulin are used in combination, adjusting the dosage of insulin and reconsideration of the meal composition (carbohydrate content) are needed [2, 5].

Adverse reactions

Adverse reactions appeared in 60.0% of patients. They occurred predominantly as gastrointestinal symptoms. As reported by other researchers [4, 11], most of these adverse reactions were gradually reduced or eliminated during the study. The incidence was not especially high in light of the results of a placebo-controlled double-blind study of NIDDM patients in Japan [6]. This study found gastrointestinal adverse reactions in 19.8% of placebo-treated patients. These gastrointestinal symptoms were considered to be based on the pharmacological action of acarbose. Patient compliance was satisfactory, suggesting that these adverse reactions were not so serious as to interfere with the use of acarbose. Systemic pruritus appeared in one case, which lead to discontinuation of the drug. Whether it was directly related to acarbose treatment or not was unclear.

Based on these results, we concluded that acarbose can be used also in combination with insulin without causing clinically important safety problems.

Global utility rating

The global utility rating of acarbose was assessed by considering both the global improvement rating and the overall safety rating. Acarbose was assessed as at least "useful" in 31.1% of patients, and as at least "slightly useful" in 75.6% of patients. These results were comparable to a placebo-controlled double-blind comparative study of NIDDM patients [6]. The available findings thus suggest that acarbose is useful as a new ancillary drug for IDDM patients controlled with insulin.

Conclusion

Administration of acarbose to insulin-controlled IDDM patients produced the following results:

(1) Blood glycohemoglobin levels were reduced, and postprandial hyperglycemia was reduced. This lead to improvement in blood glucose control.
(2) Insulin consumption was slightly but significantly reduced.
(3) The incidence of hypoglycemic episodes tended to increase, but the symptoms were satisfactorily treated with symptomatic interventions. Hypoglycemic symptoms were not serious and did not persist in any of the cases.
(4) Adverse reactions appeared in 60% of patients. Most of them were gastrointestinal symptoms, and did not interfere with the continuation of the study. They tended to be reduced spontaneously during the study. The treatment of 5 patients (11.1%) was discontinued before completion because of adverse reactions. The reactions were promptly eliminated after the drug was discontinued.
(5) From these results, we conclude that acarbose is a useful and safe adjunct drug for treating IDDM.

Acknowledgement

For this study, full support was given by the Research Groups for Self-Monitoring of Blood Glucose (members: Y. Ikeda, A. Tsuruoka, K. Izumi, Y. Omori, T. Kitagawa, M. Kondo, T. Sato, A. Takeda, I. Hibi, K. Matsuoka, K. Murakami).

References

[1] Caspary, W. F. et al.: Inhibition of human intestinal α-glucosidehydrolases by a new complex oligosaccharide. Res. Exp. Med. *175* (1979) 1–6.
[2] Damoiseaux, Ph. et al.: Effect of acarbose on blood glucose profile of totally insulin-dependent diabetic patients. Acta Clinica Belgica *38* (1983) 5–11.

[3] Dimitriadis, G. D. et al.: α-Glucosidase inhibition improves postprandial hyperglycemia and decreases insulin requirements in insulin-dependant diabetes mellitus. Metabolism *34* (1985) 261 – 265.
[4] Dimitriadis, G. et al.: Effects of prolonged (6 months) α-Glucosidase inhibition on blood glucose control and insulin requirements in patients with insulin-dependent diabetes mellitus. Horm. Metabol. Res. *18* (1986) 253 – 255.
[5] Gérard, J. et al.: Improvement of metabolic control in insulin dependent diabetics treated with the α-Glucosidase inhibitor acarbose for two months. Diabetologia *21* (1981) 446 – 451.
[6] Goto, Y. et al.: Utility of BAY g 5421 (acarbose) on NIDDM/Placebo-controlled double blind study. J. Clin. Exp. Med. *149* (7) (1989) 591 – 618.
[7] Hillebrand, I. et al.: The effect of the α-Glucosidase inhibitor BAY g 5421 (acarbose) on meal-stimulated elevations of circulating glucose, insulin and triglyceride levels in man. Res. Exp. Med. *175* (1979) 81 – 86.
[8] Ito, K. et al.: Effects of acarbose on glycemic control in insulin-dependent diabetes mellitus (IDDM) under feedback control with artificial endocrine pancreas (Biostator®). J. Japan. Diab. Soc. *32* (8) (1989) 573 – 577.
[9] Lecavalier, L. et al.: The effects of sucrose meal on insulin requirement in IDDM and its modulation by acarbose. Diabete & Metabolism *12* (1986) 156 – 161.
[10] Nakano, K. et al.: Effect of acarbose on daily profile of blood glucose in treatment of type-II diabetics. J. Japan Diab. Soc. *28* (6) (1985) 701 – 706.
[11] Sachse, G. et al.: Effect of the α-Glucosidase inhibitor BAY g 5421 on blood glucose control of sulphonylurea-treated diabetics and insulin-treated diabetics. Diabetologia *17* (1979) 287 – 290.
[12] Sailer, D. et al.: Treatment of non-insulin dependent diabetic adults with a new glycoside hydrolase inhibitor (BAY g 5421). Arzneim.-Forsch./Drug Res. *30* (II) (1980) 2182 – 2185.
[13] Suehiro, I. et al.: Effect of alpha-Glucosidehydrolases inhibitor on diabetic treatment. J. Japan. Diab. Soc. 25 (10) (1982) 1087 – 1093.
[14] Zimmet, P. et al.: Improved control in self-blood glucose monitoring insulin dependent diabetics treated with acarbose. Tohoku J. Exp. Med. *141* (Suppl.) (1983) 687 – 692.

European experience in the treatment of IDDM with acarbose in combination with insulin

S. A. Raptis

It is characteristic that postprandial hyperglycemia of insulin-dependent diabetics is particularly difficult to manage since the increase of blood glucose after the meal cannot be easily synchronized with the concentration of insulin circulating in the blood after subcutaneous administration.

We must emphasize that retardation of glucose absorption from the intestine depends on the type of food, the protein and fat content of the meal, the content of free sugars and, of course, on the presence in the intestine of inhibitors of enzymes which break down carbohydrates. Included in this category are the alpha-glucosidase inhibitors. Acarbose is the main representative and the most investigated so far. This contribution is designed to highlight the action of acarbose in the treatment of insulin-dependent diabetes mellitus and, in addition to the European literature on the subject, I will refer to some of our own studies.

For the first time in May and June of 1980 [21, 20], we reported that glucose fluctuations measured over 24 h with the help of the Artificial Endocrine Pancreas (Biostator®) can be smoothened when insulin-dependent diabetics take acarbose along with insulin. Insulin requirements in such patients decreased significantly after the first month of treatment [6, 22].

If one compares the required amount of insulin in 10 patients before, one month and 6 months after acarbose treatment, one will realize [6, 22] that the decrease of insulin requirements which were estimated by the use of the Artificial Pancreas is highly significant and ranges between 40 to 46% of the initial dose (Fig. 1). Moreover, if one monitors [6, 14] the fluctuations in all patients (Fig. 2) then one will certainly realize that blood glucose fluctuations have disappeared, the peaks of postprandial hyperglycemia are not existent, although as we had previously stated, insulin requirements were less. In 1982 Beyer and his collaborators [3] could confirm the above findings as well through the application of the Artificial Pancreas. They could verify that in all 9 investigated juvenile diabetics a significant diminution of insulin requirements occurred during a 24-hr period. The same investigators could demonstrate that the reduction of insulin requirements was very pronounced from 8 am to 8 pm while it was not evident for the next 12 hours. Perhaps this is explained by the fact that the insulin requirements of all diabetics are minimal during the night period. As it is known, the severe

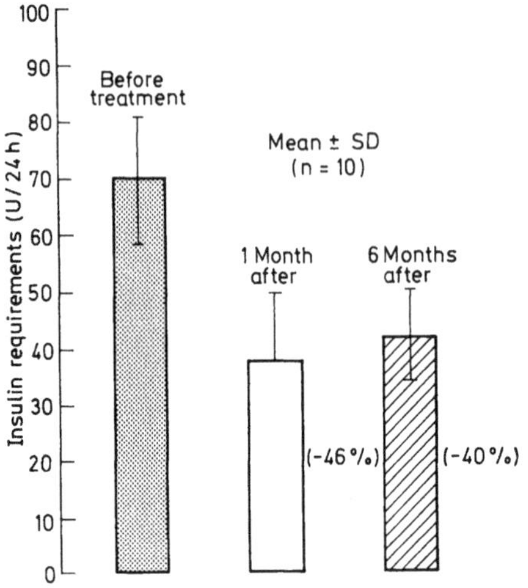

Fig. 1: Mean insulin requirements of 10 diabetic patients monitored by the Artificial Pancreas before treatment with acarbose as well as 1 and 6 months after. The differences between the values before and during treatment are statistically significant [22].

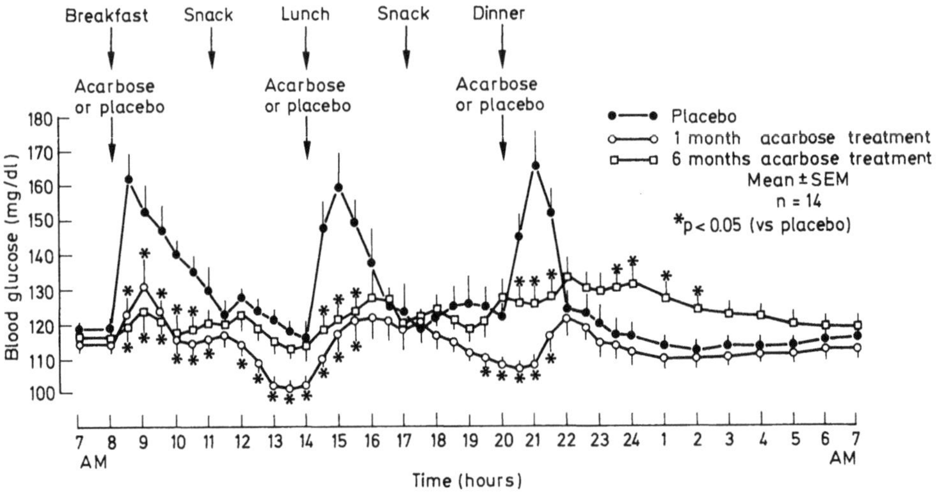

Fig. 2: Comparison of 24 hr profiles of blood glucose measured via the Artificial Endocrine Pancreas (Biostator®) in patients with insulin-dependent diabetes mellitus given acarbose or placebo [6].

fluctuations of blood glucose cause an increase of the concentration of several hormones such as catecholamines, cortisol etc. However, we could demonstrate [22] that the treatment with acarbose and the smoothening of blood glucose fluctuations after the first month led to a decrease of epinephrine and norepinephrine as well as plasma cortisol concentrations in comparison to the period before acarbose treatment. In these insulin-dependent patients the smoothening of blood glucose with the use of acarbose led to a significant fall of triglyceride concentration [22]. Quite probably this fall does not reflect anything else but the improvement in blood glucose control.

Recently in 1991, Austenat proved [2] in a double-blind cross-over study that in brittle diabetics, therapy with acarbose for a period of 12 weeks and in a dosage of 100 mg t. i. d. resulted in a significant fall in blood cholesterol and triglycerides. The other parameters of liver enzymes did not show any statistically significant difference. In the same insulin-treated brittle diabetics, therapy with acarbose resulted in a statistically significant reduction of the mean amplitude of glycemic excursions (MAGE), while the glycosylated hemoglobin did not show any difference since it was already at normal levels without acarbose. However, when acarbose was interrupted, HbA_{1c} significantly increased. In a well documented study in 1981, Gérard and his co-workers [11] from Lefèbvre's group were able to prove that daily blood glucose, the standard deviations of mean daily blood glucose and the mean amplitude of glycemic excursions (MAGE) in insulin-dependent diabetics showed a statistically significant decrease during treatment with acarbose.

In another study, Austenat [2] proved in insulin-dependent obese diabetics that glycosylated hemoglobin showed a small decrease as well. Before and after acarbose the values were within normal limits but a statistically significant decrease in insulin-requirements was evident in patients who were treated with conventional insulin therapy.

In comparison, in a similar study by the group of Pagano in Turin [15] where the regulation of the diabetics with insulin was less good, glycosylated hemoglobin showed a statistically significant decrease and insulin requirements were reduced by 35%. Not only glucose, but also blood lactate and pyruvate showed a decrease in insulin-dependent diabetics after acute administration of acarbose, as was shown by Walton et al. [25] from the group of Alberti, in 1979.

Not only the long-term but also the short-term administration of acarbose to insulin-dependent diabetics was capable to create only lower postprandial glucose values, not fasting values, after a three day course of a regimen with either acarbose or placebo as Petzoldt and co-workers [16] showed in a cross-over study in 11 diabetics. In insulin-dependent diabetics who were hospitalized for one month under a strict diet, Katsimantis and his co-workers [14] could clearly demonstrate that not only blood glucose fell but they also had to decrease the amount of administered insulin as the patients were experiencing frequent bouts of hypoglycemia. Long-term management (1 year) not only led to a fall of postprandial blood glucose but also of the fasting glucose [1].

In a multi-center study conducted by Shuman in 1980 [23], acarbose was administered for 12 weeks to 100 insulin-dependent diabetics and to 495 type II diabetics. The regimen initially consisted of 3 × 50 mg daily and after 2 weeks, acarbose dosage was increased to 3 × 200 mg daily. At the end of the treatment period both in the group of insulin-dependent diabetics as well as in the other groups, a fall in the postprandial hyperglycemia by 20–26% was noted in comparison to the period before the acarbose treatment. Moreover, in 1980, Willms and his co-workers [26] could document both in brittle diabetics and in insulin-dependent patients that acarbose administration significantly lowered the mean and the maximal blood glucose values as well as the integrated blood glucose response in comparison to placebo. Therefore, acarbose has its indication even in the rare cases of brittle diabetes. In a double-blind crossover study, Hillebrand and co-workers [13] administered acarbose or placebo for a period of 7 days to 10 type I diabetics with high glucosuria. The daily excretion of glucose in the urine decreased by an average of 80% during the period that patients were taking acarbose in comparison to the placebo period. Moreover Aubell et al. (1983) [1] could document in a multi-center study under conditions of private practice that the addition of acarbose to the insulin therapy led to the disappearance of glucose from the urine in 50% of cases. In a double-blind 4 week crossover study, Edmonds and his co-workers [10] administered acarbose to insulin-dependent diabetics on home blood glucose monitoring. In this case also, acarbose could lower the postprandial increases of blood glucose in comparison to the placebo period.

Henrichs and his co-workers [12] in Germany administered 200–300 mg of acarbose per day divided into 3 equal sized doses for a period of 12 weeks to 11 juvenile diabetics aged 11 to 17 years in addition to their diet and insulin. Subsequently, the same group received a placebo for an equal period of time. During acarbose therapy the insulin requirements as well as the HbA_1 levels decreased significantly.

Finally, Viviani and his co-workers [24] clearly demonstrated in a double-blind cross over study that in all occasions when acarbose was added to the insulin treatment of insulin-dependent diabetics, blood glucose levels were significantly lower than with insulin and placebo. The number of hypopglycemic episodes with acarbose was more frequent, so that the patients had to take sugar more frequently. However, the level of blood glucose remained lower under acarbose treatment. Normally these patients should lower the units of s.c.-injected insulin.

In 1985 my co-worker Dimitriadis [9] attempted to investigate whether acute acarbose administration had any effect on blood glucose control of insulin-dependent diabetics. Insulin was administered to these diabetic patients as a 30 min subcutaneous infusion which began either 30 min before the meal or immediately before the commencement of the meal. Each time, 1 tablet of acarbose was administered to the patients in a dose of 100 mg orally, or a placebo was given.

The administration of acarbose induced a significant decrease in values of plasma xylose in these insulin-dependent diabetic patients in comparison to placebo (Fig. 3). From these results it is obvious that acarbose administration influences postprandial carbohydrate absorption and as we have shown so far, the local action of the drug on the intestine constitutes the main mechanism by which this inhibitor improves postprandial hyperglycemia. Of course it must be emphasized that this experiment applies only to the acute administration of the inhibitor.

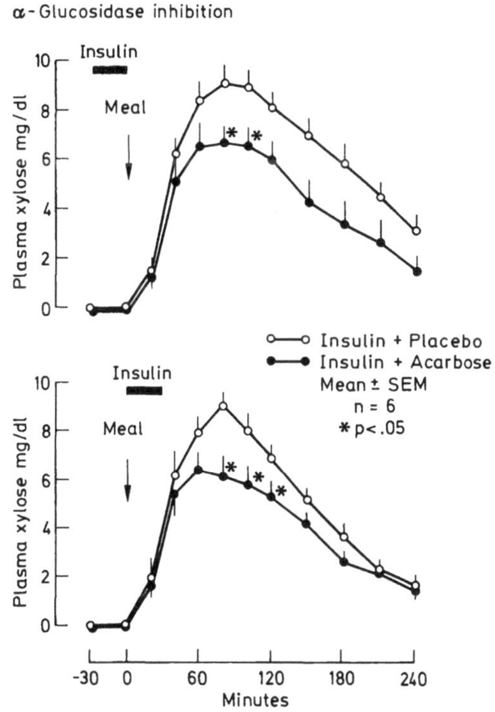

Fig. 3: Postprandial plasma xylose concentrations in patients with insulin-dependent diabetes mellitus following a 30-minute subcutaneous infusion of insulin begun 30 minutes (A) or immediately prior to meal ingestion (B) with concomitant administration of acarbose or placebo [9].

The postprandial concentrations of blood glucose, insulin, glucagon and gastrointestinal polypeptide in these insulin-dependent diabetics after the administration of acarbose in the dose of 100 mg or placebo are shown in Figure 4. In these experiments, the 30 min subcutaneous insulin infusion began 30 min before the administration of a mixed meal. As we can see, after the administration of placebo blood glucose increased about 170 mg% on the average and at 4 hours it did not return to the levels before the meal. In contrast, after the administration of acarbose blood glucose did not increase more than 130 mg% on the average and these levels were statistically lower than the respective values after the administration of placebo. After 4 hours, blood glucose had already come back to the level before the meal. In other words we can say that by administering acarbose we obtained lower postprandial levels of blood glucose with less insulin. As we can observe (Fig. 4), the postprandial concentrations of glucagon and

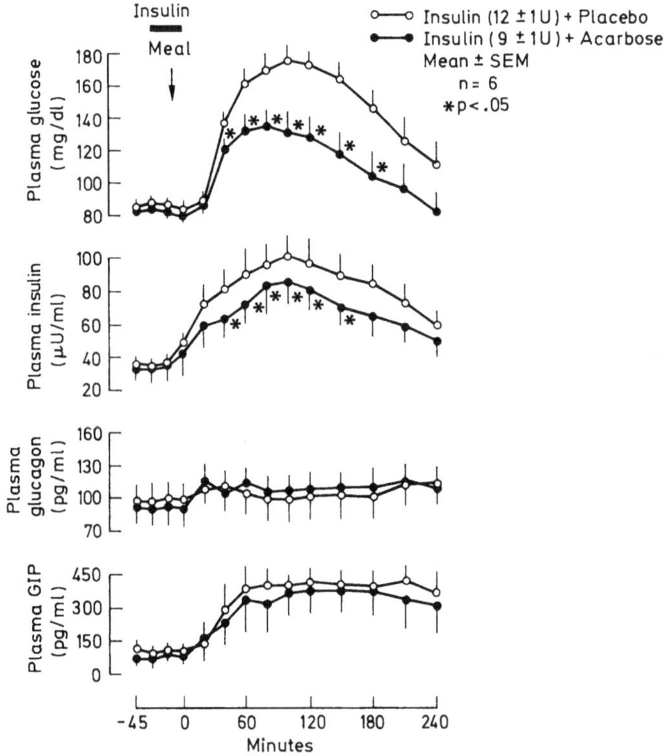

Fig. 4: Postprandial plasma glucose, insulin, glucagon, and gastrointestinal inhibitory polypeptide (GIP) concentrations in patients with insulin-dependent diabetes mellitus following a 30-minute subcutaneous infusion of insulin begun 30 minutes preprandially with concomitant administration of acarbose or placebo [9].

gastrointestinal polypeptide did not differ significantly between the administration of acarbose or placebo in our patients.

The postprandial concentrations of glucose, insulin, glucagon and gastrointestinal polypeptide in the same patients after the administration of acarbose in the same dose as previously or placebo is demonstrated in Figure 5. The only difference, however, was that the 30 min subcutaneous insulin infusion was initiated immediately before the meal. As we can see when the placebo was administered, the postprandial concentrations of blood glucose were higher than 190 mg% but when acarbose was administered these concentrations were significantly lower. In this case as in the previous experiments, the insulin that was administered as a subcutaneous infusion when acarbose had been given before the meal was less

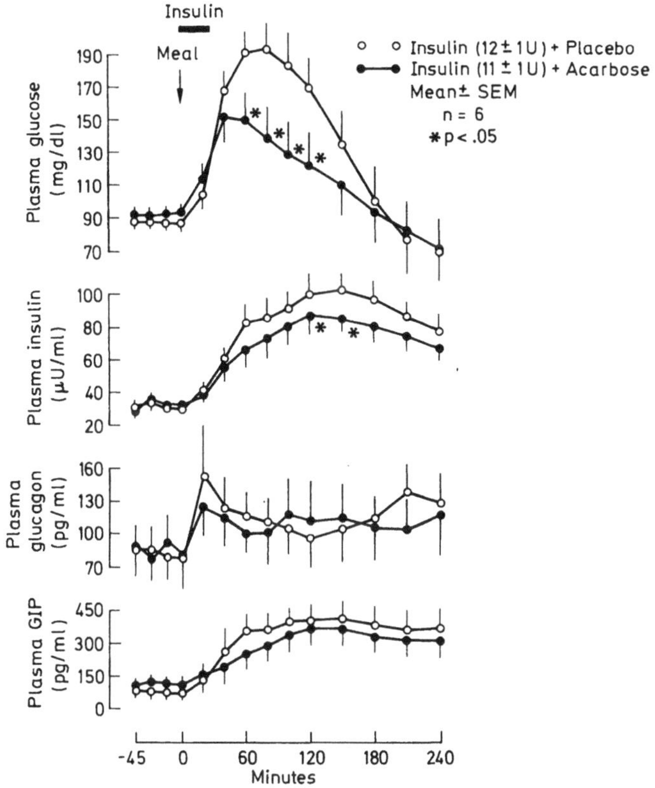

Fig. 5: Postprandial plasma glucose, insulin, glucagon, and gastrointestinal imhibitory polypeptide (GIP) concentrations in patients with insulin-dependent diabetes mellitus following a 30-minute subcutaneous infusion of insulin begun immediately prior to food ingestion with conconmitant administration of acarbose or placebo [9].

than that when the placebo had been given. For this reason insulin levels in the circulation after acarbose administration were lower than the respective values after the administration of placebo.

As seen in Figure 4 after the administration of acarbose or placebo, no difference existed regarding the postprandial concentrations of glucagon or gastrointestinal polypeptide.

So, in conclusion we can say that in patients with insulin-dependent diabetes mellitus, the administration of an inhibitor of alpha-glucosidase such as acarbose along with insulin diminishes postprandial hyperglycemia. The same improvement in postprandial hyperglycemia was observed when insulin was administered 30 min before the meal and when insulin was given immediately before the meal. This fact has a practical significance in that the administration of this inhibitor might allow patients to inject insulin immediately before the meal so that there is no need to wait for 30 or more minutes before eating.

It should be pointed out that the acarbose treatment does not at all affect intravenous glucose tolerance, while it evidently diminishes the postprandial hyperglycemia [8].

Our studies clearly demonstrate that prolonged administration of the alpha-glucosidase inhibitor acarbose in insulin-dependent diabetic subjects improve their glucose tolerance. Postprandial blood glucose increases as well as insulin requirements estimated by the Biostator® are both significantly reduced following acarbose treatment.

The artificial endocrine pancreas is an objective indicator of insulin requirements and has been widely used for this purpose, although insulin infused by this device may exceed diurnal insulin secretion observed in normal subjects. The present results of improved glucose tolerance along with an insulin sparing effect of acarbose, are consistent with those of previous studies in normal or diabetic volunteers. The effect of acarbose on plasma glucose and insulin increments after food ingestion have been attributed to the delay (in small doses) or partial inhibition (in larger doses) of starch and sucrose digestion, leading to the slower entrance of glucose into the circulation. With the dose used in diverse experiments a degree of malabsorption was most probably present in the beginning of the investigation. It should be noted, however, that the symptoms (flatulence, borborygmi) became milder during continuous administration of acarbose and the inhibitor was better tolerated. This could be explained by the progressive increase of alpha-glucosidase activity in the lower part of the small intestine following initial inhibition of these enzymes in the upper part of the small intestine by acarbose.

In order to explain the effect of acarbose on the gastrointestinal tract, the decrease of plasma concentrations of various gastrointestinal hormones and the increase of plasma somatostatin levels by this inhibitor should also be mentioned [17, 18].

According to all the published evidence [19], there is no longer any doubt that the alpha-glucosidase inhibitor, acarbose, is established as an innovation in the treatment for patients suffering from type I diabetes. Research efforts in this field were never stopped, but were actually continued in the development of two more alpha-glucosidase inhibitors (BAY 1099 and BAY 1248). Both of these compounds proved to be potent in insulin-dependent diabetics and appeared to exert, as was published by our group in 1986 [7] and 1988 [4] after a short and a prolonged

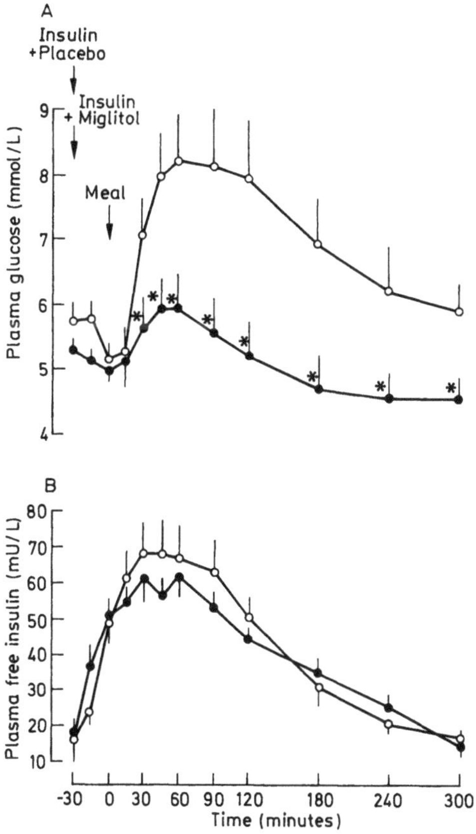

Fig. 6: Postprandial plasma glucose (A) and plasma free insulin (B) concentrations in patients with insulin-dependent diabetes mellitus after subcutaneous injection of insulin given 30 min before food ingestion with concomitant administration of miglitol (•) or placebo (o). $p < 0.05$ vs control subjects with paired Student's test. Values are means ± SE; n = 12 [5].

administration, an improvement of glycemic control, a reduction of insulin requirements measured via the Artificial Endocrine Pancreas and an absence of malabsorption.

From those 2 inhibitors of the second generation, Bay 1099 with the generic name miglitol, was further investigated by our group recently [5]. This inhibitor (Fig. 6) is more effective with insulin than insulin therapy alone, in controlling postprandial hyperglycemia in patients with type I diabetes and permits (in the same way as acarbose) insulin to be administered just before the meal (Fig. 7).

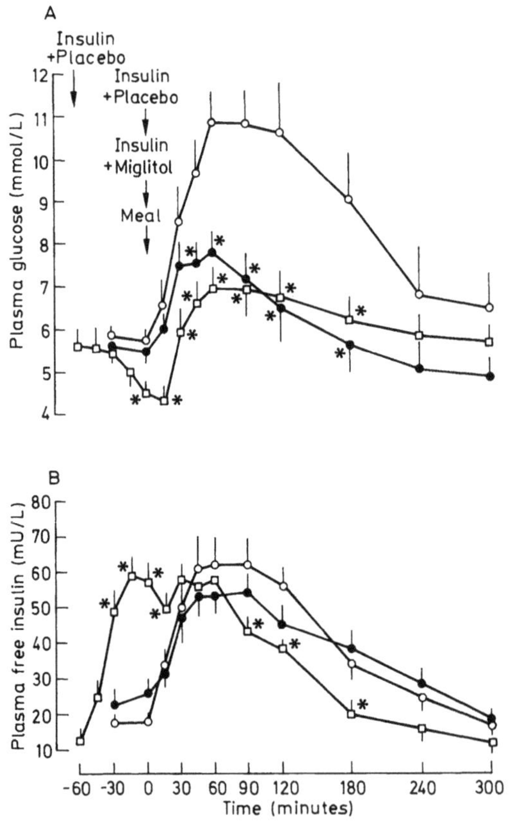

Fig. 7: Postprandial plasma glucose (A) and plasma free insulin (B) concentrations in patients with insulin-dependent diabetes mellitus after subcutaneous injection of insulin given 1 h (□) or immediately before meal ingestion with concomitant administration of miglitol (●) or placebo (○). $p < 0.05$ vs control subjects with paired Student's test. Values are means ± SE; n = 12 [5].

Acknowledgements

This work was supported by grants from the Ministry of Health-Welfare and Social Insurance Athens, Greece and the Alexander S. Onassis Foundation, Vaduz Liechtenstein.

References

[1] Aubell, R., K. Boehme, P. Berchtold: Blood glucose concentrations and glycosuria during and after one year of acarbose treatment. Arzneimittelforschung *33* (II) 9 (1983) 1314–1318.

[2] Austenat, E.: Neuere Therapie Studien mit Acarbose bei Typ-I-Diabetikern. Akt. Endokr. Stoff. *12* (1991) 19–24.

[3] Beyer, J., G. Schulz, H. Jaeger et al.: Improvement of carbohydrate tolerance in insulin-dependent diabetics after administration of an α-glucosidase inhibitor demonstrated by artificial pancreas. In: W. Creutzfeldt (ed.): Acarbose – Effects on Carbohydrate and Fat Metabolism, pp. 451–454. Excerpta Medica, Amsterdam 1982.

[4] Dimitriadis, G., E. Hatziagelaki, S. Ladas et al.: Effects of prolonged administration of two new α-glucosidase inhibitors on blood glucose control, insulin requirements and breath H_2 excretion in patients with type I diabetes mellitus. Eur. J. Clin. Invest. *18* (1988) 33–38.

[5] Dimitriadis, G., E. Hatziagelaki, E. Alexopoulos et al.: Effects of α-Glucosidase Inhibition on Meal Glucose Tolerance and Timing of Insulin Administration in Patients with Type I Diabetes Mellitus. Diabetes Care *14* (1991) 393–398.

[6] Dimitriadis, G., C. Karaiskos, S. Raptis: Effects of Prolonged (6 Months) α-Glucosidase Inhibition on Blood Glucose Control and Insulin Requirements in Patients with Insulin-Dependent Diabetes Mellitus. Horm. Metabol. Res. *18* (1986) 253–255.

[7] Dimitriadis, G., S. Raptis, A. Raptis et al.: Effects of two new α-glucosidase inhibitors on glycemic control in patients with insulin-dependent diabetes mellitus. Klin. Wochenschr. *64* (1986) 405–410.

[8] Dimitriadis, G., P. Tessari, V. Go et al.: Effects of the Disaccharidase Inhibitor Acarbose on Meal and Intravenous Glucose Tolerance in Normal Man. Metabolism *31* (1982) 841–843.

[9] Dimitriadis, G., P. Tessari, V. L. W. Go, et al.: α-Glucosidase Inhibition Improves Postprandial Hyperglycemia and decreases Insulin Requirements in Insulin Dependent Diabetes Mellitus. Metabolism *34* (1985) 261–265.

[10] Edmonds, M. E., M. Doddridge, P. N. John et al.: Acarbose and postprandial glycaemia in the home blood-glucose profile. In: W. Creutzfeldt (ed.): Acarbose – Effects on Carbohydrate and Fat Metabolism, pp. 402–405. Excerpta Medica, Amsterdam 1982.

[11] Gérard, J., A. Luyckx, P. Léfèbvre: Improvement of metabolic control in insulin dependent diabetics treated with the α-glucosidase inhibitor acarbose for two months. Diabetologia *21* (1981) 446–451.

[12] Henrichs, I. A., E. Heinze, E. Kohne et al.: Improved management of juvenile diabetes by acarbose. In: W. Creutzfeldt (ed.): Acarbose – Effects on Carbohydrate and Fat Metabolism, pp. 490–493. Excerpta Medica, Amsterdam 1982.

[13] Hillebrand, I., H. E. Reis, K. Boehme et al.: The effect of the α-glucosidase acarbose on the urinary glucose excretion in poorly controlled insulin dependent diabetics. In: W. Creutzfeldt (ed.): Acarbose – Effects on Carbohydrate and Fat Metabolism, pp. 482–485. Excerpta Medica, Amsterdam 1982.

[14] Katsimantis, D., I. Hillebrand, D. Vikeli et al.: Acarbose treatment in hospitalizated diabetics. In: W. Creutzfeldt (ed.): Acarbose – Effects on Carbohydrate and Fat Metabolism, pp. 340–343. Excerpta Medica, Amsterdam 1982.

[15] Marena, S., V. Tagliaferro, A. Pagani et al.: Acarbose supplementation in the diet of Type I diabetic patients improves metabolic Control. Diabetologia *32* (1989) 312–313.

[16] Petzoldt, R., J. Vrahimis, H. D. Fink et al.: Effect of a single dose of acarbose on postprandial blood glucose values in insulin-dependent diabetics. In: W. Creutzfeldt (ed.): Acarbose – Effects on Carbohydrate and Fat Metabolism, pp. 427–432. Excerpta Medica, Amsterdam 1982.

[17] Raptis, S., G. Dimitriadis, H. Etzrodt et al.: The effects of Acarbose Treatment on release of pancreatic and gastrointestinal Hormones in Man: Results of a Randomized Double-Blind Cross Over Study. Diabetologia *21* (1981) 319.

[18] Raptis, S., G. Dimitriadis, H. Etzrodt et al.: The effects of acarbose treatment on release of pancreatic and gastrointestinal hormones in man. In: W. Creutzfeldt (ed.): Acarbose – Effects on Carbohydrate and Fat Metabolism, pp. 210–215. Excerpta Medica, Amsterdam 1982.

[19] Raptis, S., G. Dimitriadis, D. Hadjidakis: Acarbose Treatment in Insulin Dependent (Type I) Diabetes Mellitus. In: W. Creutzfeldt (ed.): Acarbose for the Treatment of Diabetes Mellitus, pp. 141–152. Springer-Verlag, Berlin – Heidelberg – New York 1987.

[20] Raptis, S., G. Dimitriadis, K. Karaiskos et al.: Long-term effects of an α-glucosidase inhibitor on catecholamine levels and insulin requirements as assessed by the artificial beta-cell (Abstract). Diabetes *29* (Suppl. 2) (1980) 41A.

[21] Raptis, S., G. Dimitriadis, K. Karaiskos et al.: Langzeitbehandlung mit einem Glykosidhydrolasen-Inhibitor. Effekte beim täglichen Insulinbedarf, Cortisol, Triglyzeridspiegel und biochemischen Laborprofil bei Diabetikern. Akt. Endokrin. Stoff. *1* (1980) 195–196.

[22] Raptis, S., G. Dimitriadis, K. Karaiskos et al.: Short and long-term studies of acarbose on various metabolic parameters and insulin requirements assessed by the artificial endocrine pancreas. In: W. Creutzfeld (ed.): Acarbose-Effect on Carbohydrate and Fat Metabolism, pp. 393–401. Excerpta Medica, Amsterdam 1982.

[23] Schumann, F., K. Janssen, R. Aubell et al.: Acarbose in diabetic out-patient treatment: results of a 3-month study. In: W. Creutzfeldt (ed.): Acarbose-Effects on Carbohydrate and Fat Metabolism, pp. 367–372. Excerpta Medica, Amsterdam 1982.

[24] Viviani, G. L., L. Camogliano, M. G. Borgoglio et al.: Acarbose Treatment in insulin-dependent diabetics. A double-blind Crossover Study. Current Therap. Res. *42* (1987) 1–11.

[25] Walton, R. J., I. T. Sherif, G. A. Noy et al.: Improved metabolic profiles in insulin treated diabetic patients given alpha glucosidase hydrolase inhibitor. Br. Med. J. *1* (1979) 220–221.

[26] Willms, B., G. Sachse: Short-term effects of acarbose in insulin treated diabetics. In: W. Creutzfeldt (ed.): Acarbose-Effects on Carbohydrate and Fat Metabolism, pp. 471–473. Excerpta Medica, Amsterdam 1982.

Round table discussion on open questions and future aspects

The discussion was moderated by D. Nathan.
Participants: H. Bischoff, J. L. Chiasson, W. Creutzfeldt, J. Gerich, H. E. Lebovitz, H. Meyer, S. Raptis, T. R. Weihrauch, B. Willms

Summary of the discussion

The goal of the concluding round table discussion was to explore future directions for diabetes research and treatment. The focus of the discussion was not only diabetes, but also the constellation of risk factors for macrovascular disease that occur both in diabetes and in the absence of significant glucose intolerance. The important discussion points were:

1. to define the borders between non-insulin-dependent diabetes mellitus (NIDDM) and the so-called Syndrome X, or to determine that a continuum of risk factors for macrovascular disease in both renders the distinction unnecessary.
2. to develop therapies that can be widely implemented across various populations either to interfere with the development of Syndrome X or to interfere with macrovascular disease and other risk factors that accompany it. The risk factors are multiple and multiplicatively contribute to macrovascular disease.
3. to determine whether insulin or pro-insulin levels are in fact causally related to the development of these macrovascular complications.
4. to determine the extent to which glucose levels are directly related to complications and based on the evidence to decide whether to treat them.
5. to determine the role of acarbose in treating diabetes.

What is the best and scientifically proven therapy for a 50 year old, otherwise healthy, but grossly obese and hyperinsulinemic type II diabetic patient who, after several attempts, shows no complicance to a diet or physical activity program?

One approach is to try an agent which does not raise insulin levels and which helps to control the glucose level such as acarbose and use it as a first-line monotherapy drug. Then perhaps add or substitute metformin. The combination of metformin and acarbose is also effective. Even without regarding the possibility of cardiovascular disease, there is no reason to treat this patient with insulin or sulfonylureas just to get the blood glucose down. The other end of the spectrum is to argue that the basis of any therapy is diet. Without adherence to a diet it is impossible to improve the quality or extent of this patient's life. To treat this patient with anything unless he/she complies with a diet is useless. The opposite response is to claim that it is not fair to assume that a dramatic effect cannot occur without trying and to treat the patient with everything to start.

Given this range, it is necessary to examine individual situations more closely. For example, if the patient's fasting glucose level is normal and his/her hemoglobin A_{1c} is 8% and the postprandial glycemia is about 10 mmol, then metformin and acarbose are equally effective.

However with a fifty-year-old patient it is necessary to look for contraindications, in which case acarbose is safer.

Control of the blood glucose is also an issue to be discussed in this context. If one can believe that control – glycemic control measured by its effects on the lipids or by its direct effects – is of benefit, then the doctor is obligated to treat the patient. The debate is whether or not to treat with insulin to gain control of the blood glucose. Some feel strongly that insulin levels are detrimental and cause complications, others disagree. One possibillity is to treat the patient with intensive insulin for two to three weeks to gain optimal control of glycemia and then switch to oral treatment. Another is to bring him/her into the hospital and gain control by putting them on a 600 or 700 kcal. diet rather than give insulin. The blood glucose will come down and the insulin sensitivity will improve. The insulin approach has the advantage that it takes control in 24 hours whereas a diet takes 2 to 2½ days.

The issue becomes more complex as one considers the potential link between hyperinsulinemia and multiple complications including cardiovascular disease. If insulin plays a role in atherogenesis, it must be together with high glucose, not low glucose. Others argue that the analogy between an insulin-treated, poorly controlled diabetic patient and cases of hyperinsulinemia which occur in the presence of insulin resistance and normal glucose levels is not valid. The disturbance of lipids in the poorly controlled diabetic probably has a different basis than the risk profile evident in the pre-type II diabetic. Thus the risk factor profile in type II diabetics who are insulin treated may differ from the pattern for chronic hyperinsulinemia with normal glucose metabolism. Studies testing the relationship of insulin therapy to cardiovascular risk factors have been done, but the results have been either inconclusive or have yet to be published. With regard to the threat of high insulin levels, the connection between hyperinsulinism in type II diabetes and risk factors has not absolutely been determined. In fact, patients often need insulin to control their hyperglycemia.

What is the clinical relevance of impaired glucose tolerance (IGT) and should IGT be treated?

There is a spectrum of opinions on IGT. One possibility is not to treat it at all because it may not be a disease; it has never been proven definitively that impaired glucose tolerance produces an increase in cardiovascular disease. It is, however associated with increased cardiovascular disease. Another argument is that it is an important risk factor, or that it can be a marker for other risks such as cardiovascular disease, hyperlipidemia, obesity and hypertension. These physicians argue that the IGT category describes moderately or at least increased cardiovascular risk. The question then is whether the limits for treating hyperlipidemia or hypertension should not be extended to IGT as well. Still others feel that measuring insulin is much more important than measuring blood glucose in making decisions about which people to treat with which oral agents. One of the main conclusions from the discussion is that at this time there is not enough data to support treatment of IGT. No one has been able to demonstrate a direct link between glucose levels themselves and cardiovascular disease.

The question is whether to wait until the patient at risk develops hypertension or hyperlipidemia and treat those individually, or to monitor insulin levels or to use glucose intolerance as a marker of increased risk and treat it independent of other risk factors.

Have you done a meta-analysis for assessment of the efficacy and tolerance of acarbose?

The overall durability experienced in tests of acarbose is 65%. The leading side effects are flatulence and meteorism in 65%. Diarrhea was experienced in 40%, abdominal pain in 7.6%, hypoglycemia in 9.4%.

Since the major demonstrated impact of acarbose has been on postprandial glucose levels, does that suggest a group of patients who will most benefit from acarbose monotherapy? Is there any evidence that a decrease in postprandial glucose levels by themselves will lead to fewer long-term complications?

Often it depends on the aim of the therapy for a particular patient. If the type II diabetic patient cannot be successfully treated with diet alone, then acarbose is a plausible first choice. In patients with relatively modest hyperglycemia, the older patient, and the patient with high postprandial blood glucose levels, acarbose is indicated for monotherapy. Metformin can be substituted if failure occurs. In case of further failure, sulfonylurea can be used. Care needs to be taken to ensure that a patient not be treated for a number of years with acarbose without regard to the complications that may ensue because of a lack of control.

What are the guidelines for treating type I diabetics with acarbose?

Acarbose can lower postprandial glucose in insulin-dependent diabetics (IDDM). It is not possible to titrate the acarbose dose for patients who are used to titrating their insulin doses based on algorithms. The role of acarbose in IDDM treatment has not clearly been determined.

Do patients change their diet when they are treated with acarbose to reduce the side effects and interfere with their therapy?

No, patients do not change their diets by themselves in reaction to side-effects. Diet does in fact contribute a large part to acarbose treatment. There is some dispute as to whether calories or carbohydrates affect acarbose treatment. However, compliance to diet is a large problem. The best diet plan for each individual patient is difficult to determine. In any case, the patient should be encouraged to eat regular meals – not to skip a meal and overdo the next one.

Do diabetic patients have more severe intestinal problems related to mild gastroenteropathy? Does acarbose exacerbate this tendency?

No complications or increase of impaired gastric emptying or delayed gastric emptying have been shown in connection with acarbose.

Is there any change in intestinal bacteria after long-term use of acarbose?

There are some changes in the bacterial flora and especially in the lactobacillus.

Are insulin and/or pro-insulin levels causally related to macrovascular complications?

The issue of the potential risk factors with pro-insulin, split-pro-insulin and insulin was raised. There has been a recent controversy as to whether insulin and/or pro-insulin levels are causally related to the development of macrovascular complications. If this connection were to be established, then the use of insulin, which lowers pro-insulin/insulin ratios, and sulfonylureas which increase this ratio would require re-evaluation. The discussion was brief and the main conclusion was that more information needs to be available in order to properly discuss the subject.

The participants of the final round table discussion debated many aspects of the future for diabetes research and treatment. There was a spectrum of opinions on the proper treatment of diabetes both in general and as applied to specific situations. As to the question of insulin or pro-insulin levels in relation to the development of macrovascular complications, opinions were equally varied. The primary conclusion was that, in order to determine definitively the relationship, more data are necessary.

IV Abstracts

A multi-center, double-blind, placebo-controlled study of the long-term efficacy and safety of acarbose (BAY g 5421) in the treatment of obese patients with NIDDM treated by diet alone

R. F. Coniff

After a 6-week lead-in, 212 demographically comparable patients were randomized: 107 to placebo and 105 to acarbose. The patients were then titrated in a step-wise fashion at 3 to 6-week intervals from 50 mg t. i. d. to 300 mg t. i. d. for a total duration of 24 weeks on study treatment. This was followed by a 6-week lead-out period.

Mean changes from baseline

	Placebo	Acarbose
HbA_{1c} in %	0.53 (A)	−0.06
FBS in mg/dl	10.53 (A)	−5.11
60′ BS in mg/dl	19.26 (A)	−30.55
90′ BS in mg/dl	12.45 (A)	−39.08
120′ BS in mg/dl	12.45 (A)	−37.95
Glucose AUC mg-min/dl	1366.11 (A)	−4560.39
Glucose Cmax mg/dl	14.72 (A)	−40.31
Glucose rise mg/dl	5.17 (A)	−29.29

change is % change
(A): significantly different from acarbose

Acarbose was superior to placebo in affecting all glycemic efficacy variables. Notably, the placebo group significantly deteriorated glycemic control on diet alone which acarbose was able to prevent. Tolerability was good despite a high gastrointestinal adverse drug reaction profile related to the drug's mechanism of action.

A multi-center, double-blind, placebo-controlled study of long-term efficacy and safety of acarbose (BAY g 5421) and sulfonylureas in the treatment of NIDDM inadequately controlled by maximal doses of sulfonylureas (SFU)

R. F. Coniff, R. J. Innerfield

After 6-week lead-in, 167 demographically comparable NIDDM patients poorly controlled on maximal doses of SFU were randomized: 81 to placebo and 86 to acarbose. Patients were titrated step-wise from 50 mg to a maximum of 300 mg t. i. d. at 6-week intervals for a total duration of 24 weeks on study treatment. This was followed by a 6-week lead-out.

Mean changes from baseline

	Placebo	Acarbose
HbA_{1c} in %	0.18 (A)	−0.23
FBG in mg/dl	6.00	4.54
60′ BG in mg/dl	6.15 (A)	−27.29
90′ BG in mg/dl	−0.54 (A)	−28.63
120′ BG in mg/dl	−3.92 (A)	−26.92
Glucose AUC mg-min/dl	677.90 (A)	−2824.92
Glucose Cmax mg/dl	1.32 (A)	−28.73
Glucose rise mg/dl	0.12 (A)	−30.41
FP insulin	23.71	14.51
60′ insulin	20.32	3.53
90′ insulin	20.57 (A)	−7.91
120′ insulin	28.71	0.84
Insulin AUC	20.31 (A)	−5.15

change is % change
(A): significantly different from acarbose

A multi-center, double-blind, comparative study of the long-term efficacy and safety of acarbose (BAY g 5421) vs. placebo in the treatment of patients with insulin requiring type II diabetes mellitus

F. X. Pi-Sunyer

This is a report of a 36-week, outpatient, multi-center (7), double-blind, placebo-controlled, stratified by HbA_{1c}, randomized, parallel group (acarbose vs. placebo) forced titration study. It consists of a 6-week pretreatment (run-in) period, a 24-week treatment period, and a 6-week post treatment period (run out). Acarbose was started at 50 mg and raised at each subsequent 6-wk visit to 100, 200, and finally 300 mg (unless the patients reported intolerable side-effects). The stratification for HbA_{1c} was: Stratum I less than 6.3% and Stratum II 6.3% or greater (normal 3.6 – 4.9%).

Primary criteria of efficacy were: (1) reduction in glycosylated hemoglobin (HbA_{1c}) levels from baseline, (2) reduction in daily insulin requirements (dosage) from baseline. Secondary criteria for efficacy were: (1) reduction from baseline in fasting glucose levels, (2) reduction from baseline in postprandial glucose levels, following a meal tolerance test, as manifested by, (a) reduction from baseline in the area under the postprandial plasma glucose concentration-time curve (AUC), from 60 to 120 min, (b) reduction from baseline in plasma glucose at each postprandial timepoint, (c) reduction from baseline in maximal postprandial glucose level (Cmax), (3) reduction from baseline in serum lipid levels (total cholesterol and triglycerides), (4) reduction from baseline in reported episodes of hypoglycemia.

The demographic characteristics of the population (drug vs. placebo) showed the groups to be comparable with regard to age (mean age 59 years), gender (54% male), race (71% caucasian), body mass index (31), and years since diagnosis (12 years).

Since there were few significant drug by stratum interactions the intended analysis by stratum was deemed unnecessary. All continuous efficacy analyses were based on both strata combined, with a main effect for stratum included. 110 placebo and 107 acarbose patients were valid for safety analysis; 104 placebo and 103 acarbose patients were valid for efficacy analysis. Mean changes from baseline in all efficacy variables at double-blind endpoint, for patients valid for analysis of efficacy, are shown in the following table.

Mean changes from baseline	Placebo	Acarbose
HBA_{1c} in %	−0.17*	−0.57
Total daily insulin dose in units	1.19*	−7.14
Fasting plasma glucose in mg/dl	11.86*	−4.55
60 min plasma glucose in mg/dl	6.08*	−34.72
90 min plasma glucose in mg/dl	7.75*	−47.10
120 min plasma glucose in mg/dl	6.03*	−44.16
Plasma glucose AUC mg-min/dl	1177.33*	−3676.79
Plasma glucose CMAX mg/dl	4.07*	−42.05
Plasma glucose RISE mg/dl	−6.03*	−30.10
No. of hypoglycemic episodes	−1.63	−0.30
Total serum triglycerides in mg/dl	22.73	4.16
Total serum cholesterol in mg/dl	−4.88	0.46
HDL serum cholesterol in mg/dl	0.70	−0.07
LDL serum cholesterol in mg/dl	−7.48	0.79

change is % change
*: significantly different from acarbose

With regard to adverse events, 46% of the placebo patients and 80% of the acarbose patients reported one or more adverse events while taking study medication, a highly significant difference. This difference occurred solely in the digestive system. 13% of the placebo vs. 33% of the acarbose group reported diarrhea; 35% of the placebo vs. 76% of the acarbose group reported flatulence. These were significantly different at the $p < 0.05$ level.

In conclusion, in this long-term placebo-controlled study of insulin-requiring type II diabetes patients, while there was a significantly greater incidence of adverse events in the acarbose treated patients, the great majority were gastrointestinal in nature and not serious. With regard to efficacy, acarbose was shown to significantly improve glycemic control while also significantly reducing daily insulin requirements.

Prospective, multi-center studies of the efficacy and safety of acarbose (BAY g 5421) in the treatment of type I diabetes mellitus

D. S. Schade

The safety and efficacy of acarbose (BAY g 5421) was studied in two large, prospective multi-center clinical trials in the United States, involving approximately 500 patients. The protocol of both studies was similar, i. e., a 24 week placebo-controlled, randomized parallel design in which half the patients received placebo and half a forced titration dose of acarbose (50 mg to 300 mg). This treatment period was preceded by a 6 week observation period and also followed by a 6 week no treatment period. The patients were all type I diabetic adults in general good health.

The combined results of both clinical trials demonstrated that acarbose significantly reduced both HBA_{1c} (by 0.22%) and total daily insulin requirements (by 5.7 units per day). In addition, glucose excursion post meal was significantly improved as assessed by the decreased area under the curve (−5,536 mg-min/dl). No significant changes in plasma lipids were observed, and no serious adverse events were caused by acarbose. Gastrointestinal side-effects (flatulence and diarrhea) were the most common manifestations of acarbose therapy.

These two studies demonstrate that acarbose can improve glucose control in type I diabetic patients, Its side effects were mild and it was well tolerated by the majority of patients. Acarbose appears as a clinically useful addition to the therapeutic regimen in type I diabetic patients.

Two multi-center, double-blind, placebo-controlled studies of efficacy and safety of acarbose treatment of type I diabetes

P. Holander, R. F. Coniff

Acarbose, an alpha-glucosidase inhibitor, because of it's effect on postprandial (PP) glucose may serve as an adjunct therapy in IDDM. In this study, two groups of IDDM patients were treated with identical protocols. After a 6-week lead-in demographically compatible patients were randomized. Drug was titrated in a step-wise fashion at 3 to 6-week intervals from 50 mg t. i. d. to 300 mg t. i. d. for a total of 24 weeks on study treatment. This was followed by a 6-week lead-out period. Insulin adjustment was done per individual investigator.

Mean changes from baseline

Protocol (PR)	D86-005		D86-053	
	Placebo	Acarbose	Placebo	Acarbose
No. of patients	116	103	122	114
Daily insulin dose in units	3.15 (A)	−5.41	−0.49	−3.38
HbA_{1c} in %	0.06	0.10	0.18 (A)	−0.30
FBS in mg/dl	13.88	11.39	−0.37 (A)	−26.75
60′ BS on mg/dl	16.09 (A)	−19.57	0.62 (A)	−57.96
90′ BS on mg/dl	15.68 (A)	−31.54	−11.69 (A)	−58.58
120′ BS on mg/dl	16.16 (A)	−31.75	−12.44 (A)	−53.60
Glucose AUC mg-min/dl	1385.66	−2185.8	−445.56 (A)	−7947.94
Glucose Cmax mg/dl	18.89 (A)	−31.38	−6.28 (A)	−60.36
Glucose rise mg/dl	2.21 (A)	−30.96	−3.36 (A)	−26.22
Hypoglycemic events	−1.64	−2.00	−2.87	−2.19

change is % change
(A): significantly different from acarbose

Acarbose lowered PP glucose in both groups. Interestingly investigators on PR D86-053 did not lower insulin dose which resulted in lower HbA_{1c} and FBS, whereas in PR D86-005 insulin dose was significantly reduced with no change in HbA_{1c} or FBS. Tolerability was good despite a high gastrointestinal adverse drug reaction profile. These findings support a role for acarbose as an adjunct therapy in IDDM.

Clinical study of reduced postprandial hyperglycemia by acarbose and glycemic impact of fructose and sucrose in insulin therapy

J. Wernecke, M. Dreyer, R. Fisch, G. Michels, M. Lührs, H. G. Dammann

Introduction

Glucosidase inhibitors are new therapeutics which reduce the function of intestinal brush-border glucosidase by competition. This leads finally to a decreased carbohydrate digeston and a diminished postprandial serum level of glucose and insulin [3, 8]. Acarbose, a pseudotetrasaccharide, has proven to have a certain benefit on glucose metabolism in diabetics in a number of clinical studies. This glucosidase inhibitor reduced the amount of insulin and sulphonylurea necessary for a sufficient diabetic therapy [4].

Fructose is often used instead of saccharose as a sugar substitute in the diet of diabetics. Although saccharose as a disaccharide is effected by acarbose, fructose as a monosaccharide is not. Therefore, one may ask whether the diet rules for patients taking acarbose must be changed.

Patients and methods

This study was an unicentric, double-blind, placebo-controlled, randomized fourfold cross-over study (latin square: 4 × 1 day treatment, interrupted by days of wash-out every two days).

Patients

12 patients with a mean age of 33 ± 11 years were randomized. Mean Broca Index was 1.0 ± 0.1, mean body weight was 70 ± 8 kg and mean height was 172 ± 10 cm. 9 patients were females. Duration of diabetes varied from 1 to 28 years (median = 13.5 years). Mean daily dosage was 42 ± 10 U/d.

Criteria of inclusion

- insulin-dependent diabetes mellitus
- HbA_{1c} < 9%
- duration of diabetes > 12 months
- age between 20 and 75 years
- Broca Index < 1.3
- constant diet
- creatinine < 2 mg/dl

Randomization

Each of the patients went through each of the treatment combinations (acarbose/placebo) and got each of the two test meals (fructose/sucrose). The sequence of these four combinations was fixed by chance in three latin squares each with four patients.

Study timing

Blood glucose was measured on treatment days before the meal and 30, 60, 90, 120, and 180 min postprandial.

At the beginning of the study blood was taken from each patient and measured for HbA_{1c}, creatinine, GOT, GPT, hemoglobin and erythrocytes. Before each test meal fasting-blood glucose, blood pressure and heart rate were measured.

After ingestion of the test meals, postprandial blood glucose levels were measured and events documented. During the study, diet and insulin dosage at each test meal was constant. The insulin bolus of each patient was given at a fixed time prior to the test meal.

Test meal

The test meal was baked with fructose or saccharose as a cake and was frozen for later use. One single test meal contained two slices of 55 g = 4 BE.

- 7.6 g protein
- 23.0 g fat
- 47.8 g carbohydrates (containing 20.2 g saccharose or fructose)

Results

The fasting blood sugar levels of all the four test groups varied between 184 and 202 mg/dl. Mean blood sugar levels 90 min after a test meal were 278 mg/dl for placebo + saccharose, 228 mg/dl for placebo + fructose, 208 mg/dl for acarbose + saccharose and 183 mg/dl for acarbose + fructose (Fig. 1).

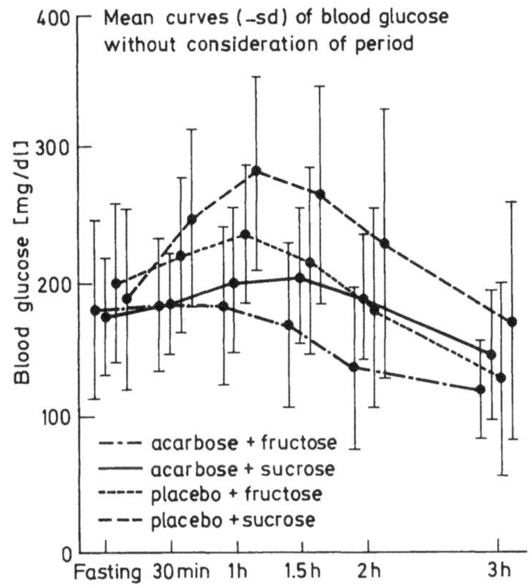

Fig. 1: Time dependency of blood glucose levels after test meals.

After three hours plasma levels for glucose were 168 mg/dl for placebo + sucrose, 141 mg/dl for placebo + fructose, 142 mg/dl for acarbose + sucrose and 125 mg/dl for acarbose + fructose. Variance analysis of the maximal postprandial blood glucose level showed a significant reduction in the combination acarbose + test meal ($p < 0.0001$).

Also differentiation in orthogonal contrasts resulted in a significant difference between acarbose and placebo with a very low postprandial blood glucose level for acarbose.

In comparison to fructose-sucrose, the mean maximal blood glucose levels after 2 hours for fructose were also much lower (276/223 mg/dl) than those for sucrose (415/267 mg/dl; placebo/acarbose). Because of a high interindividual variation this difference between fructose and sucrose was not statistically significant.

Side-effects like gastrointestinal complications which occurred in other studies with acarbose were not evident. There were no drop-outs in this study. All vital signs and other laboratory parameters were estimated to be in normal ranges. So acarbose was well tolerated by the patients.

Discussion

The high fasting blood glucose levels reflect the strong hyperglycemic effect of higher morning demand of insulin and fastly decreasing effect of the last given dose of long acting insulin on the preceding evening. Additionally, this reflects the low body activity level in the schoolish atmosphere of our diabetes training center.

The significant decrease of postprandial blood glucose levels by acarbose confirmed the data of former clinical investigations [4, 5]. If these lower postprandial blood glucose levels also lead to a better metabolic control in the long run has still to be proven. Preliminary investigations seem to confirm this hope [6, 9].

The absolute difference between mean postprandial blood glucose levels after fructose- or sucrose-test meal and equal doses of prandial insulin injection confirms the investigations of Chantelau et al. [2] and our recommendation to reduce the prandial insulin dose in case of meals with high amount of low GI carbohydrates. The Glycemic Index [7] should be a basis for prandial insulin substitution. The extremely individual variation and the resulting loss of significance in comparing meals with fructose or sucrose shows that, in daily insulin therapy, other factors are more important [1]. On the other hand, the fructose test meal contained only 20 g pure fructose. If one accounts only a third of this for the insulin dosage in comparison with the full amount of 47 g carbohydrates, the difference of the insulin dose would not be extreme. Only if you choose pure or high amounts of fructose food like fruit salads should the difference be big enough. Therefore, a reduction of the insulin dose for fructose containing meals is advisable for safety reasons especially in the case of large fructose meals.

Type II diabetics, who use fructose-containing diet products, need not to change to a diet with complex carbohydrates under the treatment with acarbose.

References

[1] Beattle, V. A. et al.: Brit. Med. J. *296* (1988) 1147–1149.
[2] Chantelau, E. et al.: Aktuelle Ernährungsmedizin *10* (1985) 231–240.
[3] Creutzfeld, W.: MMW *31/31* (1990) 475–490.
[4] Fölsch, U. R.: Diab. Nutr. Metab. *3* (1990) 63–68.
[5] Hanefeld, M. et al.: Diab. Nutr. Metab. *3* (1990) 51–57.
[6] Hoffmann, J.: MMW *132* (1990) 49–51.
[7] Jenkins, D. J. et al.: Am. J. Clin. Nutr. *34* (1981) 362–366.
[8] Müller, L., Puls, W.: Excerpta Medica (1990) 288–308.
[9] Rodler, M. et al.: Diabetes et Metab. *14* (1988) 12–14.

6 months monotherapy of NIDDM with acarbose or glibenclamide

M. Spengler, G. Hänsel, K. Boehme

Introduction

NIDDM insufficiently controlled with diet alone needs additional treatment with oral antidiabetic drugs. Sulphonylureas have been considered standard therapy for many years. Acarbose represents a new therapeutic principle with antihyperglycemic properties. It acts by inhibiting intestinal α-glucosidases resulting in a delayed absorption of dietary carbohydrates and a reduction of the blood glucose response.

Aim of the study

The aim of this study was to investigate the efficacy of 6 months monotherapy with acarbose versus glibenclamide on metabolic control of dietarily treated NIDDM patients.

Study design

Multicentered, randomized, 2-arm group comparison study with 20 blocks of 4 patients each.

Dosage

Acarbose:	weeks 1 – 2: 3 × 50 mg per day weeks 3 – 24: 3 × 100 mg per day
Glibenclamide:	1 – 3 × 3.5 mg per day, individually according to metabolic control (mean daily dose at beginning: 1.2 ± 0.6, in week 24: 1.8 ± 0.6 tablets)

Inclusion criteria

Male and female NIDDM outpatients, insufficiently treated with diet alone; blood glucose fasting ≥ 7.8 mmol/l and 1 hour p. p. ≥ 10.0 mmol/l; duration of diabetes ≥ 2 months, age 40 – 70 years; Broca-index ≤ 1.3.

Description of treatment groups (Tab. 1)

Table 1: Description of treatment groups (means ± s. d.)

	Acarbose n = 26	Glibenclamide n = 29
Age [years]	59 ± 5	60 ± 7
Sex [♂]	11 = 42%	11 = 38%
Weight [kg]	76 ± 10	73 ± 10
Height [cm]	171 ± 7	170 ± 7
Broca-index	1.07 ± 0.12	1.06 ± 0.11
Diabetes since [years]	1.0 (median)	0.7 (median)
Diet [kJ/day]	7006 ± 1167	6755 ± 1262

55 out of 72 included patients were valid for efficacy analysis. 11 patients did not fulfill the inclusion criteria, 6 were drop-outs.

Efficacy (Tab. 2, 3, Fig. 1)

Table 2: Baseline (day 0) and after 24 weeks (end) geometric means; 1 s-range

		Acarbose n = 26	Glibenclamide n = 29
Blood glucose [mmol/l]			
fasting	day 0	8.6; 7.5 – 9.9	8.6; 7.5 – 10.5
	end	6.7; 5.3 – 8.6	6.6; 5.8 – 7.4
1 h p.p.	day 0	11.3; 9.6 – 13.3	11.4; 9.1 – 14.2
	end	8.7; 6.8 – 11.1	8.2; 7.1 – 9.5
HbA_1 [%]	day 0	10.8; 9.6 – 12.3	11.0; 9.6 – 12.5
	end	8.5; 7.2 – 10.1	8.7; 7.6 – 9.9

No statistically significant differences in blood glucose and HbA_1 between acarbose and glibenclamide treatment were detected.

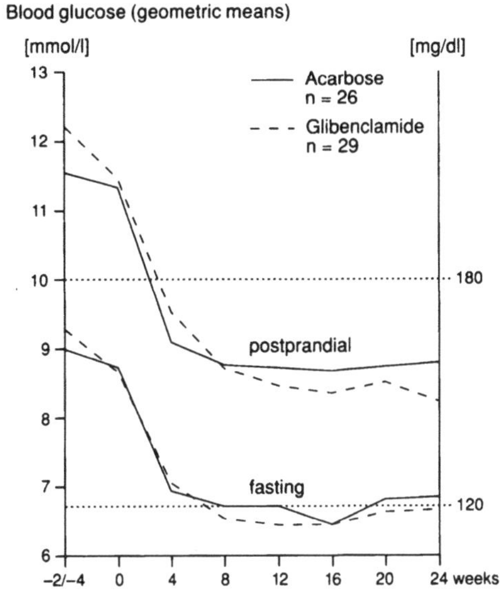

Fig. 1: Mean courses of fasting and postprandial blood glucose.

Table 3: Percentage of patients [%] within normal, tolerable and not tolerable HbA_1-range before (0) and after 24 weeks of treatment

	Acarbose		Glibenclamide	
HbA_1-range	0	24	0	24
Normal range 5 – 8%	0	35	0	24
Tolerable range > 8 – 10%	31	50	24	59
Not tolerable > 10%	69	15	76	17

Tolerability

Neither treatment revealed any influence on safety parameters. The tolerability of both treatments was good. Intestinal symptoms caused by enhanced colonic carbohydrate fermentation were reported by 58% of the patients within the first weeks of acarbose treatment. This number continuously decreased with the duration of treatment. At the end of the study, only 2 patients = 6% reported meteorism. No hypoglycemia was seen under both treatments.

Conclusion

Blood glucose fasting and 1 hour postprandial and HbA_1 of NIDDM patients, insufficiently controlled with diet alone, were markedly improved by long-term monotherapy with acarbose as well as with glibenclamide. Patients with HbA_1-values above 10%, classified as "not tolerable", dropped under acarbose from 69% at the beginning to 15% after 24 weeks of treatment, under glibenclamide from 76% to 17%.

The study results demand further controlled studies including a placebo arm and additional measurements such as postprandial insulin and insulin sensitivity.

Decreased insulin requirement and postprandial insulin plasma concentrations under treatment with the α-glucosidase inhibitor acarbose

H. Hobler, M. Spengler

Introduction

Hyperinsulinism is a common feature in NIDDM patients and probably a pathogenic factor in macroangiopathy. Acarbose treatment delays carbohydrate absorption by inhibiting intestinal α-glucosidases and thus affecting postprandial blood glucose and insulin levels. The dosages recommended for antidiabetic treatment range from 50 to 200 mg acarbose t. i. d.

Results

In *healthy volunteers* given acarbose 200 mg t. i. d. immediately prior to standardized meals, the area under the curve (AUC) of postprandial insulin (IRI) concentration in blood (0 – 360 min post applicationem) was reduced by 33% compared to placebo ($p < 0.02$) (Fig. 1). This insulin-saving effect was not substantially dependent on the carbohydrate (CHO) content (43% or 60%) of the standardized food intake [1].

In *NIDDM patients* (Fig. 2) given acarbose 100 mg t. i. d. without any additional antidiabetic medication, the decrease of the 1 h postprandial insulin and glucose blood concentrations persisted during long-term treatment (6 months) [5].

In *NIDDM patients* ($n = 8$), acarbose 200 mg t. i. d. reduced breakfast postprandial increase of gastroinhibitory polypeptide (GIP) blood concentration (60 min p. appl. Acarbose mean = 243 (SD = 98) pg/ml versus placebo mean = 365 (SD = 103) pg/ml). Glucagon plasma concentrations were not affected by acarbose treatment [4].

In *IDDM patients* (Fig. 3), the insulin requirement under acarbose (50, 100 or 200 mg as single dose) decreased by 25 – 65% as measured by an artificial pancreas (Biostator) [2]. In accordance with these results a decrease of 24 h insulin requirement of 40 – 46% (Biostator) in IDDM-patients ($n = 19$) under treatment with 200 mg t. i. d. acarbose was described [3].

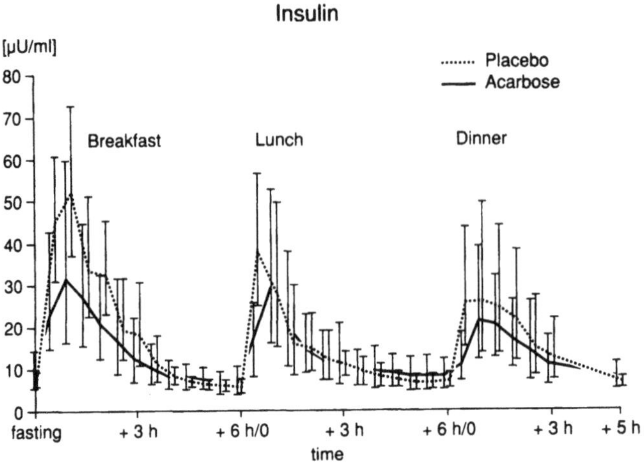

Fig. 1: Effects of 200 mg acarbose compared to placebo on the insulin release after standardized diet containing 43% carbohydrates in 12 volunteers per treatment group.
Data are expressed as geometric means geometric SD [1].

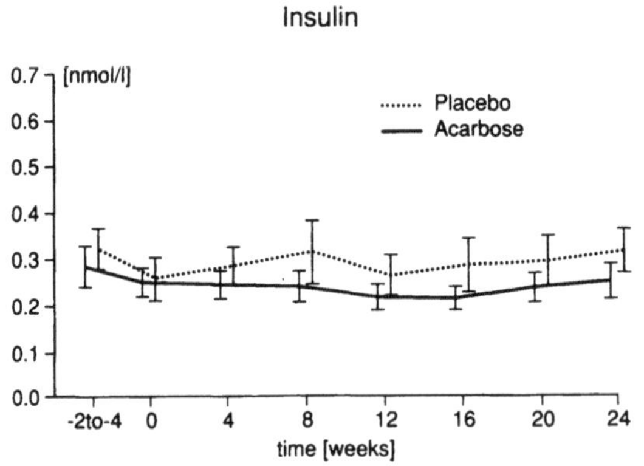

Fig. 2: 1 h postprandial insulin concentrations in long-term treatment with 100 mg acarbose t. i. d. versus placebo in 47 NIDDM patients per treatment group.
Data are expressed as means with 95% confidence limits [5].

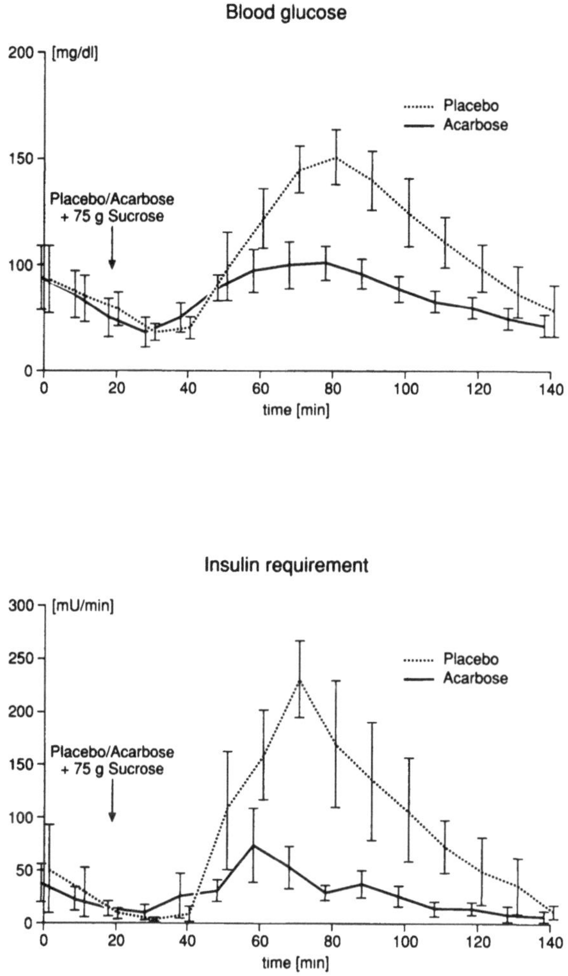

Fig. 3: Effects of 75 g of sucrose with placebo versus 75 g of sucrose with 200 mg acarbose on blood glucose levels and insulin requirements (Biostator) in 5 IDDM patients. Data are expressed as means ± SEM. * = $p < 0.05$, and ** = $p < 0.025$ compared to placebo [2].

Conclusions

Concentrations of insulin in the blood and insulin requirement are reduced with acarbose treatment at the dosage recommended for the treatment of diabetes mellitus.

References

[1] Seiberling, M., M. Toeller, A. R. Baunack et al.: Does the amount of carbohydrates of a meal influence the effects of Acarbose on the insulin- and blood glucose response? Naunyn-Schmiedeberg's Archives of Pharmacology *339* (1989) (Suppl.) R 76.

[2] Chiasson, J. L.: Effects of sucrose meal on insulin requirements in IDDM and its modulation by Acarbose. In: W. Creutzfeldt (ed.): Acarbose for the treatment of Diabetes Mellitus, p. 177. Springer Verlag, Berlin 1988.

[3] Raptis, S., G. Dimitriadis, K. Karaiskos et al.: Long term effect of an α-glucosidase inhibitor on insulin requirements and catecholamine levels assessed by the artificial β-cell. Diabetes *29* (1980) (Suppl. 2) 41A.

[4] Berger, W., H. Hobler, M. Wargenau: unpublished data.

[5] Schulze, J., S. Fischer, M. Hanefeld et al.: 25. Deutscher Diabetes-Kongreß, Düsseldorf 1990.

Long-term treatment of BAY g 5421 (acarbose) in non-insulin-dependent diabetes mellitus

Yoshio Goto, T. Toyota, S. Oikawa, Y. Maruhama, M. Tamura, K. Komatsu, H. Fujiya, R. Abe, H. Kikuchi

Summary

Efficacy and safety of acarbose in non-insulin-dependent diabetes mellitus (NIDDM) were determined under a long-term test period of up to 1 year in a single-blind multi-clinical study. Postprandial blood glucose (PBG) and HbA_{1c} levels were significantly decreased, fasting blood glucose (FBG) and triglyceride levels tended to decrease in the 60 cases evaluated. Adverse abdominal reactions were reported frequently, but they were not severe and about half of them disappeared during the test period. Acarbose was concluded to be effective in controlling NIDDM patients with diet therapy in a long-term treatment.

Introduction

Though many clinical studies of BAY g 5421 (acarbose) have been reported in Japan and other countries, a majority of the studies are conducted under 8 – 12 weeks test period. In this study, effectiveness and safety of acarbose were evaluated in a 6 – 12 month test period for non-insulin-dependent diabetes mellitus (NIDDM) patients of poor control with diet therapy alone.

Subjects and methods

One hundred mg of acarbose was administered normally 3 times daily in 95 NIDDM patients with diet therapy alone (Tab. 1) for at least 6 months and up to 1 year. Doses of acarbose could be reduced to 50 mg in cases in which patients did not tolerate it well. Drugs affecting blood glucose, HbA_{1c} or lipids were prohibited.

Table 1: Background of subjects

Items		No. of cases
Total number of subjects		95
Sex	male	43
	female	52
Age	Mean ± S. E.	59. 0 ± 1.1
In-/Out-patients	in-patients	2
	out-patients	86
	others	7
BMI	< 20	8
	$20 \leqq \sim < 23$	26
	$23 \leqq \sim < 25$	24
	$25 \leqq \sim < 27$	18
	$27 \leqq$	19
	Mean ± S. E.	24.5 ± 0.4
Complications	without	21
	with	74
	diabetic retinopathy	19
	diabetic nephropathy	7
	diabetic neuropathy	14
	hypertension	37
	hyperlipemia	27
	heart disease	10
	disturbance of hepatic functions	10
	obesity	3
	cataract	2
	others	21
Treatment before the observation period	without	18
	with	77
	diet therapy alone	65
	diet therapy + SU agents	12
	SU agents alone	0

Results

At the end 60 cases were evaluated for efficacy and safety, and 35 cases were evaluated for safety according to the inclusion criteria for evaluation. The mean days of administration were 276.5 ± 12.4 (mean ± S. E.) in the 95 cases.

Efficacy

PBG and HbA_{1c} level were significantly decreased (Fig. 1; PBG 1 hr: 261.8 ± 7.6 → 206.4 ± 6.4 mg/dl, HbA_{1c}: 7.5 ± 0.2 → 6.7 ± 0.2%, Fig. 2, 3) and acarbose showed no tachyphylaxis during the test period (Fig. 2). Fasting blood glucose levels tended to decrease (Fig. 1; 148.0 ± 3.6 → 141.5 ± 4.6 mg/dl), body weight declined by only 0.7 kg, though the reduction was significant (Fig. 4). No significant change was observed in blood glucose, insulin and C-peptide plasma levels after 75 g OGTT (Fig. 5) and in lipids (Fig. 6).

Safety

Flatulence and abdominal fullness were mostly reported, but they were not so severe and about half of them disappeared during the test period (Tab. 2, Fig. 7).

Table 2: Adverse drug reactions (n = 95)

Symptoms	No. of cases (%)	Severity		
		Severe	Moderate	Mild
Flatulence	54 (56.8)	4	21	29
Abdominal distension	42 (44.2)	4	11	27
Meteorism	36 (37.9)	2	11	23
Defecation frequency increased	15 (15.8)		5	10
Loose stool	15 (15.8)		4	11
Diarrhea	6 (6.3)		2	4
Abdominal pain	4 (4.2)		2	2
Others	10 (10.5)	2	4	4
No. of matters	183			

Incidence of ADRs 67.4% (64/95 cases)
Discontinued 5.3% (5/95 cases)

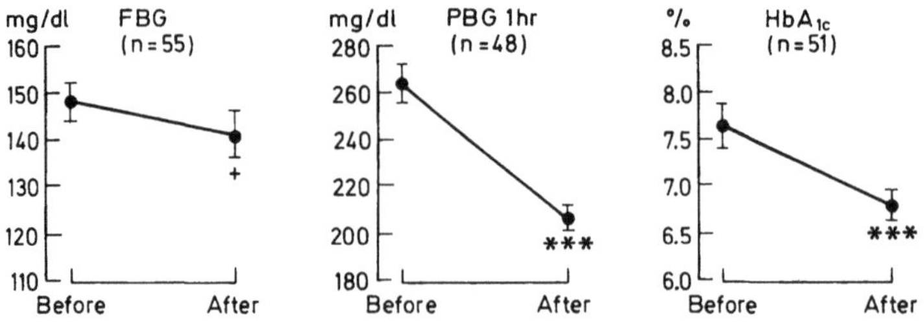

Fig. 1: Changes in FBG, PBG and HbA_{1c}.
Mean $\pm$ S.E., Paired *t*-test, †: $p < 0.1$, ***: $p < 0.001$.

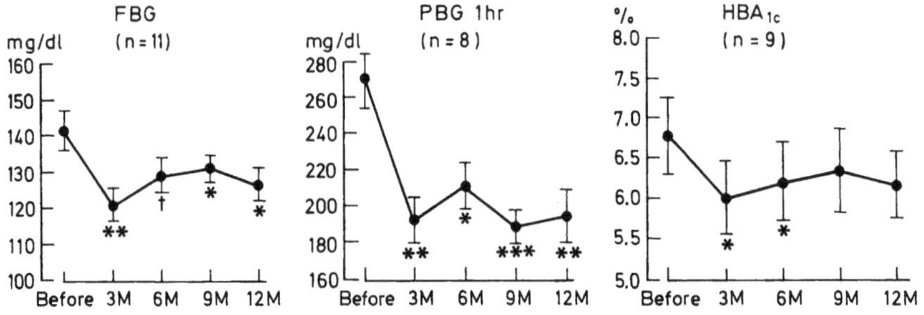

Fig. 2: Transition of FBG, PBG and HbA_{1c}.
Mean $\pm$ S.E., Paired *t*-test, †: $p < 0.1$, *: $p < 0.05$, **: $p < 0.01$, ***: $p < 0.001$.

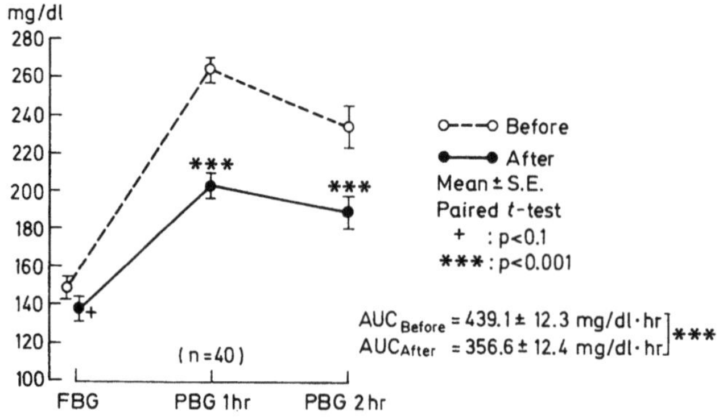

Fig. 3: Changes in area under the curve.

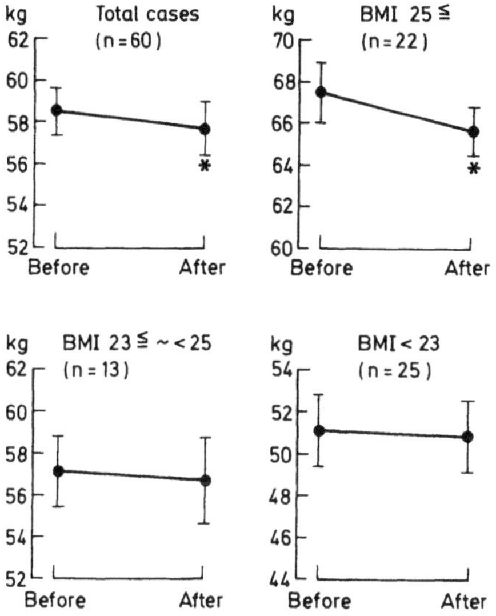

Fig. 4: Changes in body weight.
Mean ± S.E., Paired *t*-test, *: $p < 0.05$.

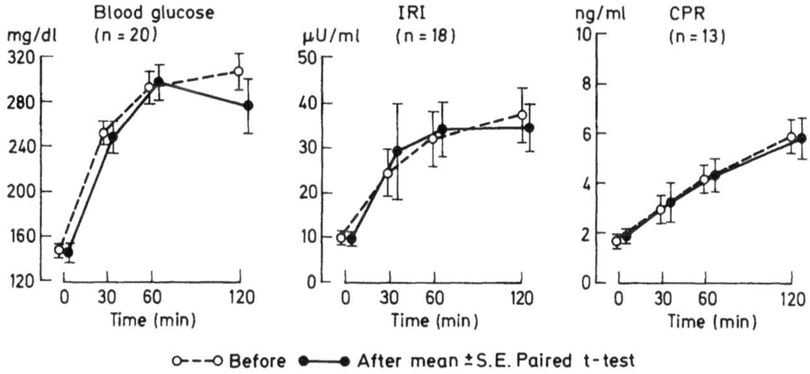

Fig. 5: Changes in blood glucose, insulin and C-peptide plasma levels after 75 g OGTT.

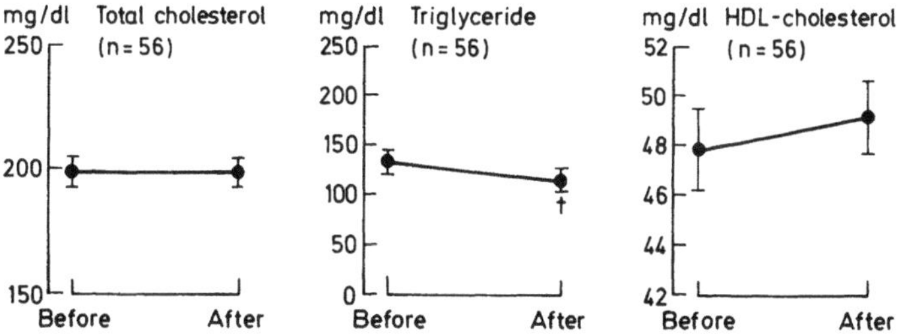

Fig. 6: Changes in serum lipids.
Mean ± S.E., Paired *t*-test, †: $p < 0.1$.

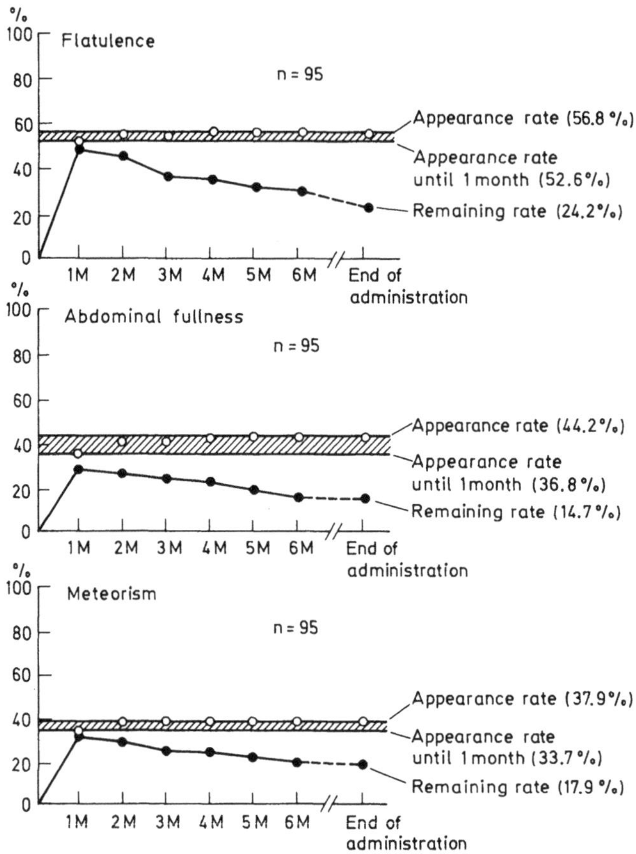

Fig. 7: Disappearance of intestinal symptoms
o: Appearance rate of intestinal symptoms (accumulation)
●: Remaining rate of intestinal symptoms (accumulation)
("Appearance rate" – "Disappearance rate").

Global utility rating

Treatment of 78.5% of the patients was evaluated "useful" by physicians (Tab. 3).

Table 3: Global utility rating

<table>
<tr><th>Very useful</th><th>Useful</th><th>Slightly useful</th><th>Useless</th><th>Undesirable</th><th>Total</th></tr>
<tr><td>13</td><td>23</td><td rowspan="2">15</td><td rowspan="3">13</td><td rowspan="3">1</td><td rowspan="3">65</td></tr>
<tr><td colspan="2">55.4%</td></tr>
<tr><td colspan="3">78.5%</td></tr>
</table>

Conclusion

Acarbose is effective in controlling blood glucose levels in NIDDM patients and is tolerated in long-term treatment.

Clinical efficacy and tolerability of acarbose in IDDM treatment

H. de la Calle, F. Escobar, D. Figuerola, E. Gíl, J. L. Herrera-Pombo, A. Jiménez, A. de Leiva, L. F. Pallardo, F. Piñón, J. Soler, J. Tebar, V. A. Vázquez

Introduction

Acarbose is a competitive and reversible α-glucosidase inhibitor that decreases postprandial glucose and insulin levels.

Previous studies in IDDM as well as NIDDM patients have shown that acarbose significantly decreases the postprandial glucose and insulin levels, thus leading to a better metabolic control.

The objective of this study was to evaluate the efficacy and tolerability of acarbose in the treatment of insulin-dependent diabetics on diet plus insulin. The treatment period lasted for three months and the main evaluation parameters were postprandial glucose as well as glycosylated hemoglobin levels.

Material and methods

A multi-center, randomized double-blind placebo-controlled study was conducted and 137 patients (61% female) were included. They were all IDDM patients, aged between 20 and 50 (27 ± 7) years and with a Broca-index below 1,30 (0.98 to 0.12). Informed consent was obtained from all participants.

During the first 3 months of treatment patients received randomly acarbose (50 mg t. i. d. during the first month and 100 mg t. i. d. during the following 2 months) or placebo. After a 1 month placebo wash-out period a 3 months treatment with acarbose or placebo followed.

Clinical and analytical controls were performed monthly and consisted of adverse events check-list, hypoglycemic crisis and glycosylated hemoglobin assessment, fasting blood glucose, cholesterol, and triglyceride measurements.

Postprandial glucose levels (0 – 120 minutes) after standard breakfast were measured at the start and at the end of each treatment period.

ANOVA was used for statistical analysis. Comparability of groups (age, weight, height, sex, fasting glucose and HbA_1 levels) was assessed also by ANOVA.

Results

The results of the study are shown in Figures 1 – 5. Statistical significant differences were reached on HbA_1 ($P = 0.0005$) and postprandial glucose ($P = 0.007$).

102 patients reported adverse effects (mostly intestinal symptoms). Only 12 patients (10 with acarbose) withdrew from the study due to adverse effects.

Discussion

The results of this study show the efficacy of acarbose in reducing HbA_1 levels and postprandial glucose in IDDM patients. These results are in agreement with those from the literature. In our study, fasting glucose levels, although decreased, did not reach statistical significance. Neither did cholesterol nor triglycerides. In contrast, postprandial glucose levels showed a clinical and statistical significant decrease. No body weight reductions and no insulin dosage changes were observed. Adverse reactions appear quite frequently, although only 10 patients withdrew due to intestinal side-effects. The frequency of them depends on the dosage and tend to decrease during the course of therapy.

In summary, the results indicate that acarbose is a useful drug in the treatment of IDDM patients reducing significantly postprandial glucose as well as glycosylated hemoglobin.

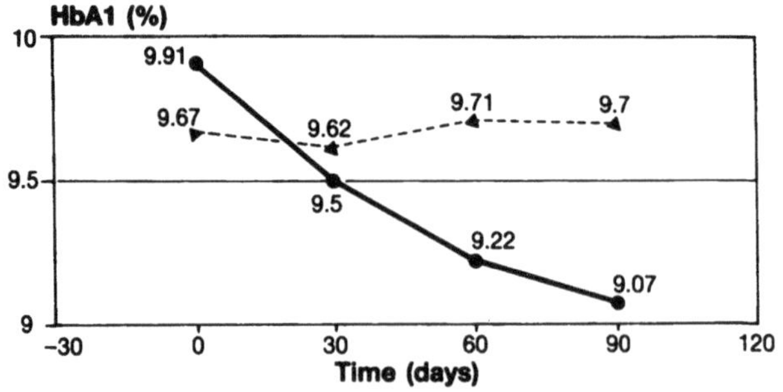

Fig. 1: Mean HbA_1 levels (0, 30, 60 and 90 days) in IDDM patients treated with acarbose (solid line) or placebo (dashed line).

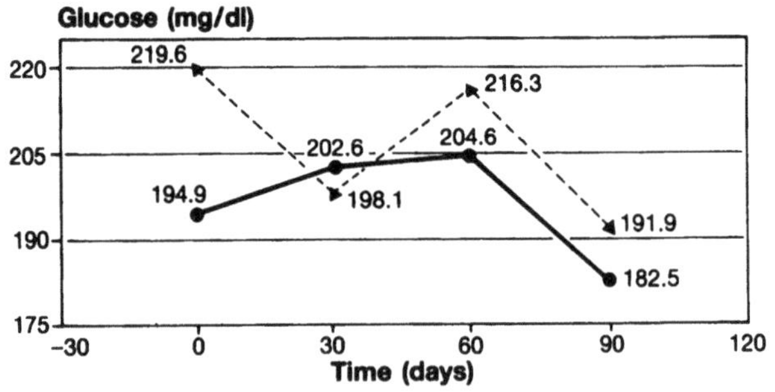

Fig. 2: Fasting glucose levels (0, 30, 60 and 90 days) in IDDM patients treated with acarbose (solid line) or placebo (dashed line).

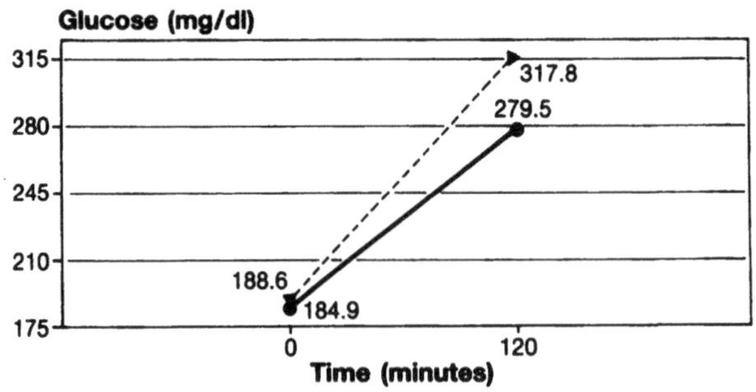

Fig. 3: Postprandial glucose levels (after standard breakfast) in IDDM patients treated with acarbose (solid line) or placebo (dashed line).

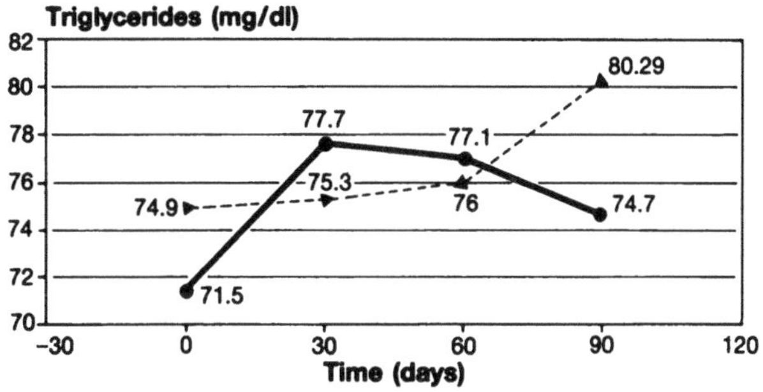

Fig. 4: Triglyceride levels (0, 30, 60 and 90 days) in IDDM treated with acarbose (solid line) or placebo (dashed line).

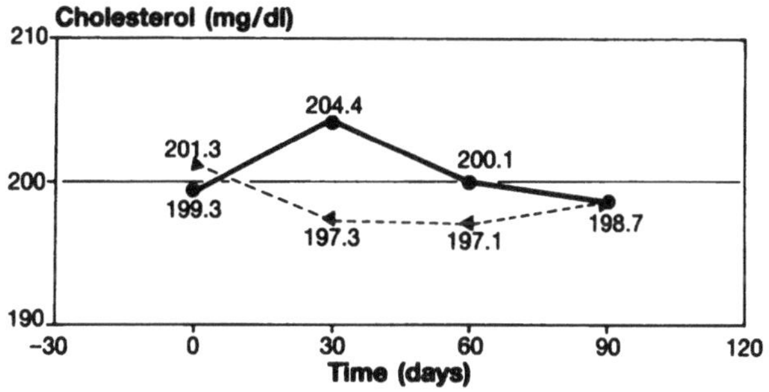

Fig. 5: Cholesterol levels (0, 30, 60, and 90 days) in IDDM treated with acarbose (solid line) or placebo (dashed line).

Effects of acarbose on the glycemic index of different foods

A. Calle, C. Rodríguez, E. Gíl

Introduction

Acarbose is a complex oligosaccharide from bacterial origin that inhibits the intestinal brush border α-glucosidases and, consequently delays the absorption of diet carbohydrates and smoothen the glycemic and insulinemic response.

It is well known that the glycemic increases after the consumption of different food is not always the same, even when the quantity of carbohydrates is identical. The glycemic index (GI) stratifies foods according to postprandial glucose rises. A diet of low GI is specially recommended for the treatment of diabetics.

The aim of this study was to evaluate the effect of acarbose – 100 mg single dose – on the glycemic response after 50 g carbohydrates from different foods (white bread, lentils, potatoes and rice), and to compare it with placebo.

Materials and methods

In a randomized, double-blind, cross-over study, 9 healthy volunteers (7 male, 2 female), aged between 18 and 46, with a body mass index of 22,7 (18 – 24), consumed different test meals on two different occasions (one with 100 mg acarbose, one with placebo). Following each single administration, a three-day wash-out period followed. All volunteers gave his/her consent to participate in the study. Meals consisted of a 50 g carbohydrate portion of either white bread (98 g), lentils (80 g), polished white rice (63 g), or potatoes (250 g). Volunteers were asked to take one tablet with the first bite of each meal and blood samples were drawn at time: – 10, 0, 30, 45, 60, 90, 120, 150 and 180 minutes. Glucose and insulin levels were analyzed and Area Under the Curve (AUC) as well as GI were obtained.

Data are presented as means ± SD. ANOVA test was used to analyze intragroup differences and the U-Mann-Whitney-test for the intergroup differences.

Results

Results from the study are shown in Tables 1 and 2 as well as in Figure 1.

Table 1: Blood glucose and insulin responses (AUC) after consumption of 50 g carbohydrates

Parameter	Meal	AUC/Placebo	AUC/Acarbose	P
	Bread	3502 ± 1390	1542 ± 1162	
Glucose	Potatoes	2399 ± 1600	1698 ± 1163	< 0.0.5
(mg-min/dl)	Lentils	1160 ± 1024	465 ± 412	
	Rice	3857 ± 1565	1909 ± 977	
	Bread	3501 ± 1390	956 ± 670	
Insulin	Potatoes	1211 ± 609	1203 ± 1354	< 0.05
(mcU. min/ml)	Lentils	1038 ± 747	333 ± 312	
	Rice	2523 ± 1368	509 ± 604	

Table 2: Glycemic index (GI) of different meals

	GI Placebo	GI Acarbose
Bread	100%	55%
Potatoes	72%	64%
Lentils	34%	12%
Rice	118%	72%

Discussion

The results demonstrate that the addition of 100 mg acarbose to different foods with a high content of carbohydrates significantly reduced both the AUC (glucose and insulin) and the GI of these foods. Our results confirm the great inequality in the extent to which different carbohydrate sources raise the blood glucose and indicate that single carbohydrate exchanges based on chemical analysis do not predict the physiological response.

In our study, the administration of 100 mg acarbose did not cause important symptoms of malabsorption. Tolerance was good, and only meteorism was described, which suggests that this dosage does not produce malabsorption.

Acarbose significantly decreased the GI of different foods in healthy volunteers. It may have an important role in the modification of absorption of carbohydrates. Low GI foods are especially appropiate for diabetic patients; as acarbose reduces this index, it could be useful in the management of these patients.

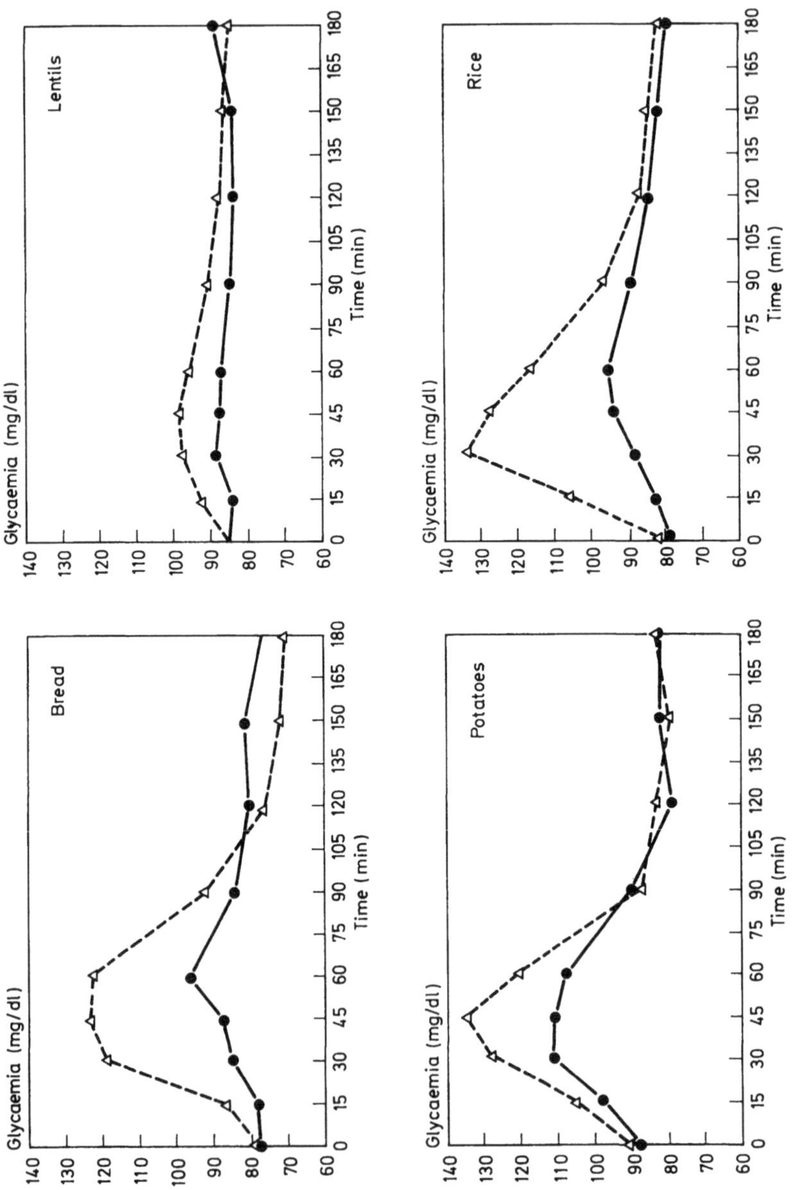
Bread
Lentils
Potatoes
Rice
Glycaemia (mg/dl)
Glycaemia (mg/dl)
Glycaemia (mg/dl)
Glycaemia (mg/dl)
140 130 120 110 100 90 80 70 60
140 130 120 110 100 90 80 70 60
140 130 120 110 100 90 80 70 60
140 130 120 110 100 90 80 70 60
Time (min)
Time (min)
Time (min)
Time (min)
0 15 30 45 60 75 90 105 120 135 150 165 180
0 15 30 45 60 75 90 105 120 135 150 165 180
0 15 30 45 60 75 90 105 120 135 150 165 180
0 15 30 45 60 75 90 105 120 135 150 165 180

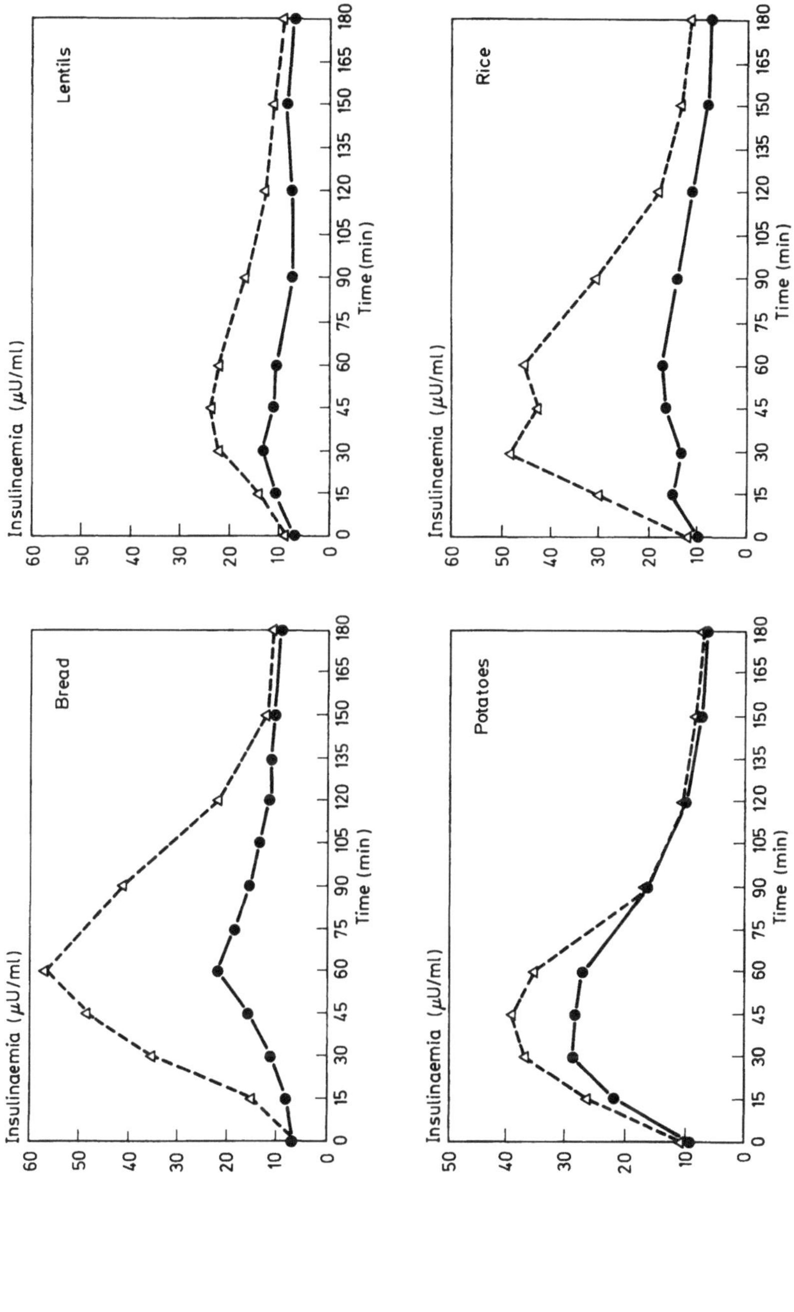

Fig. 1: Blood glucose (insulin) increments after consumption of 50 g carbohydrates portion of different meals with acarbose (solid line) or with placebo (dotted line).

Effects of acarbose on the release of gastrointestinal, pancreatic and hypophysial hormones including somatostatin in type II diabetics

G. Rohr, I. Schmidt, U. Schwedes, K. H. Usadel, Chr. Norenberg, M. Spengler

Introduction

Acarbose, a pseudotetrasaccharide, was recently shown to be effective in improving of metabolic control in type I as well as in type II diabetics. In many cases, insulin- or sulphonylurea-treatment could be reduced. Acarbose leads to a delay of the digestion of carbohydrates via inhibition of glucosidases at the brush border of the small intestine. During acarbose treatment, the serum concentration of gastrointestinal or pancreatic hormones may be changed. Raptis and coworkers found a strong increase of plasma-somatostatin. It was postulated that this increase was involved in the improvement of diabetes control.

Aim of the study

In this study, the effect of acarbose on the plasma concentration of gastrointestinal, pancreatic and hypophyseal hormones was determined, especially on somatostatin. The influence on diabetes control was investigated. The tolerability and safety of the drug was monitored.

Methods

The study was designed as a double-blind, randomized group comparison versus placebo.

Patients

- 2 × 14 type II diabetics, male or female
- pretreatment with diet only or diet and sulphonylurea
- diabetic control: blood glucose fasting ≥ 150 mg/dl
2 h pp ≥ 180 mg/dl

- duration of diabetes > 6 months
- age ≥ 40 years
- Broca-index ≤ 1.3

Exclusion criteria

- secondary failure of sulphonylurea treatment
- treatment with biguanides
- myocardial infarction < 6 months
- malignant tumors
- acute or chronic enteropathy, febrile conditions
- severe impairment of live or kidney function

Criteria for evaluation (Tab. 1)

- somatostatin (3 h-AUC, main target variable)
- blood glucose, fasting and postprandial
- insulin, C-peptide, glucagon, gastrin, GIP, ACTH, TSH, HGH, T_3 and T_4

Table 1: Profile evaluation

min	Serum-glucose -insulin -C-peptide	GIP glucagon gastrin	Somato-statin	ACTH TSH HGH	T_3 T_4
−60			•		
0	•	•	•	•	•
15	•	•	•		
30	•	•	•		
45	•	•	•		
60	•	•	•	•	
90	•	•	•		
120	•	•	•		
180	•	•	•	•	•

Treatment

- standard breakfast on day 1, followed by measurement of profiles; after that, start of treatment with 3 × 100 mg acarbose (BAY g 5421) or placebo
- duration of treatment 7 days
- test drugs: BAY g 5421-active substance 100 mg
  BAY g 5421-placebo 100 mg

- dosage: 3 × 100 mg for 7 days, measurement of profiles on day 8 after standard breakfast and 2 × 100 mg-tablets
- diet: standardized diet containing 50% carbohydrates, 30% fat, 20% protein

Statistical methods

- analysis of covariance for main target variable (somatostatin 3 h-AUC) and secondary variables

Results

Somatostatin (main target variable)

The postprandial profiles for somatostatin (3 h-AUC) showed no significant treatment-induced differences between acarbose and placebo (Tab. 2, Fig. 1). Somatostatin decreased slightly under placebo and increased slightly under acarbose.

Table 2: Somatostatin (geom. mean (1 s-range)) [pg/ml]

	Acarbose		Placebo	
	day 1	day 8	day 1	day 8
–60 min	3.9 (1.8)	4.9 (1.7)	4.4 (2.4)	5.0 (1.8)
fasting	4.9 (2.0)	6.5 (1.5)	3.8 (2.1)	4.0 (1.9)
1 h pp	3.8 (1.5)	4.6 (1.9)	4.6 (2.4)	3.5 (2.1)
2 h pp	4.0 (1.5)	3.7 (1.9)	3.6 (1.7)	3.0 (1.8)
3 h pp	3.0 (1.7)	3.8 (1.9)	3.9 (1.8)	3.0 (1.9)
AUC	12.8 (1.4)	14.0 (1.5)	14.4 (1.7)	10.6 (1.6)

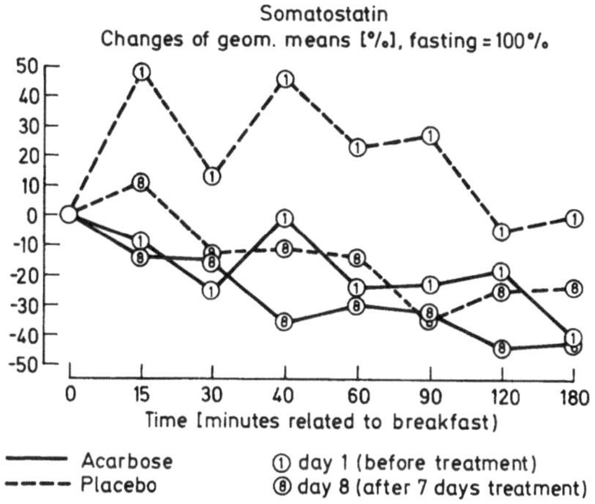

Fig. 1

Glucose

Fasting blood glucose decreased under acarbose by 28 mg/dl (= 14%), under placebo by 4 mg/dl (= 2%). The 3 h-AUC after breakfast was lowered by 22%, under placebo by 6% (Tab. 3, Fig. 2).

Table 3: Blood glucose (mean ± SD) [mg/dl]

	Acarbose		Placebo	
	day 1	day 8	day 1	day 8
fasting	204 ± 36	176 ± 38	195 ± 46	191 ± 59
1 h pp	288 ± 51	230 ± 42	279 ± 43	260 ± 58
2 h pp	31'8 ± 45	242 ± 39	311 ± 66	291 ± 78
3 h pp	315 ± 57	230 ± 43	279 ± 64	269 ± 81
AUC	868 ± 122	677 ± 120	828 ± 145	780 ± 189

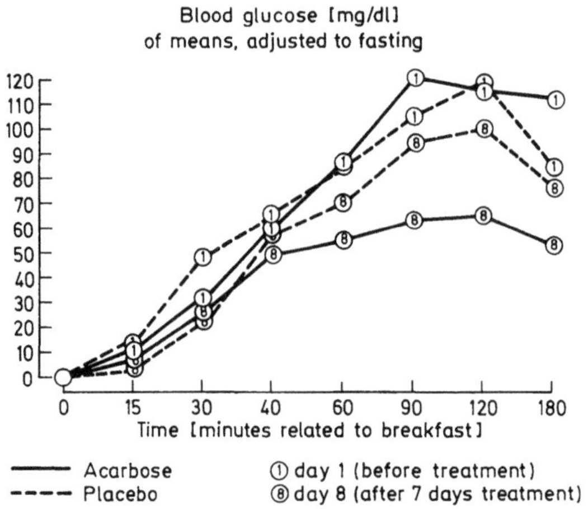

Fig. 2

Further results

Insulin, C-peptide, glucagon and gastrin remained unchanged. GIP was slightly less under acarbose (Figs. 3–6).

The postprandial profiles for ACTH, TSH, HGH, T_3 and T_4 showed no treatment-induced differences between acarbose and placebo.

Regarding tolerability, there were no remarkable differences between acarbose and placebo.

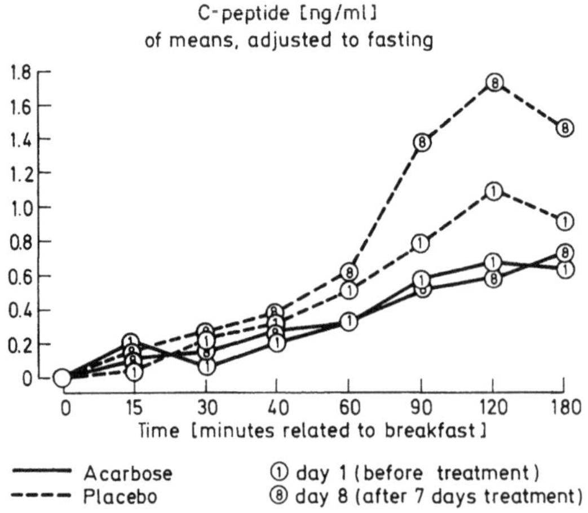

Fig. 3

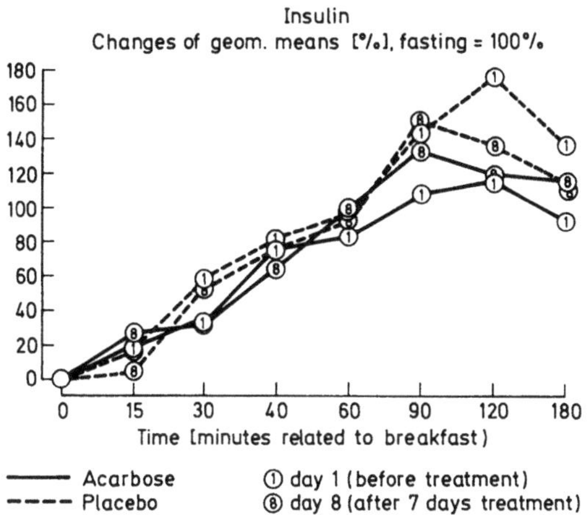
Insulin
Changes of geom. means [%], fasting = 100%
180
160
140
120
100
80
60
40
20
0
0
15
30
40
60
90
120
180
Time [minutes related to breakfast)
Acarbose
Placebo
① day 1 (before treatment)
⑧ day 8 (after 7 days treatment)

Fig. 4

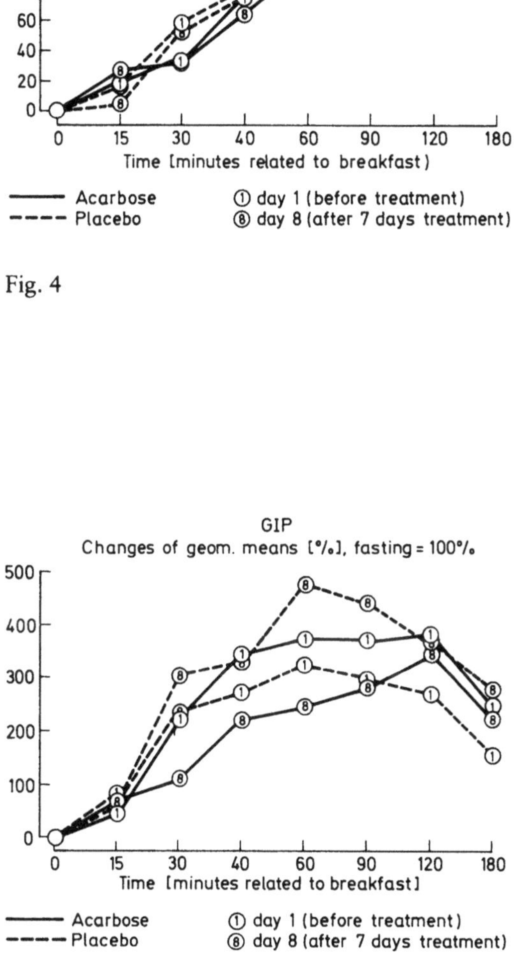
GIP
Changes of geom. means [%], fasting = 100%
500
400
300
200
100
0
0
15
30
40
60
90
120
180
Time [minutes related to breakfast]
Acarbose
Placebo
① day 1 (before treatment)
⑧ day 8 (after 7 days treatment)

Fig. 5

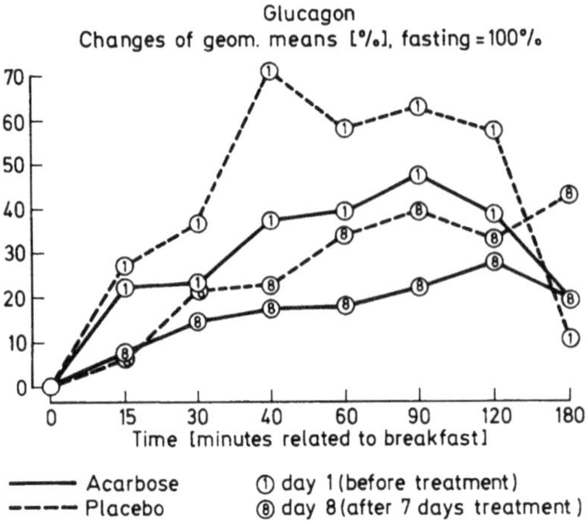

Fig. 6

Discussion

The results of Raptis and co-workers could not be confirmed: There are no treatment-induced differences between acarbose and placebo regarding serum somatostatin levels after 7 days of treatment of type II diabetics with either acarbose or placebo. As there were also no treatment-induced differences in hormone profiles of C-peptide, insulin, GIP, glucagon, ACTH, TSH, HGH, T_3 or T_4 either, there is no evidence for risks with respect to hormonal regulation by acarbose treatment.

As the glucose control was significantly improved in the acarbose group compared to placebo and as there were no remarkable differences regarding tolerability, acarbose seems to be a useful drug in the treatment of type II diabetes.

Conclusions

- Postprandial profiles of blood glucose were decreased by acarbose compared to placebo.
- The postprandial profiles for somatostatin (3 h-AUC) as well as for ACTH, TSH, HGH, T_3 and T_4 showed no treatment-induced differences between acarbose and placebo.
- Insulin, C-peptide, glucagon and gastrin remained unchanged, GIP was slightly less under acarbose.
- Regarding tolerability, there were no remarkable differences between acarbose and placebo.

References

Aubell, R., K. Boehme, P. Berchthold: Blood glucose concentrations and glucosuria during and after one year of acarbose therapy. Arzneim.-Forsch./Drug Res. *33* (9) (1983) 1314–1318.

Dimitriadis, G. D., P. Tessari, V. L. W. Go et al.: α-glucosidase inhibition improves postprandial hyperglycemia and decreases insulin requirements in insulin-dependent diabetes mellitus. Metabolism *34* (3) (1985) 261–265.

Hillebrand, I., M. Catagay, H. Schulz et al.: Efficacy and tolerability of the glucosidase inhibitor acarbose (BAY g 5421) by evaluation from the clinical data pool. Diabetes *35* Suppl. 1 (1986) 122A.

Puls, W., W. Keup, H. P. Krause et al.: Glucosidase inhibition. A new approach to the treatment of diabetes, obesity, and hyperlipoproteinaemia. Naturwissenschaften *64* (1977) 536.

Raptis, S., G. Dimitriadis, H. Etzrodt et al.: The effects of acarbose treatment on release of pancreatic and gastro-intestinal hormones in man. In: W. Creutzfeldt (ed.): Proceedings – First International Symposium on Acarbose, pp. 210–215. Excerpta Medica, Amsterdam 1982.

Raptis, S., G. Dimitriadis, C. Karaiskos et al.: Short-and-long-term studies of acarbose on various metabolic parameters and insulin requirements assessed by the artificial endocrine pancreas. In: W. Creutzfeldt (ed.): Proceedings – First International Symposium on Acarbose, pp. 393–401. Excerpta Medica, Amsterdam 1982.

Influence of acarbose on the release of gastrointestinal, pancreatic and hypophysial hormones including somatostatin in healthy volunteers

C. Rosak, B. O. Boehm, P. H. Althoff, H. Hobler, K. Boehme

Introduction

Acarbose inhibits the intestinal glucosidases in the brush border membrane of the small intestine. As a result, in healthy volunteers and in diabetics, the postprandial rise in blood glucose is reduced and delayed. This new therapeutic principle is employed successfully in more and more type II diabetics. In addition to the reduction and delay of the blood glucose increase, there is an influence on pancreatic and gastrointestinal hormones. In a study in healthy volunteers, Raptis et al. (1982) found a considerable rise in plasma-somatostatin and it was speculated that a causal relationship between this increase and the beneficial therapeutic effect of acarbose might exist.

It was the aim of this study to investigate the effect of an administration of acarbose or placebo prior to a standardized meal on somatostatin levels and on other, hitherto uninvestigated kinetics of hormones.

Study design

In a double-blind, randomized cross-over study, 10 male, healthy volunteers took 200 mg of acarbose or placebo prior to a standardized meal. The average age of these volunteers was 24 ± 4 years, the mean Broca index was 0.94 ± 0.04.

The standardized meal consisted of 75 g white bread, 15 g margarine, ¾ BE jam for diabetics, 40 g curd (20% fat), and max. 300 ml tea (mallow or mint).

Blood samples were taken at −60, 0, 15, 30, 45, 60, 90, 120 and 180 min postprandial.

Blood glucose, insulin, C-peptide, gastrointestinal polypeptide, glucagon, gastrin, somatostatin, ACTH, TSH, HGH, prolactin, T_3 and T_4 were determined.

The statistical evaluation of somatostatin (main target criterion) was based on the analysis of covariance.

Results

The administration of acarbose prior to the standardized meal led to a lower increase in the blood glucose level compared with the administration of placebo (Fig. 1).

This is paralleled by a lower increase (both AUC and maxima) of serum insulin and C-peptide as well as by a lower secretion of gastrointestinal polypeptide (GIP) and gastrin under acarbose administration as demonstrated by the correlation diagrams of the respective areas under the curve (Fig. 2).

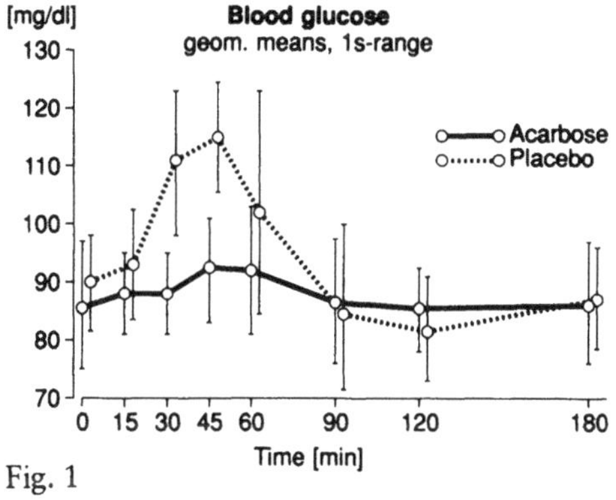

Fig. 1

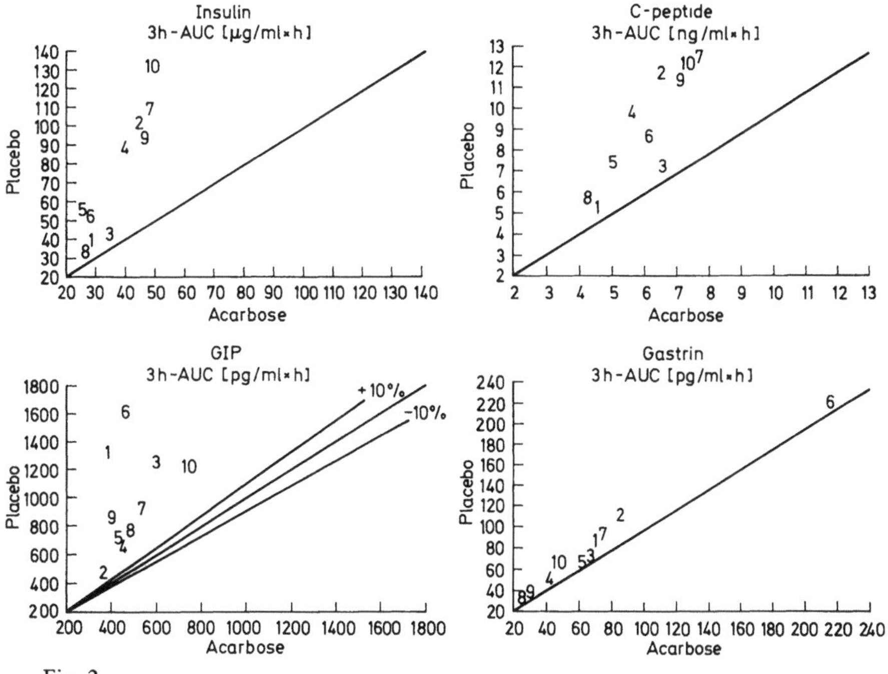

Fig. 2

Serum-somatostatin was the main target parameter of this study. After analysis of covariance no significant difference between acarbose and placebo treatment was detected for the postprandial AUC ($p \leq 0.5$) and maxima ($p \leq 0.6$ (Fig. 3). Furthermore, no changes were seen for glucagon, ACTH, HGH, prolactin, TSH and T_3 and T_4.

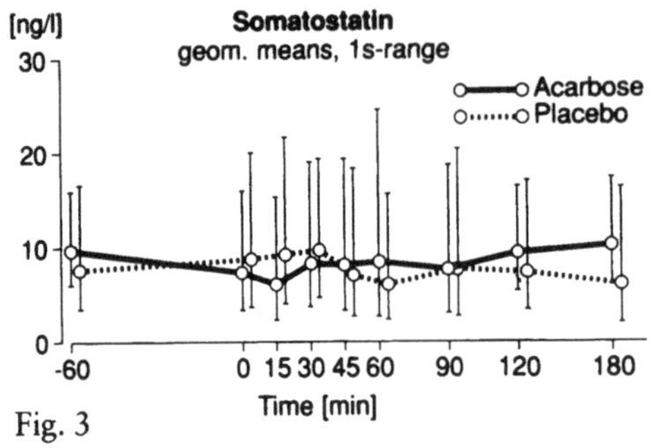

Fig. 3

Discussion and conclusion

In this placebo-controlled cross-over study in healthy volunteers with a single application of 200 mg acarbose prior to a standardized breakfast, it should in particular be investigated whether, apart from its largely known influence on the release of gastrointestinal hormones, acarbose possibly affects somatostatin concentrations in the blood and, additionally, the release of anterior pituitary and thyroid hormones. As could be expected, blood glucose values were markedly lower under acarbose treatment. The same holds true for insulin, C-peptide, GIP and, with restrictions, for the gastrin values. An influence on glucagon concentration could not be verified.

For blood concentrations of somatostatin as well as for the anterior pituitary and thyroid hormones investigated, no changes were found.

Altogether, from these investigations in healthy volunteers, a clinically relevant influence of acarbose could neither be established on serum-somatostatin-concentrations nor on the release of the anterior pituitary and thyroid hormones investigated.

Acarbose: an intestinal tract α-glucosidase inhibitor – pharmacological effects on insulin and glycemia in response to a sucrose load

K. Tawara, N. Mochizuki, A. Donkai, Y. Hikima

Introduction

Acarbose (BAY g 5421) shows prominent inhibitory effects on intestinal α-glucosidases [1] when orally administered with carbohydrate-rich meals, and consequently reduces and/or delays glucose absorption [2].

In this report, dose dependency of inhibitory effects of acarbose on plasma glucose and serum insulin increments were examined after sucrose loading in healthy subjects. Safety and tolerability were also examined.

Material and methods

Fifty, 100 and 200 mg of acarbose and placebo were given orally after an overnight fast to 12 healthy subjects with 75 g of sucrose in a 4-way crossover design (Tab. 1). Plasma glucose and serum insulin were measured before and 0.5, 1, 1.5, 2, 3, 4 hours after sucrose loading. Peak increments (C max) of plasma glucose and serum insulin profiles were measured. AUCs of plasma glucose increment and serum insulin increment were calculated using the trapezoidal method.

Table 1: Allocation design

Group	Volunteer No.	Time period			
		I	II	III	IV
A	1 ~ 3	Placebo tab. × 1	50 mg tab. × 1	50 mg tab. × 2	50 mg tab. × 4
B	4 ~ 6	50 mg tab. × 1	50 mg tab. × 2	50 mg tab. × 4	Placebo tab. × 1
C	7 ~ 9	50 mg tab. × 2	50 mg tab. × 4	Placebo tab. × 1	50 mg tab. × 1
D	10 ~ 12	50 mg tab. × 4	Placebo tab. × 1	50 mg tab. × 1	50 mg tab. × 2

Results

Dose dependency

Inhibitory effects of acarbose on both C_{max} and AUC of plasma glucose and serum insulin were dose-dependent. There was the highest correlation between the dose and the inhibition in AUC of serum insulin increment ($r = 0.934$, $p < 0.001$) (Fig. 1–4).

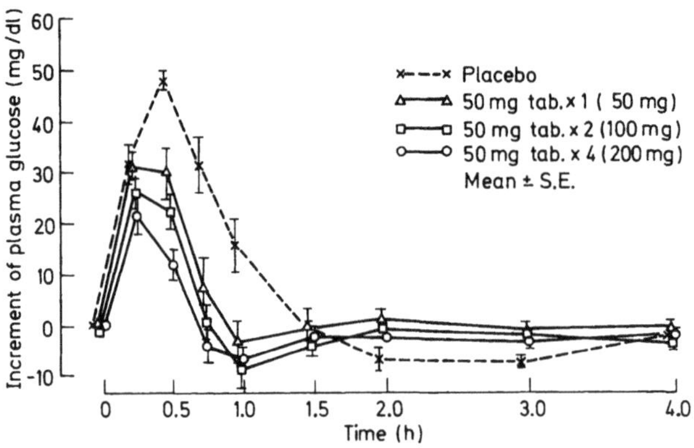

Fig. 1: Plasma glucose level increments after single oral administration of 75 g sucrose without (×) and with 50 mg (△), 100 mg (□) or 200 mg (○) BAY g 5421 in 12 healthy volunteers.

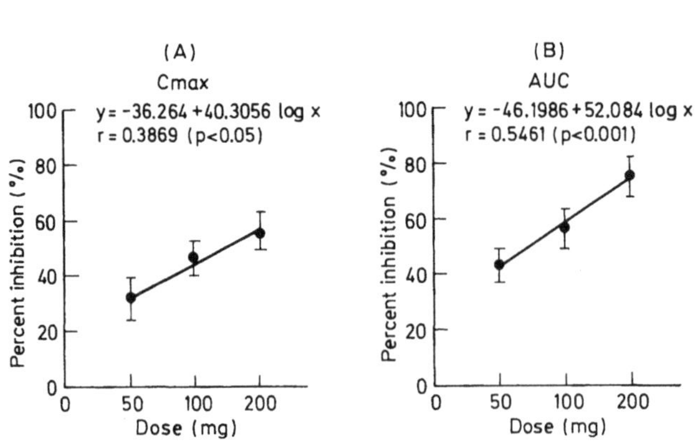

Fig. 2: Relationship between inhibitory effects of BAY g 5421 on plasma glucose and doses.

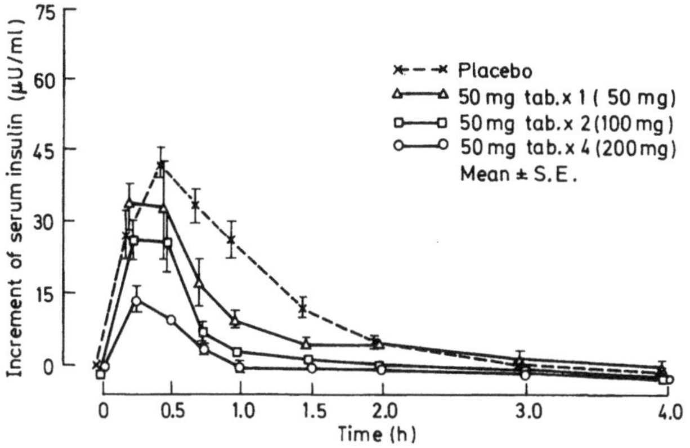

Fig. 3: Serum insulin level increments after single oral administration of 75 g sucrose without (×) and with 50 mg (△), 100 mg (□) or 200 mg (○) BAY g 5421 in 12 healthy volunteers.

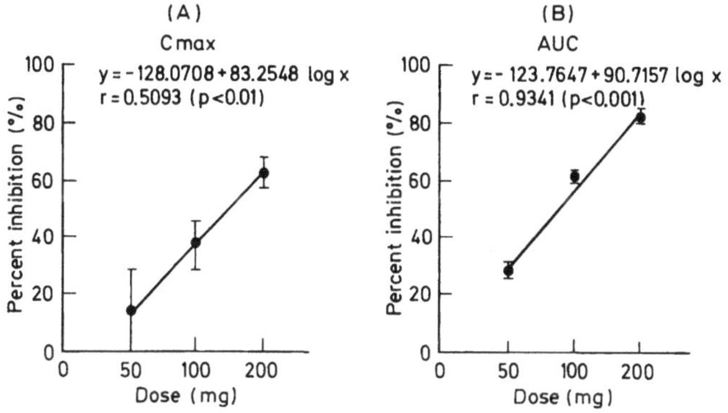

Fig. 4: Relationship between inhibitory effects of BAY g 5421 on serum insulin and doses.

Side-effects

Although almost all the subjects reported occasional diarrhea, flatulence and abdominal fullness, these symptoms were self-limiting and well tolerated. There was no abnormality in clinical laboratory findings.

References

[1] Caspary, W. F., F. Graf: Inhibition of human intestinal α-glucosidehydrolases by a new complex oligosaccharide. Resp. Exp. Med. (Berl.) *175* (1979) 1 – 6.

[2] Caspary, W. F., H. Kalisch: Effect of α-glucosidehydrolase inhibition on intestinal absorption of sucrose water and sodium in man. Gut *20* (1978) 750 – 755.

Assessment of efficacy and tolerability of acarbose (Glucobay®) by clinical data pool

M. Spengler, M. Cagatay

Introduction

In the course of the clinical development worldwide more than 8000 patients have been treated with acarbose. All their data have been collated in the clinical data pool and can be used for synoptic assessment of efficacy and tolerability.

A total of 8476 patients is documented including 8281 diabetics (2028 IDDM and 6253 NIDDM patients). Efficacy is judged in diabetics, tolerability in all patients (chapter 1).

In addition, efficacy and tolerability are judged using all placebo-controlled studies with 2462 acarbose- and 2384 placebo-treated patients (chapter 2).

1. Total clinical data pool (Tab. 1–3)

Demographic data of diabetics

Table 1

variable (* = median)		NIDDM	IDDM
Number of patients		6253	2028
Age (years)*		62	49
Female (%)		59	58
Broca-index*	male	1.09	0.97
	female	1.27	1.15
Duration of diabetes (months)*			
	male	72	126
	female	80	144
Duration of acarbose therapy (months)*		3	2
Acarbose dose (mg/day)*		300	300
SU-treated patients (%)		62	–
Biguanide-treated patients (%)		1	–
Insulin-treated patients (%)		5	100
Patients under acarbose monotherapy (%)		29	–

Efficacy

Table 2

variable (median)	NIDDM n	NIDDM pre	NIDDM end	IDDM n	IDDM pre	IDDM end
Blood glucose (mg/dl)						
fasting	3737	165	147	1092	191	170
1 h pp morning	2557	242	192	752	261	210
2 h pp morning	3300	230	187	1016	250	199
HbA_1 (%)*	833	9.9	8.7	183	10.1	9.4
HbA_{1c} (%)*	558	7.1	6.6	298	7.1	6.8
Urinary glucose (g/24 h)	1159	2.7	0.0	507	12.0	3.1
Body weight (kg)	4564	72	71	1419	67.5	67

* treatment for $\geq$ 2 months

Tolerability

No difference between pre- and end-values (means as well as medians) for clinicochemical and hematological laboratory values could be found. Deviations from initial values outside the normal range were seen in individual cases. The results do not indicate undesirable effects to be expected under acarbose treatment.

Table 3: Patients with adverse events and drop-outs (%)

Total	57.9		
Flatulence/meteorism	51.4		
Diarrhoea	12.5		
Abdominal pain	4.6	acarbose mono	0.1
Hypoglycemia	3.6	acarbose + insulin	2.9
Nausea	1.8	acarbose + SU	0.6
Constipation	1.7		
Drop-outs overall	13.0		
Drop-outs due to intestinal symptoms	3.2		

2. Placebo-controlled studies (Tab. 4–6, Fig. 1, 2)

Demographic data

Table 4

variable (* = median)		NIDDM Acarbose	NIDDM Placebo	IDDM Acarbose	IDDM Placebo
Number of patients		1689	1612	692	693
Age (years)*		59	58	36	36
Female (%)		53	52	48	48
Broca-index*	male	1.12	1.13	0.96	0.96
	female	1.34	1.33	1.09	1.09
Duration of diabetes (months)*					
	male	65	67	121	127
	female	72	72	136	132
Duration of acarbose/ placebo therapy (months)*		3	2.5	3	3.2
Acarbose/placebo dose (mg/day)*		300	300	300	300
SU-treated patients (%)		41	37	–	–
Biguanide-treated patients (%)		1.2	1.4	–	–
Insulin-treated patients (%)		9	9	100	100
Patients under acarbose Monotherapy (%)		37	36	–	–

Efficacy

Table 5

	NIDDM				IDDM			
	Acarbose		Placebo		Acarbose		Placebo	
variable (median)	pre	end	pre	end	pre	end	pre	end
Blood glucose (mg/dl)								
fasting	170	158	167	169	189	177	175	182
1 h pp morning	250	210	251	251	263	227	272	275
2 h pp morning	240	207	235	233	271	229	257	273
HbA_1 (%)*	9.4	8.7	9.3	9.3	9.9	9.0	9.5	9.3
HbA_{1c} (%)*	6.9	6.3	7.0	7.0	6.6	6.5	6.5	6.6
Urinary glucose (g/24 h)	2.8	0.0	1.8	2.0	26.1	11.6	15.3	23.3
Body weight (kg)	74.0	74.0	74.5	74.0	67.0	66.1	66.5	66.4

* treatment for ≥ 2 months

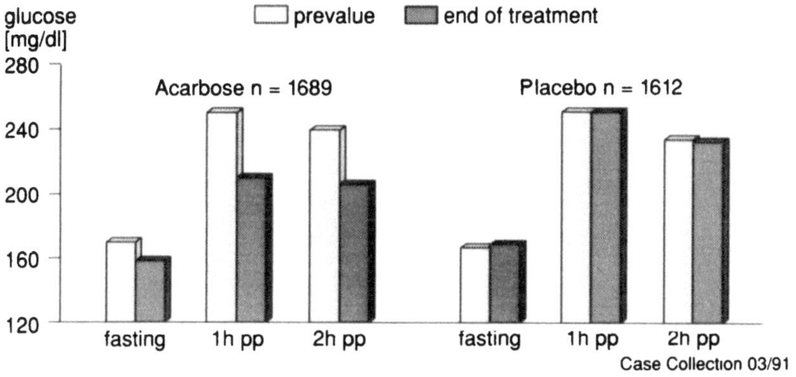

Fig. 1: Mean blood glucose values (median) in NIDDM treated with acarbose or placebo.

Tolerability

No differences between pre- and end-values (means as well as medians) for clinico-chemical and hematological laboratory values could be found in both treatment groups (Fig. 1, Tab. 5). Deviations from initial values outside the normal range were seen in individual cases in the acarbose and placebo groups. Correlation diagrams for individual pre- and end-values of aspartate aminotransferase are shown as an example in Figure 2.

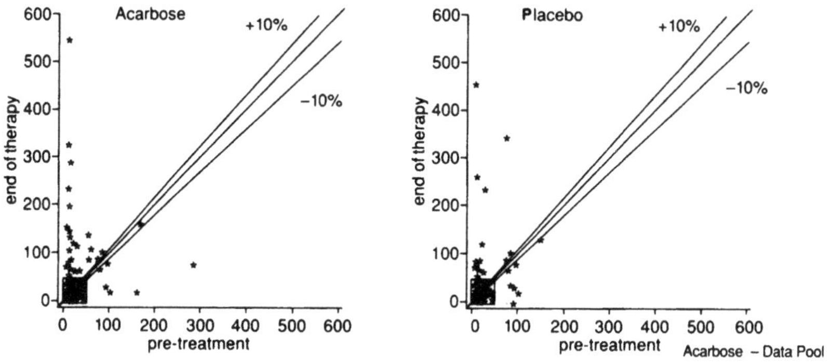

Fig. 2: Aspartate aminotransferase [U/l] (× 16,67 = nkat/l).

Table 6: Patients with adverse events and drop-outs [%]

	Acarbose	Placebo
Total	63.1	35.8
Flatulence/meteorism	54.9	20.3
Diarrhoea	14.1	4.5
Abdominal pain	7.6	3.1
Hypoglycemia	9.4	8.1
Nausea	2.4	1.6
Constipation	2.2	2.8
Headache	1.4	1.6
Drop-outs overall	15.0	12.0
Drop-outs due to intestinal symptoms	3.4	1.0

Conclusion

The beneficial effect of acarbose in the treatment of diabetics has been demonstrated in numerous studies. Summarized data from the clinical data pool on fasting and postprandial blood glucose, on glycated hemoglobin and on urinary glucose show the same results.

Assessment of laboratory safety variables of more than 8000 patients does not indicate any harmful potency of acarbose. There is no hint of a hypoglycemic potential in acarbose treatment.

The patterns of the adverse events of acarbose in the patients in the total data pool and in placebo-controlled studies are comparable.

The total rate of patients with adverse events is 63% in acarbose and 36% in placebo-treated patients, mainly flatulence (55 resp. 20%) and diarrhoea (14 resp. 5%).

The overall drop-out rate is 15% under acarbose and 12% under placebo. Drop-outs for intestinal symptoms, the typical result of increased colonic carbohydrate fermentation by acarbose, are rare.

Long-term tolerability of acarbose

M. Spengler, H. Hobler, M. Cagatay

Introduction

Under acarbose treatment, colonic fermentation can be enhanced by passing undigested carbohydrates into the large bowel, thus causing meteorism, flatulence, smoothing of stool consistency and diarrhoea. In this context, the following questions have arisen:

1. Do intestinal symptoms persist under long-term treatment with acarbose?
2. Does long-term treatment with acarbose cause any changes in electrolyte absorption?
3. Does long-term treatment with acarbose influence any safety parameters?

Based on the clinical data pool and on single studies answers to these questions can be given.

Intestinal symptoms

530 patients were treated for at least 300 days with a median daily dose of 300 mg acarbose. 71% of these patients reported adverse reactions. The most frequent symptoms were flatulence in 66% and diarrhoea in 21% of the patients.

These figures, however, do not provide any information with regard to the time course of these symptoms. Therefore, over a 10 months period, the rate of patients with at least one report of any adverse reaction within an interval of two months is shown in Figure 1.

The decrease in the rate of adverse reactions in the course of treatment (total from 53.4% within 0 – 2 months to 24.3% within > 8 – 10 months, flatulence from 47.7% to 23.8%, diarrhoea from 4.9% to 0%) is confirmed by a low total drop-out rate (7%). No patient dropped out due to adverse reactions.

Taking into account the occurrence of intestinal symptoms under placebo treatment, the data of a placebo-controlled, long-term study give additional information (Fig. 2).

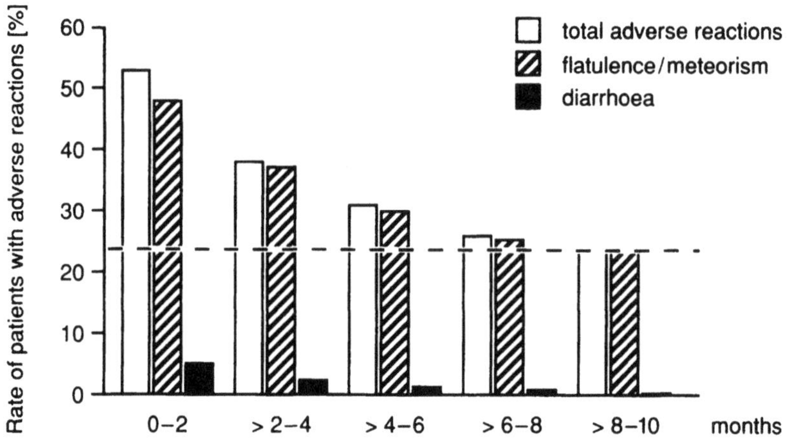

Fig. 1: Time course of adverse reactions under acarbose long-term treatment. Rate of patients with at least one report of adverse reactions within two months intervals (from clinical data pool).

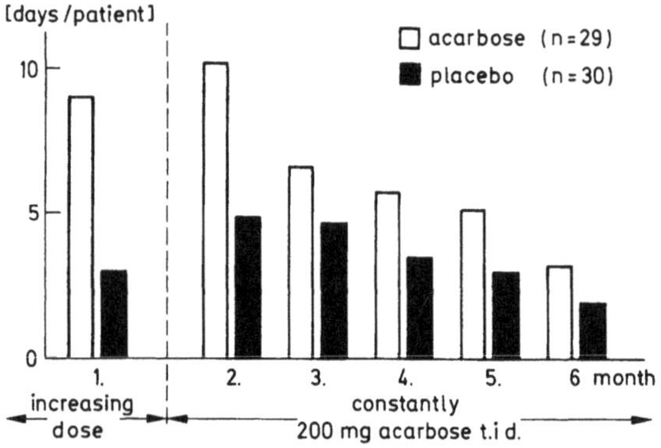

Fig. 2: Intestinal symptoms (meteorism, flatulence, diarrhoea) within monthly intervals, mean number of days per patient (study no. BAY g 5421/0583).

Electrolyte absorption

A subgroup of the clinical data pool (n = 79, median age 64 years, 52% female) was treated for at least 700 days with a median daily dose of 300 mg acarbose. Evaluation of serum electrolyte concentrations (sodium, potassium, calcium, iron) showed no indications of electrolyte malabsorption. There was no connection between fluctuations in serum sodium, potassium or calcium levels and the occurrence of diarrhoea. Examples for calcium and iron levels before and after treatment are given as a correlation diagram (Fig. 3).

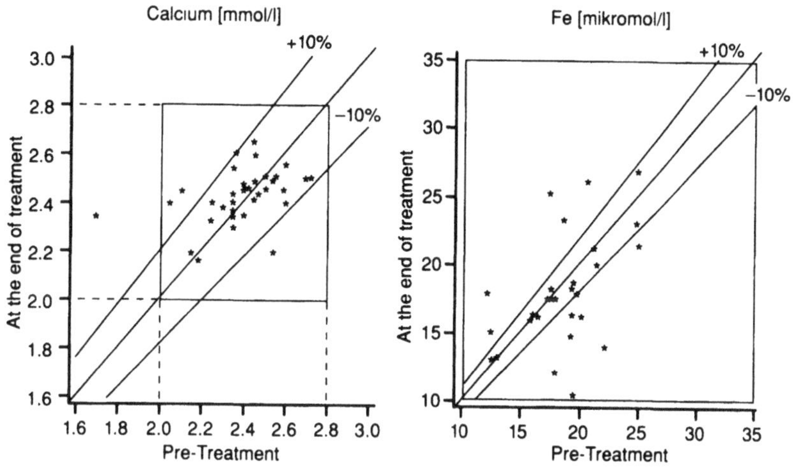

Fig. 3: Serum calcium and iron levels before and after treatment in patients (Ca: n = 70, Fe: n = 30) treated for at least 700 days with acarbose (from clinical data pool).

Safety parameters

Data of patients from the clinical data pool treated for at least 300 days (n = 530, 83% NIDDM, median dose 300 mg/day) were analysed (Tab. 1).

The mean clinico-chemical and hematological laboratory variables revealed no evidence of intolerance. Only in individual cases deviations in values after treatment from pretreatment values were seen (in both directions).

Table 1: Median change of safety parameters under long-term treatment with acarbose ($\geq$ 300 days). Comparison of prevalues (Pre) and values at the end of treatment (End).

Variable	n	Pre	End
AST (SGOT) [U/l]	482	12	12
ALT (SGPT) [U/l]	484	14	14
Gamma-GT [U/l]	476	19	21
Alc. phosphatase [U/l]	441	116	119
Urea [mmol/l]	432	6.22	6.33
Creatinine [µmol/l]	485	81.33	85
Uric acid [µmol/l]	479	315.20	312.30
Bilirubin [µmol/l]	468	12	11
Total protein [g/l]	432	72	71
Hemoglobin [mmol/l]	484	9.06	9.01
Erythrocytes [T/l]	483	4.70	4.68
Leucocytes [G/l]	484	6.60	6.50
Platelets [G/l]	435	210.00	202.00

Conclusion

Acarbose is a well tolerated drug:

1. Intestinal symptoms caused by increased colonic carbohydrate fermentation are tolerated and decreased with the duration of treatment. Adverse reactions are no reason for drop-outs under long-term treatment.
2. Long-term treatment with acarbose does not cause changes in electrolyte plasma levels.
3. Long-term treatment with acarbose does not influence the median clinico-chemical and hematological laboratory variables.

Assessment of efficacy and tolerability of acarbose in diabetic patients 5 – 16 years of age

M. Spengler, M. Cagatay

Introduction

The registration of acarbose in Germany and other countries does not include treatment of children due to scarce data available up to now. On the other hand, both pediatricians and diabetologists have shown great interest in improving the metabolic control of diabetic children with acarbose, especially with respect to the flattening of their oscillating daily blood glucose curve.

In designing controlled studies with acarbose in children, previous experiences may be helpful. The pooled data for children between 5 and 16 years of age treated with acarbose so far are summarized here (from clinical data pool).

Demographic data (Tab. 1)

Table 1

		n	mean	s. d.
Age [years]		65	12.7	2.6
Weight [kg]	male	24	42.3	14.3
	female	33	43.4	9.7
Height [cm]	male	25	151	18
	female	34	151	11
Broca-Index	male	24	0.9	0.1
	female	33	0.9	0.1
Duration of diabetes [months]	male	26	62	46
	female	34	60	32
Diet	energy [kcal]	27	2200	260
	carbohydrates [g]	27	223	49
	fat [g]	16	86	14
	protein [g]	16	111	15

Dosage and duration of treatment (Tab. 2, 3)

Table 2: Dosage scheme of acarbose

Mean daily dose [mg]	Number of patients: total	applications per day: 2	3	5	6	7
50 – 150	23	9	14	–	–	–
>150 – 300	34	5	16	–	13	–
>300 – 450	1	–	–	–	–	1
>450 – 600	5	–	3	2	–	–
Total	63	14	33	2	13	1

Most of the patients (90%) received daily doses of between 50 and 300 mg. The most frequent mode of application was 3 times daily (52%), followed by 2 times (22%) and 6 times daily (21%).

Table 3: Duration of acarbose treatment

Duration (days)	Number of patients
1 – 34	22
35 – 74	24
75 – 104	15
105 – 135	2
>135	2

Efficacy

The pooled efficacy data are shown in Figure 1. A slight drop in the median fasting blood glucose by 8 mg/dl (–4%), a remarkable reduction in the median 2 hours postprandial blood glucose by 49 mg/dl (–19%) and in the median HbA_{1c} by 1.1% point (–11%) is seen. The median urine glucose excretion was reduced from 24.8 g/24 h to 11 g/24 h.

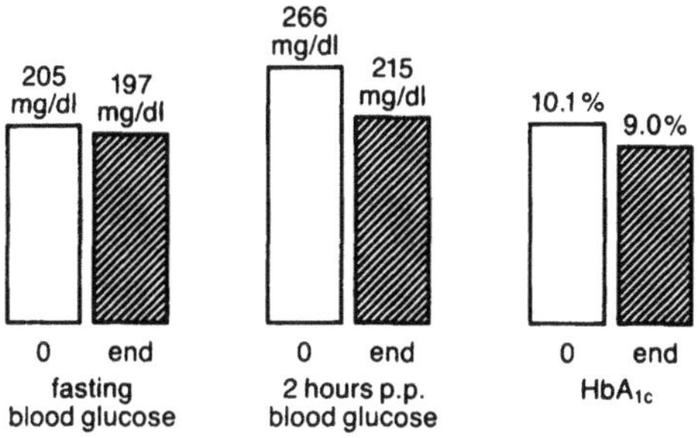

Fig. 1: Efficacy of acarbose treatment on fasting and postprandial blood glucose and HbA_{1c} (median values, before (0) and at the end (end) of treatment in diabetic children.

Tolerability

The tolerability was comparable to that in adults, represented by the total group of the data pool. 50.7% of the children and 57.9% of all patients reported side-effects. 41% of the children and 54.9% of all patients reported intestinal symptoms, mainly flatulence (Fig. 2). The clinico-chemical and hematological laboratory tests did not provide any evidence of intolerance. 6.9% of the children withdrew prematurely from the treatment (13% of all patients), 2.7% because of intestinal side-effects (3.2% of all patients).

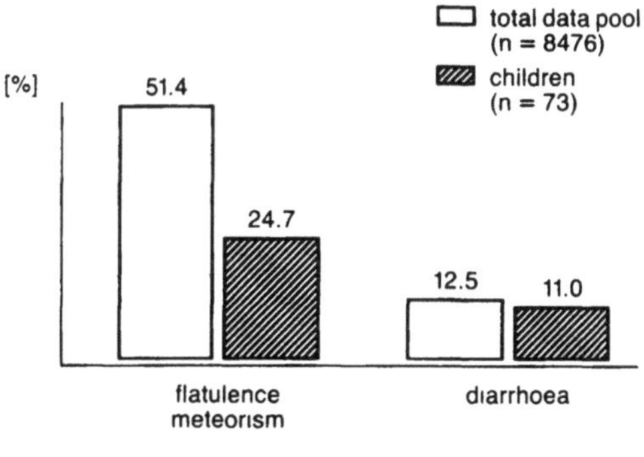

Fig. 2: Rate of patients with intestinal side-effects.

Conclusion

The first results of acarbose in diabetic children show efficacy concerning the postprandial blood glucose, HbA_{1c}, and the urine glucose excretion. There is neither evidence for a difference in tolerability in children compared to adults nor of any major risk of acarbose treatment. The intestinal symptoms are tolerated, shown in the low drop-out rate of 2.7%.

Effect of acarbose repeated dosing on antipyrine test in healthy volunteers

J. L. Pinquier, J. Y. Pello, E. Rey, D. De Lauture, P. D'Athis, G. Strauch, G. Olive, I. Morer, F. Prunièras

Introduction

Most drug interactions are linked to hepatic metabolism induction [2]. The aim of our study was to investigate the acarbose potential of induction using antipyrine test. This classical test could determine quantitatively the effect of a drug administration on hepatic drug metabolizing capacity [5].

Materials and methods

Twelve healthy male volunteers (age: 20 – 25 years, mean 22.8 and weight: 62 – 78 kg, mean 70.8) received 500 mg of oral antipyrine after an overnight fast, before and after oral acarbose 100 mg t. i. d. for 10 days. Antipyrine was measured in plasma following extraction by chloroform, using a sensitive and specific HPLC method with phenacetin as internal standard at selected times. Pharmacokinetic parameters were estimated for each subject.

Statistical analysis used ANOVA for Cmax, $t_{1/2}$, AUC (Area under curve) and MRT (Mean residence time), and Friedman test for tmax. The difference between means were given with symmetrical confidence intervals calculated by Westlake's method [6] for Cmax, $t_{1/2}$, AUC and MRT.

Results (Tab. 1, Fig. 1)

Table 1: Antipyrine pharmacokinetic parameters before and after oral acarbose 100 mg t.i.d. for 10 days. Results are given as means ± SD. Symmetrical confidence intervals were calculated by Westlake's method. *: $p < 0.05$ (ANOVA)

	Before acarbose	After administration	Symmetrical confidence intervals
Cmax (mg/l)	10.83 ± 1.17	11.14 ± 1.70	10.3%
tmax (h)	1.09 ± 0.29	1.09 ± 0.29	–
$t^{1/2}\beta$ (h)	10.58 ± 1.70	9.97 ± 1.89	12.5%
AUC ∞ (mg/l, h)	157.6 ± 32.9	149.5 ± 31.3	11.5%
CI (l/h)	3.34 ± 0.89	3.52 ± 0.97	13.6%
MRT (h)	15.05 ± 2.41	13.92 ± 2.72	12.6%*

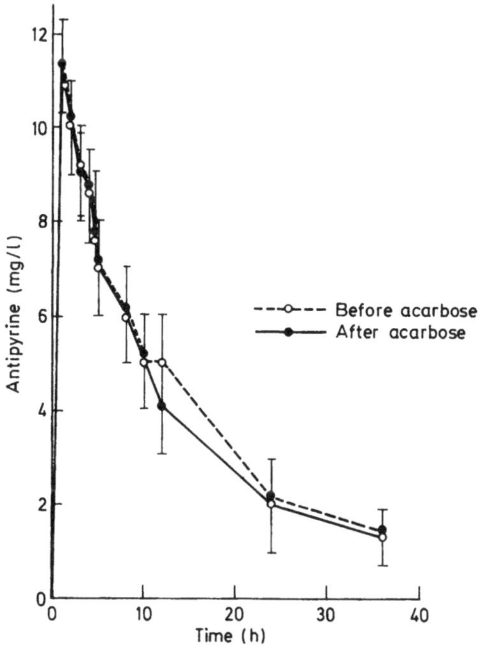

Fig. 1: Mean antipyrine plasma levels following the oral administration of 500 mg antipyrine, before and after oral acarbose 100 mg t.i.d. for 10 days.

Discussion

This study demonstrates that acarbose does not induce hepatic drug metabolizing capacity. Slight changes in antipyrine clearance, $t_{1/2}$ and MRT were found after acarbose administration. Only those for MRT were statistically significant.

These modifications in antipyrine pharmacokinetic could be linked to spontaneous fluctuations and are not clinically relevant. For example, phenytoin induces a clear increase of antipyrine clearance by 91% after administration for two weeks [4].

After acarbose oral administration, a very small amount of unchanged drug and approximately 35% of the metabolites formed in the gut are absorbed [1]. A modification of antipyrine clearance could result from a direct hepatic effect, or from the pharmacodynamic changes in carbohydrate absorption at gut level. As a matter of fact, antipyrine half-life has been found to be modified by the content of carbohydrate in the diet; decreased or increased with low or high content respectively [3].

Our study shows that possible acarbose interactions with other drugs would not be linked to a modification of hepatic drug metabolizing capacity. Whether interaction through other mechanisms could occur needs to be answered by well designed interaction studies.

References

[1] Clissold, S. P., C. Edwards: Acarbose. A preliminary review of its pharmacodynamic and pharmacokinetic properties, and therapeutic potential. Drugs *35* (1988) 214–243.

[2] Guillet, P., C. Caulin: A strategy for the identification of clinically significant drug interactions. In: G. Strauch, J. M. Husson (eds.): Recent trends in clinical pharmacology III, pp. 93–108. INSERM Vol. 186. Paris 1990.

[3] Kappas, A., K. E. Anderson, A. H. Conney et al.: Influence of dietetary protein and carbohydrate on antipyrine and theophylline metabolism in man. Clin. Pharmacol. Ther. *20* (1976) 643–653.

[4] Shaw, P. N., J. B. Houston, M. Rowland: Antipyrine metabolite kinetics in healthy volunteers during multiple dosing of phenytoin and carbamazepine. Br. J. Clin. Pharmacol. *20* (1985) 611–618.

[5] Vesell, E. S.: The antipyrine test in clinical pharamcology: conceptions and misconceptions. Clin. Pharm. Ther. *26* (1979) 275–286.

[6] Westlake, W. J.: Symmetrical confidence intervals for bioequivalence trials. Biometrics *32* (1976) 741–744.

Bei Fragen zur Produktsicherheit wenden Sie sich bitte an:
If you have any questions regarding product safety,
please contact:

Walter de Gruyter GmbH
Genthiner Straße 13
10785 Berlin
productsafety@degruyterbrill.com